FUNCTIONAL IMMUNO
NUTRITIONAL IMMUNOMODULATION

Presentation Slides Part 1:
Introduction to the Use of Nutrition and Functional Medicine
in the Prevention and Treatment
of Chronic Inflammation, Allergy, Autoimmunity...
and the FIND SEX Acronym.

DR. ALEX VASQUEZ

- Doctor of Osteopathic Medicine, graduate of University of North Texas Health Science Center, Texas College of Osteopathic Medicine (2010)
- Doctor of Naturopathic Medicine, graduate of Bastyr University (1999)
- Doctor of Chiropractic, graduate of Western States Chiropractic College (1996)
- Director of the Medical Board of Advisors (2011-present), Researcher and Lecturer (2004-2010), Biotics Research Corporation in Rosenberg, Texas
- Adjunct Faculty (2004-2005, 2010-present) and Forum Consultant (2003-2007), The Institute for Functional Medicine in Gig Harbor, Washington
- Adjunct Professor of Pharmacology, Program Director for Master of Science in Nutrition and Functional Medicine, University of Western States in Portland, Oregon
- Former Adjunct Professor of Orthopedics (2000) and Rheumatology (2001), Bastyr University in Kenmore, Washington
- Private practice in Seattle, Washington (2000-2001), Houston, Texas (2001-2006), Portland, Oregon (2011-present)
- Author of approximately 100 articles and letters published in *Annals of Pharmacotherapy, The Lancet, Nutritional Perspectives, BMJ—British Medical Journal, Journal of Manipulative and Physiological Therapeutics, JAMA—Journal of the American Medical Association, The Original Internist, Integrative Medicine, Holistic Primary Care, Nutritional Wellness, Dynamic Chiropractic, Alternative Therapies in Health and Medicine, JAOA—Journal of the American Osteopathic Association, Evidence-based Complementary and Alternative Medicine, Journal of Clinical Endocrinology and Metabolism*, and *Arthritis & Rheumatism*: Official Journal of the American College of Rheumatology

OPTIMALHEALTHRESEARCH.COM

Vasquez A. <u>Functional Immunology and Nutritional Immunomodulation. Presentation Slides Part 1</u>. Portland, Oregon; Integrative and Biological Medicine Research and Consulting, LLC.

The intended audiences for this book are health science students and doctorate-level clinicians. This book has been written with every intention to make it as accurate as possible, and each section has undergone peer-review by an interdisciplinary group of clinicians. In view of the possibility of human error and as well as ongoing discoveries in the biomedical sciences, neither the author nor any party associated in any way with this text warrants that this text is perfect, accurate, or complete in every way, and we disclaim responsibility for harm or loss associated with the application of the material herein. Information and treatments applicable to a specific *condition* may not be appropriate for or applicable to a specific *patient*; this is especially true for patients with multiple comorbidities and those taking pharmaceutical medications with multiple adverse effects and drug/nutrient/herb interactions. Given that this book is available on an open market, lay persons who read this material should discuss the information with a licensed healthcare provider before implementing any treatments and interventions described herein.

See website for updated information: www.OptimalHealthResearch.com

Table of Contents	*Page*
Preamble	
Introduction, Concepts, Patient Assessments, Laboratory, Evaluations, Musculoskeletal Emergencies	1
Presentation Slides Part 1: Introduction to the Use of Nutrition and Functional Medicine in the Prevention and Treatment of Chronic Inflammation, Allergy, Autoimmunity…and the FIND SEX Acronym.	134
Article Reprint	284

Dedications: I dedicate this book to the following people in appreciation for their works, their direct and indirect support of this work, and for their contributions to the advancement of true healthcare.

- **To the students and practitioners of chiropractic and naturopathic medicine**, those who continue to learn so that they can provide the best possible care to their patients.
- **To the researchers** whose works are cited in this text.
- **To Drs Alan Gaby, Jeffrey Bland, Ronald LeFebvre, Robert Richard, and Gilbert Manso,** my most memorable and influential professors and mentors.
- **To Dr Bruce Ames**[1] **and the late Dr Roger Williams**[2], for helping us to view our individuality as biochemically unique.
- **To Dr Chester Wilk**[3,4] **and important others** for documenting and resisting the organized oppression of natural, non-pharmaceutical, non-surgical healthcare.[5,6,7]
- **To Jorge Strunz and Ardeshir Farah,** for artistic inspiration

Acknowledgments for Peer and Editorial Review: Acknowledgement here does not imply that the reviewer fully agrees with or endorses the material in this text but rather that they were willing to review specific sections of the book for clinical applicability and clarity and to make suggestions to their own level of satisfaction. Credit for improvements and refinements to this text are due in part to these reviewers; responsibility for oversights remains that of the author.

- 2012 Edition of Migraine Headaches, Hypothyroidism, and Fibromyalgia: Holly Furlong DC
- 2011 Edition of *Integrative Chiropractic Management of High Blood Pressure and Chronic Hypertension*: Barry Morgan MD, Holly Furlong DC, Kris Young DC, Erika Mennerick DC, and Bill Beakey DOM
- 2011 Edition of *Integrative Medicine and Functional Medicine for Chronic Hypertension*: Erika Mennerick DC, Holly Furlong DC, JoAnn Fawcett DC, Ileana Bourland MSOM LAc, James Bogash DC, Bill Beakey
- 2010 Edition of *Chiropractic Management of Chronic Hypertension*: Joseph Paun MS DC, Joe Brimhall DC, David Candelario OMS4 (TCOM c/o 2010), James Bogash DC, Bill Beakey DOM, Robert Richard DO
- 2009 Edition of *Chiropractic and Naturopathic Mastery of Common Clinical Disorders*: Heather Kahn MD, Robert Richard DO, James Leiber DO, David Candelario (UNT-HSC TCOM DO4)
- 2007 Edition of *Integrative Orthopedics*: Barry Morgan MD, Dennis Harris DC, Richard Brown DC (DACBI candidate), Ron Mariotti ND, Patrick Makarewich MBA, Reena Singh (SCNM ND4), Zachary Watkins DC, Charles Novak MS DC, Marnie Loomis ND, James Bogash DC, Sara Croteau DC, Kris Young DC, Joshua Levitt ND, Jack Powell III MD, Chad Kessler MD, Amy Neuzil ND
- 2006 Edition of *Integrative Rheumatology*: Amy Neuzil ND, Cathryn Harbor MD, Julian Vickers DC, Tamara Sachs MD, Bob Sager BSc MD DABFM (Clinical Instructor in the Department of Family Medicine, University of Kansas), Ron Mariotti ND, Titus Chiu (DC4), Zachary Watkins (DC4), Gilbert Manso MD, Bruce Milliman ND, William Groskopp DC, Robert Silverman DC, Matthew Breske (DC4), Dean Neary ND, Thomas Walton DC, Fraser Smith ND, Ladd Carlston DC, David Jones MD, Joshua Levitt ND
- 2004 Edition of *Integrative Orthopedics*: Peter Knight ND, Kent Littleton ND MS, Barry Morgan MD, Ron Hobbs ND, Joshua Levitt ND, John Neustadt (Bastyr ND4), Allison Gandre BS (Bastyr ND4), Peter Kimble ND, Jack Powell III MD, Chad Kessler MD, Mike Gruber MD, Deirdre O'Neill ND, Mary Webb ND, Leslie Charles ND, Amy Neuzil ND

[1] Ames BN, Elson-Schwab I, Silver EA. High-dose vitamin therapy stimulates variant enzymes with decreased coenzyme binding affinity (increased K(m)): relevance to genetic disease and polymorphisms. *Am J Clin Nutr*. 2002 Apr;75(4):616-58 http://www.ajcn.org/cgi/content/full/75/4/616
[2] Williams RJ. Biochemical Individuality: The Basis for the Genetotrophic Concept. Austin and London: University of Texas Press; 1956
[3] Wilk CA. Medicine, Monopolies, and Malice: How the Medical Establishment Tried to Destroy Chiropractic. Garden City Park: Avery, 1996
[4] Getzendanner S. Permanent injunction order against AMA. *JAMA*. 1988 Jan 1;259(1):81-2 http://optimalhealthresearch.com/archives/wilk.html
[5] Carter JP. Racketeering in Medicine: The Suppression of Alternatives. Norfolk: Hampton Roads Pub; 1993
[6] Morley J, Rosner AL, Redwood D. A case study of misrepresentation of the scientific literature: recent reviews of chiropractic. *J Altern Complement Med*. 2001 Feb;7(1):65-78
[7] Terrett AG. Misuse of the literature by medical authors in discussing spinal manipulative therapy injury. *J Manipulative Physiol Ther*. 1995 May;18(4):203-10

Format and Layout: The format and layout of this book is designed to efficiently take the reader though the clinically relevant spectrum of considerations for each condition that is detailed. Important topics are given their own section within each chapter, while other less important or less common conditions are only described briefly in terms of the four "clinical essentials" of 1) definition/pathophysiology, 2) clinical presentation, 3) assessment/diagnosis, and 4) treatment/management. Each expanded section which details the more important/common conditions maintains a consistent format, taking the reader through the spectrum of primary clinical considerations: definition/pathophysiology, clinical presentations, differential diagnoses, assessments (physical examination, laboratory, imaging), complications, management, and treatment. As my books have progressed, I am increasingly using an article-by-article review format (especially in the sections on management and treatment) so that readers have more direct access to the information so as to understand and *incorporate* more deeply what the research actually states; the goal and general approach here is to use a *representative sampling* of the research literature.

References and Citations: Citations to articles, abstracts, texts, and personal communications are footnoted throughout the text to provide supporting information and to provide interested readers the resources to find additional information. Many of the cited articles are available on-line for free, and when possible I have included the website addresses so that readers can access the complete article.

Peer-review and Quality Control: Peer-review is essential to help ensure accuracy and clinical applicability of health-related information. Consistent with the importance of our goals, I have employed several "checks and balances" to increase the accuracy and applicability of the information within my textbooks:

- Reliance upon authoritative references: Nearly all important statements are referenced to peer-reviewed biomedical journals or authoritative texts, such as *The Merck Manual* and *Current Medical Diagnosis and Treatment*. Each citation is provided by a footnote at the bottom of each page so that readers will know quickly and easily exactly from where the information was obtained.
- Extensive cross-referencing: Readers will notice, if not be overwhelmed by, the number of references and citations. Many important statements have several references. Many references (especially textbooks) are referenced several times even on the same page. The purpose of this extensive referencing is three-fold: 1) to guide you to additional information, 2) to help me (as writer) stay organized, and 3) to help you and me (the practicing physicians) employ this information with confidence.
- Periodic revision: All of my books will be updated and revised on an *as-needed* basis. New information is added; superfluous information removed. Inspired by the popular text *Current Medical Diagnosis and Treatment* which is updated every year, I want my books to be accurate, timely, and in pace with the ever-growing literature on natural medicine. Any significant errors that are discovered will be posted at OptimalHealthResearch.com/updates; please check this page periodically to ensure that you are working with the most accurate information of which I am aware.
- Peer-review: The peer-review process for my books takes several forms. First, colleagues and students are invited to review new and revised sections of the text before publication; every section of the book that you are holding has been independently reviewed by health science students and/or practicing clinicians from various backgrounds: allopathic, chiropractic, osteopathic, naturopathic. Second, you - the reader - are invited to provide feedback about the information in the book, typographical errors, syntax, case reports, new research, etc. If your ideas truly change the nature of the material, I will be glad to acknowledge you in the text (with your permission, of course). If your contribution is hugely significant, such as reviewing three or more chapters or helping in some important way, I will be glad to not only acknowledge you, but to also send you the next edition at a discount or courtesy when your ideas take effect. Third, I keep abreast of new literature by constantly perusing new research and advancements in the health sciences. Having been successful in three separate doctoral programs in the health sciences, I have learned not only to master large amounts of material but to also separate and integrate different viewpoints as appropriate. I also "field test" my protocols with patients in the various clinical arenas in which I work and also with professionals and academicians via presentations and

critical dialogue. By implementing these quality control steps, I hope to create a useful text and advance our professions and our practices by improving the quality of care that we deliver to our patients.

How to Use This Book Safely and Most Effectively: Ideally, these books should be read cover-to-cover within a context of coursework that is supervised by an experienced professor. For post-graduate professionals, they might consider forming a local "book club" and meeting for weekly or monthly discussions to check their understandings and share their clinical experiences to refine the application of clinical knowledge, perceptions, and skills. Virtual groups and internet forums—specifically the forum hosted by the Institute for Functional Medicine at www.FunctionalMedicine.org—can provide access to an assembly of international professional peers wherein sharing of clinical questions and experiences are synergistic. Throughout this book, references are amply provided and are often footnoted with hyperlinks providing full-text access. This book is intended for licensed doctorate-level healthcare professionals with graduate and post-graduate training.

Notice: The intention and scope of this text are to provide doctorate-level clinicians with useful information and a familiarity with available research and resources pertinent to the management of patients in an integrative primary care setting. Specifically, the information in this book is intended to be used by licensed healthcare professionals who have received hands-on clinical training and supervision at accredited health science colleges. Additionally, information in this book should be used in conjunction with other resources, texts, and in combination with the clinician's best judgment and intention to "*first, do no harm*" and second to provide effective healthcare. Information and treatments applicable to a specific *condition* may not be appropriate for or applicable to a specific *patient* in your office; this is especially true for patients with multiple comorbidities and those taking pharmaceutical medications with multiple adverse effects and drug/nutrient/herb interactions. In my books and articles, I describe treatments—manual, dietary, nutritional, botanical, pharmacologic, and occasionally surgical—and their research support for the clinical condition being discussed; each practitioner must determine appropriateness of these treatments for his/her individual patient and with consideration of the doctor's scope of practice, education, training, skill, and—occasionally—the appropriateness of "off label" use of medications and treatments. This book has been carefully written and checked for accuracy by the author and professional colleagues. However, in view of the possibility of human error and new discoveries in the biomedical sciences, neither the author nor any party associated in any way with this text warrants that this text is perfect, accurate, or complete in every way, and we disclaim responsibility for harm or loss associated with the application of the material herein. With all conditions/treatments described herein, each physician must be sure to consider the balance between what is best for the patient and the physician's own level of ability, expertise, and experience. When in doubt, or if the physician is not a specialist in the treatment of a given severe condition, referral is appropriate. These notes are written with the routine "outpatient" in mind and are not tailored to severely injured patients or "playing field" or "emergency response" situations; consult your First Aid and Emergency Response texts and course materials for appropriate information. These notes represent the author's perspective based on academic education, experience, and post-graduate continuing education and are not inclusive of every fact that a clinician may need to know. This is not an "entry level" book except when used in an academic setting with a knowledgeable professor who can explain the concepts, tests, physical exam procedures, and treatments; this book requires a certain level of knowledge from the reader and familiarity with clinical concepts, laboratory assessments, and physical examination procedures.

Updates, Corrections, and Newsletter: When and if omissions, errata, and the need for important updates become clear, I will post these at the website: OptimalHealthResearch.com/updates.html. A reader might access this page periodically to ensure staying informed of any corrections that might have clinical relevance. This book consists not only of the text in the printed pages you are holding, but also the footnotes and any updates at the website. Be alerted to new integrative clinical research and updates to this textbook by signing-up for the free newsletter at www.OptimalHealthResearch.com/newsletter.html.

<u>**Language, Semantics, and Perspective:**</u> As a diligent student who previously aspired to be an English professor, I have written this text with great (though inevitably imperfect) attention to detail. Individual words were chosen with care. I confess to knowing, pushing, and creatively breaking several rules of grammar and punctuation. With regard to the he/she and him/her debacle of the English language, I've mixed singular and plural pronouns for the sake of being efficient and so that the images remain gender-neutral to the extent reasonable. The subtitle *The art of creating wellness while effectively managing acute and chronic musculoskeletal/health disorders* was chosen to emphasize the intentional creation of wellness rather than a limited focus on disease treatment and symptom suppression. For the 2009 printing of *Chiropractic and Naturopathic Mastery of Common Clinical Disorders*, this subtitle was slightly modified from "creating" to "co-creating" to emphasize the **team effort** required between physician and patient. *Managing* was chosen to emphasize the importance of treating-monitoring-referring-reassessing, rather than merely *treating*. *Disorders* was chosen to reflect the fact that a distinguishing characteristic of *life* is the ability to habitually create *organized structure* and *higher order* from chaos and *disorder*. For example, plants organize the randomly moving molecules of air and water into the organized structure of biomolecules which eventually take shape as plant structure—fiber, leaves, flowers, petals. Similarly, the human body creates organized structure of increased complexity from consumed plants and other foods; molecules ingested and inhaled from the environment are organized into specific biochemicals and tissue structures with distinct characteristics and definite functions. Injury and disease *result in* or *result from* a lack of order, hence my use of the word "disorders" to characterize human illness and disease. A motor vehicle accident that results in bodily injury, for example, is an example of an external chaotic force, which, when imparted upon human body tissues, results in a disruption (disorder) of the normal structure and organization that previously defined and characterized the now-damaged tissues of the body. Likewise, an autoimmune disease process that results in tissue destruction is an *anti-evolutionary* process that takes molecules of higher complexity and reverts them to simpler, fragmented, and non-functional forms. From the perspective of "health" as *organized structure and meaningful function* and "disease" as *the reversion to chaos, destruction of structure, and the loss of function*, the task of healthcare providers is essentially to restore order, and to acutely reduce and proactively prevent/eliminate clinical-biochemical-biomechanical-emotional chaos insofar as it adversely affects the patient's life experience as an individual and our collective experience as an interdependent society. What is required of clinicians then is the ability first to create conceptual order from what appears to be chaotic phenomena, and then second to materialize that conceptual order into our physical world; this is our task, and no small task it is.

<u>**Integrity and Creativity:**</u> I have endeavored to accurately represent the facts as they have been presented in texts and research, and to specifically resist any temptation to embellish or misrepresent data as others have done.[8,9] Conversely, I have not endeavored to make this book appeal to the "average" student or reader; my goal is to write and teach to the students at the top of the class, thereby affirming them and pulling the other students forward and upward. While I offer *explanations*, I intentionally resist *simplifications*, except when one simplification might facilitate the comprehension of a more complex phenomenon, or when such a simplification might facilitation the conveyance of information from clinician to patient. I have allowed this text to be unique in format, content, and style, so that the personality of this text can be contrasted with that of the instructor and reader, thus enabling the learner to at least benefit from an intentionally different – and intentionally honest – perspective and approach. Students using this text with the guidance of a qualified professor will benefit from the experience of "two teachers" rather than just one.

<u>**Linearity, Nonlinearity, Redundancy, Asynchronicity:**</u> Although the overall flow of the text is highly linear and sequential, occasionally I place a conclusion before its introduction for the sake of foreshadowing and therefore for preparing the reader for what is to come. The purpose of this is not simply one of preparation for the sake of allowing the reader to know what is already lying ahead on the path, but more to begin

---

[8] **Vasquez A**. Zinc treatment for reduction of hyperplasia of prostate. *Townsend Letter for Doctors and Patients* 1996; January: 100
[9] Broad W, Wade N. *Betrayers of the Truth: Fraud and Deceit in the Halls of Science*. New York: Simon and Schuster; 1982

creating new "shelf space" in the reader's intellectual-neuronal "library" so that when the new—particularly if *neoparadigmatic*—information is encountered, a space will already exist for it; it other words: the intent is to make learning easier. Likewise, for the sake of *information retention*—or what is better understood as synaptogenesis—important points are presented more than once, either identically or variantly. Given that *"No one ever reads the same book twice"*[10] (because the "person who starts" the reading of a meaningful book is changed into the "person who finishes" the reading of that book (assuming proper intentionality and application of one's "self"), the person reading these words might consider a second glace after the first.

The Functional Medicine Matrix (version presented in 2003): In the 2009 edition of *Chiropractic and Naturopathic Mastery of Common Clinical Disorders*, I reintroduced the Functional Medicine Matrix that I originally diagramed for the Institute for Functional Medicine (IFM) in 2003; the diagram used is updated from the original, and readers should appreciate that IFM has changed the Matrix since this version was made. My perspective is that functional medicine, naturopathic medicine, and *authentic* holistic medicine share much in common in their fundamental models of health and disease. The functional medicine matrix— designed and owned by the Institute for Functional Medicine (FunctionalMedicine.org)—is unique to the discipline of functional medicine and provides a conceptual framework for understanding the complexity of health and disease.

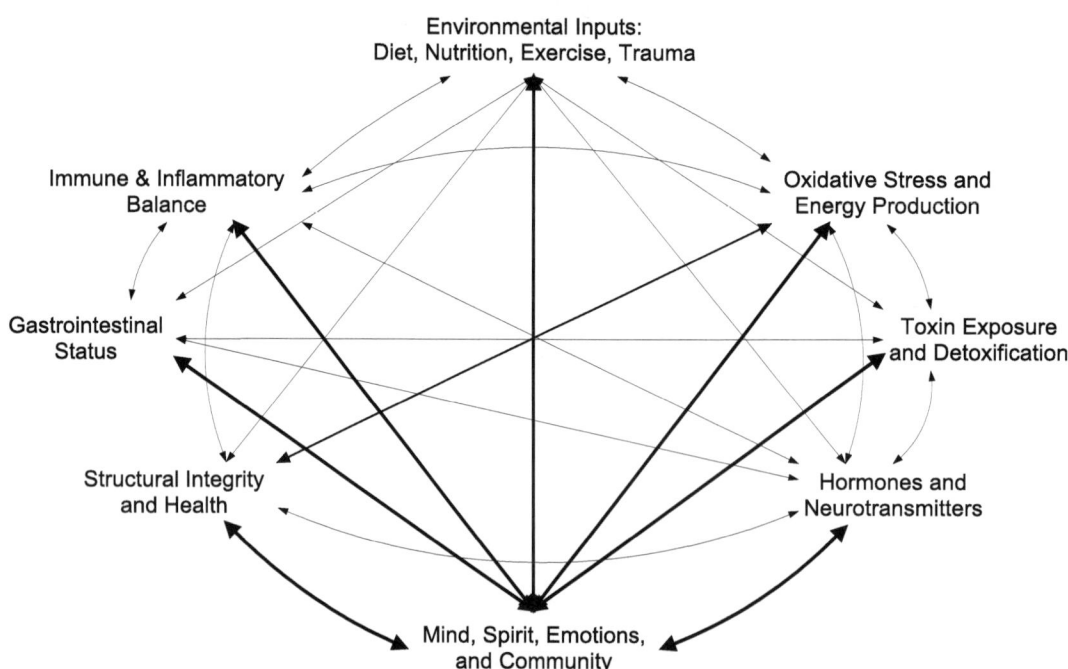

2003 Version of the Functional Medicine Matrix: Updated from the original diagram by Vasquez in 2003 for the Institute for Functional Medicine (IFM).

Distinguishing "Integrative Medicine" from "Functional Medicine"—the author's perspective[11]: The distinction of integrative medicine from functional medicine is that of *quantity* from *quality*. Integrative medicine can be understood as a quantitative extension of other already-existing healthcare models, to which additional perspectives and treatments are added; in this way, various conceptual models are "integrated" and used together in a more holistic and comprehensive approach. In contrast, functional medicine is a distinct model of health and disease that has developed an identity beyond mere integration of various models and treatments. Functional medicine is qualitatively distinct in its viewpoint of disease causation and treatment by the unique combination of emphases placed on ❶ patient-centered care (in

---

[10] Davies R. *Reading and Writing*. Salt Lake City: University of Utah Press; 1992, page 23

[11] Dr Vasquez's perspective: I have trained in functional medicine since 1994, first as a student of Jeffrey Bland PhD *et al* and later as Forum Consultant and Faculty (2003 – present in 2011) for the Institute of Functional Medicine, and I wrote three chapters in *Textbook of Functional Medicine* published by Institute of Functional Medicine. My opinions here are not necessarily currently representative of the Institute of Functional Medicine in this context.

contrast to the disease-centered care of allopathic medicine and most osteopathic medicine), ❷ detailed appreciation of the importance of the web-like interconnected nature of various organ systems[12] and psychological, physiological, and pathological processes (to a greater extent than allopathic, osteopathic, chiropractic and naturopathic medicine), ❸ its rigorous evidence-based standards, and ❹ its willingness to eagerly-yet-appropriately include *all* therapeutic options, ranging from (for example) surgical to meditative, dietary to pharmaceutical, manipulative to botanical, and antidysbiotic to psychological. In short, functional medicine can be described as an ***antiparadigmatic patient-centered discipline***, hence its therapeutic flexibility, broad applicability, and enhanced efficacy; it is antiparadigmatic due to its lack of adherence to a specific and limited set of tools (most professional disciplines are quite limited in their expertise and scope) and due to the emphasis placed on patient-centered healthcare, which first and always foremost seeks to determine the most efficient path for patient empowerment and healing.

Diseases/Conditions for Which CAM Is Most Frequently Used Among Adults - 2007

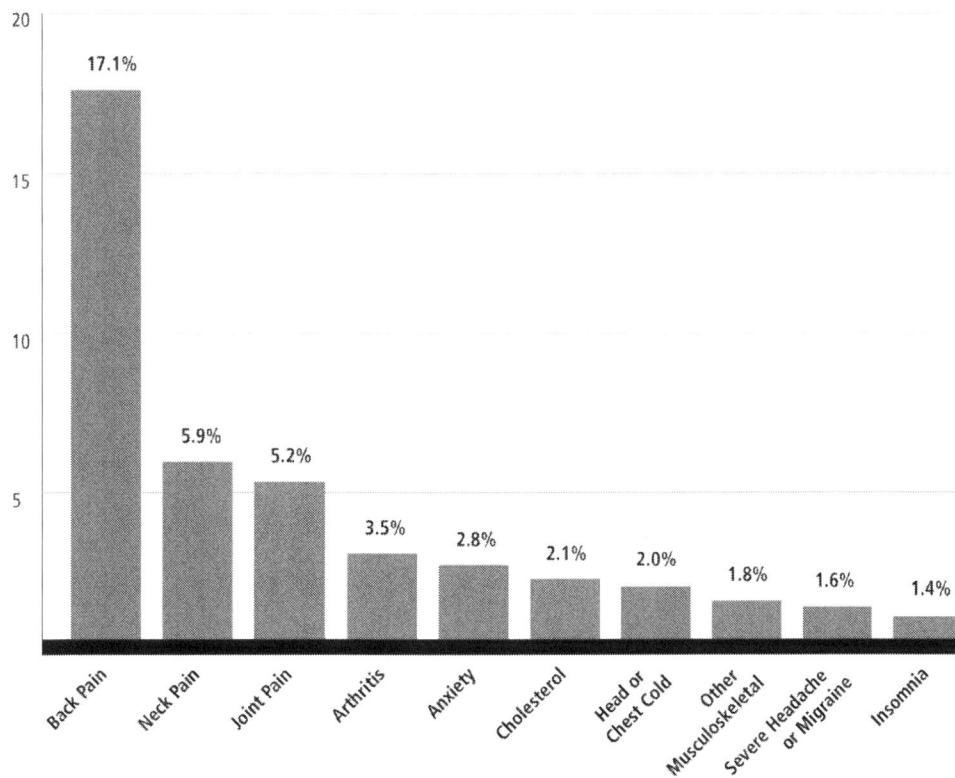

Source: Barnes PM, Bloom B, Nahin R. *CDC National Health Statistics Report #12.* Complementary and Alternative Medicine Use Among Adults and Children: United States, 2007. December 2008.

Health problems for which patients most often seek so-called CAM treatment:
Illustration from National Center for Complementary and Alternative Medicine, NIH, DHHS (http://nccam.nih.gov/news/camstats/2007/graphics.htm).

The following table provides a listing—in order of percentage—of the most common conditions seen in a general family practice of medicine, with hypertension and diabetes mellitus—two conditions highly amenable to integrative therapeutics—clearly dominating the clinical landscape.

---

[12] **Vasquez A**. Web-like Interconnections of Physiological Factors. *Integrative Medicine: A Clinician's Journal* 2006, April/May, 32-37

The Most Common Diagnoses in the Practice of General/Family Medicine

Top diagnoses	Notes and comments
1. Hypertension	5.9% of family medicine diagnoses; nearly 11 million patient visits per year.
2. Diabetes mellitus	4.1% of family medicine diagnoses; more than 7.6 million patient visits per year.
3. Acute upper respiratory infection	3.2% of family medicine diagnoses; more than 10 million patient visits per year. Most of these are caused by viral infections for which there is no direct medical treatment.
4. Sinusitis	2.5% of family medicine diagnoses; more than 10 million patient visits per year.
5. Acute pharyngitis	2.3% of family medicine diagnoses; more than 4 million patient visits per year.
6. Otitis media	2.3% of family medicine diagnoses; > 4 million patient visits per year.
7. Bronchitis	1.9% of family medicine diagnoses; > 3 million patient visits per year.
8. Back problems	1.8% of family medicine diagnoses; > 3 million patient visits per year. This is a diverse group of conditions ranging from post-traumatic to benign to developmental problems such as scoliosis. Note that back pain is listed separately below.
9. Hyperlipidemia	1.7% of family medicine diagnoses; > 3 million patient visits per year. This mostly includes the lifestyle-generated dyslipidemia epidemic, with comparably fewer cases of genotropic disorders requiring pharmacotherapy.
10. Urinary tract disorders	1.6% of family medicine diagnoses; almost 3 million patient visits per year. This can include a diverse group of problems ranging from simple and self-limited urinary tract infections to sexually transmitted diseases.
11. Allergic rhinitis	1.2% of family medicine diagnoses; > 2 million patient visits per year. A general approach to allergy treatment is included in this text.
12. Back pain	1.2% of family medicine diagnoses; > 2 million patient visits per year.
13. Abdominal or pelvic symptoms	1.1% of family medicine diagnoses; > 2 million patient visits per year. This can include a wide range of diagnoses ranging from appendicitis to dysmenorrhea. Due to the breadth and complexity, these are not covered in this text.
14. Joint pain	1.1% of family medicine diagnoses; > 2 million patient visits per year.
15. Depression or anxiety	1.1% of family medicine diagnoses; > 2 million patient visits per year.
16. Asthma	1.1% of family medicine diagnoses; almost 2 million patient visits per year. An approach to allergy treatment is included in this text, with a section on asthma.
17. Chest pain or shortness of breath	1.1% of family medicine diagnoses; almost 2 million patient visits per year. Some of these are benign musculoskeletal pain or gastroesophageal reflux while others turn out to be life-threatening conditions such as myocardial infarction, pneumothorax, pneumonia, or—rarely—aortic dissection. These are not directly covered in this text.
18. Soft tissue problems	1% of family medicine diagnoses; 1.8 million patient visits per year.
19. Acute bronchitis and bronchiolitis	1% of family medicine diagnoses; 1.8 million patient visits per year. These include bacterial and viral infections, ranging from mild to life-threatening, especially in patients with cardiopulmonary disease.
20. Skin problems	1% of family medicine diagnoses; 1.8 million patient visits per year.
21. Tendonitis	1% of family medicine diagnoses; 1.7 million patient visits per year.

Data from *Essentials of Family Medicine, 5th edition* edited by Sloane PD, Slatt LM, Ebell MH, Jacques LB, Smith MA published by Lippincott Williams & Wilkins (April 1, 2007)

Bon Voyage: All artists and scientists—regardless of genre—grapple with the divergent goals of *perfecting* their work and *presenting* their work; the former is impossible, while the latter is the only means by which the effort can create the desired effect in the world, whether that is pleasure, progress, or both. At some point, we must all agree that it is "good enough" and that it contains the essence of what needs to be communicated. While neither this nor any future edition of this book is likely to be "perfect", I am content with the literature reviewed, presented, and the new conclusions and implications which are described—many for the first time ever—in this text. Particularly for *Integrative Rheumatology* and *Chiropractic and Naturopathic Mastery*, each chapter aims to achieve a paradigm shift which distances us further from the simplistic pharmacocentric model and toward one which authentically empowers both practitioners and patients. With time, I will make future editions more complete and perhaps less polemical—but not less passionate. I hope you are able to implement these conclusions and research findings *into your own life* and into the treatment plans for your patients. In short time, I believe that we will see many of these concepts more broadly implemented. Hopefully this work's value and veracity will promote patients' vitality via the vigilant and virtuous clinicians viewing this volume. To the more attentive and thoroughgoing reader, more is revealed.

> **Authentic learning is life integration**
>
> "Ultimately, no one can extract from things—*books included*—more than he already knows. What one has no access to through experience, one has no ear for."
>
> Friedrich Nietzsche [translated by RJ Hollingdale]. *Ecce Homo: How One Becomes What One Is*. New York & London: Penguin Books; 1979, page 70

Thank you, and I wish you and your patients the best of success and health.

Alex Vasquez, D.C., N.D., D.O.
June 5, 2012

> **Work as love**
>
> "You work that you may keep pace with the earth and the soul of the earth.
> For to be idle is to become a stranger unto the seasons, and to step out of life's procession. ...
> Work is love made visible."
>
> Kahlil Gibran (1883-1930). *The Prophet*. Publisher Alfred A. Knopf, 1973

> **Newsletter & Updates**
>
> Be alerted to new integrative clinical research and updates to this textbook by signing-up for the free newsletter, sent several times per year as needed. Join at:
> www.OptimalHealthResearch.com/newsletter.html

Examples of commonly used abbreviations:

- **25-OH-D** = serum 25-hydroxy-vitamin D(3)
- **ACEi** = angiotensin-2 converting enzyme inhibitor
- **Alpha-blocker** = alpha-adrenergic antagonist
- **ARB** = angiotensin-2 receptor blocker/antagonist
- **ARF** = acute renal failure
- **BB** = beta blocker or beta-adrenergic antagonist
- **BMP** = basic metabolic panel, includes serum Na, K, Cl, CO2, BUN, creatinine, and glucose
- **BP** = blood pressure, **HBP** = high blood pressure
- **BUN** = blood urea nitrogen
- **C&S** = culture and sensitivity
- **CAD** = coronary artery disease
- **CBC** = complete blood count
- **CCB** = calcium channel blocker/antagonist
- **CE** = cardiac enzymes, generally including creatine kinase (CK), creatine kinase myocardial band (CKMB), and troponin-1, with the latter being the most specific serologic marker for acute myocardial injury; for the evaluation of acute MI, these are generally tested 2-3 times at 6-hour intervals with ECG performed at least as often.
- **CHF** = congestive heart failure
- **CHO** = carbohydrate
- **CK** = creatine kinase, historically named creatine phosphokinase (CPK)
- **CKD** = chronic kidney disease, generally stratified into five stages based on GFR of roughly <90, 90-60, 60-30, 30-15, and >15, respectively
- **CMP** = comprehensive metabolic panel, also called a chemistry panel, includes the BMP along with markers of hepatic status albumin, protein, ALT, AST, may also include alkaline phosphatase and rarely GGT; panels vary per laboratory and hospital.

- **CNS** = central nervous system
- **COPD** = chronic obstructive pulmonary disease
- **CRF, CRI** = chronic renal failure/insufficiency
- **CRP** = c-reactive protein, **hsCRP** = high-sensitivity c-reactive protein
- **CT** = computed tomography
- **CVD** = cardiovascular disease
- **CXR** = chest X-ray
- **DM** = diabetes mellitus
- **ECG** or **EKG** = electrocardiograph
- **Echo** = echocardiography
- **GFR** = glomerular filtration rate
- **HDL** = high density lipoprotein cholesterol
- **HTN** = hypertension
- **Ig** = immune globulin = antibodies of the G, A, M, E, or D classes.
- **IHD** = ischemic heart disease
- **IV** = intravenous
- **MCV** = mean cell volume
- **MI** = myocardial infarction
- **MRI** = magnetic resonance imaging, **MRI** = magnetic resonance angiography
- **PRN** = from the Latin "pro re nata" meaning "on occasion" or "when necessary"
- **PTH** = parathyroid hormone, **iPTH** = intact parathyroid hormone
- **PVD** = peripheral vascular disease
- **RA** = rheumatoid arthritis
- **RAD** = reactive airway disease, similar to asthma
- **SLE** = systemic lupus erythematosus
- **TRIG(s)** = serum triglycerides
- **UA** = urinalysis
- **US** = ultrasound

Dosing shorthand (mostly Latin abbreviations): q = each; qd = each day; bid = twice daily; tid = thrice daily; qid = four times per day; po = per os = by mouth; prn = as needed.

Chapter 1:
Review of Clinical Assessments and Concepts

Clinical Assessments and Concepts:
This review is included for students and for graduates desiring a concise overview of basic and advanced clinical concepts. Many clinical pearls are included. Reviewed herein are the three essential components of patient assessment: history, physical examination, and laboratory assessment. Additional concepts and perspectives are provided that will help facilitate risk management and optimal patient care.

<u>Topics:</u>
- **Moving past disease- and drug-centered medicine toward patient-centered health optimization: the goal is _wellness_**
- **Acute Care and Musculoskeletal Care as Opportunities for Health Optimization**
- **Clinical Assessments**
  - History taking & physical examination
  - Orthopedic/musculoskeletal examination: Concepts and goals
  - Neurologic assessment: Review
  - Laboratory assessments: General considerations of commonly used tests
    - i. _Routine tests_: Chemistry/metabolic panel, lipid panel, CBC, 25(OH)-vitamin D, ferritin, thyroid stimulating hormone, CRP, ESR,
    - ii. _Rheumatology/inflammation_: ANA (antinuclear antibodies), ANCA (antineutrophilic cytoplasmic antibodies), RF (rheumatoid factor), CCP (cyclic citrullinated protein antibodies), complement proteins, HLA-B27
    - iii. _Functional assessments_: Lactulose-mannitol assay, comprehensive stool analysis and comprehensive parasitology
- **High-Risk Pain Patients**
- **Clinical Concepts**
  - Not all injury-related problems are injury-related problems
  - Safe patient + safe treatment = safe outcome
  - Four clues to underlying problems
  - Special considerations in the evaluation of children
  - No errors allowed: Differences between primary healthcare and spectator sports
  - "Disease treatment" is different from "patient management"
  - Clinical practice involves much more than "diagnosis and treatment"
  - Risk management: A note especially to students and recent licensees
- **Musculoskeletal Emergencies**
  - Acute compartment syndrome
  - Acute red eye, including acute iritis and scleritis
  - Atlantoaxial subluxation and instability
  - Cauda equina syndrome
  - Giant cell arteritis, temporal arteritis
  - Myelopathy, spinal cord compression
  - Neuropsychiatric lupus
  - Osteomyelitis
  - Septic arthritis, acute nontraumatic monoarthritis
- **Brief Overview of Integrative Healthcare Disciplines**
  - Chiropractic
  - Naturopathic Medicine
  - Osteopathic Medicine
  - Functional Medicine

Moving past "disease and drug"-centered medicine toward patient-centered health optimization: the goal is *wellness*

Written for students and experienced clinicians, this chapter introduces and reviews many new and common terms, procedures, and concepts relevant to the management of patients with musculoskeletal disorders. Especially for students, the reading of this chapter is essential to understanding the extensive material in this book and will facilitate the clinical assessment and management of patients with various clinical presentations.

Healthcare is currently in a time of significant fluctuation and is ready for changes in the balance of power and the paradigms which direct our therapeutic interventions. For nearly a century, allopathic medicine has hailed itself as "the gold standard", and other professions have either submitted to or been crushed by their ongoing political/scientific manipulations and their continual proclamation of intellectual and therapeutic superiority[1,2,3,4,5,6,7,8,9,10,11,12,13] despite 180,000-220,000 iatrogenic *medically-induced* deaths per year (500-600 iatrogenic deaths per day)[14,15] and consistent documentation that most medical/allopathic physicians are unable to provide accurate musculoskeletal diagnoses due to pervasive inadequacies in medical training.[16,17,18,19] Increasing disenchantment with allopathic *heroic medicine* and its adverse outcomes of inefficacy, exorbitant expenses, and unnecessary death are fostering change, such that allopathic medicine has been dethroned as the leading paradigm among American patients, who spend the majority of their discretionary healthcare dollars on consultations and treatments provided by "alternative" healthcare

> **Medical iatrogenesis kills 493 Americans per day**
> "Recent estimates suggest that each year more than 1 million patients are injured while in the hospital and approximately 180,000 die because of these injuries. Furthermore, drug-related morbidity and mortality are common and are estimated to cost more than $136 billion a year."
>
> Holland EG, Degruy FV. Drug-induced disorders. *Am Fam Physician*. 1997;56(7):1781-8, 1791-2

providers.[20,21] With the ever-increasing utilization of chiropractic, naturopathic, and osteopathic medical services, we must see that our paradigms and interventions keep pace with the evolving research literature and our increasing professional responsibilities so that we can deliver the highest possible quality of care.

While we all readily acknowledge the importance of emergency care for emergency situations, those of us who advocate and practice a more complete approach to healthcare and life readily see the shortcomings of a limited and mechanical approach to healthcare, and we aspire to do more than simply fix problems. The implementation of *multidimensional* (i.e., *comprehensive* and *multifaceted*) treatment plans that address many aspects

---

[1] Wilk CA. <u>Medicine, Monopolies, and Malice: How the Medical Establishment Tried to Destroy Chiropractic</u>. Garden City Park: Avery, 1996

[2] Getzendanner S. Permanent injunction order against AMA. *JAMA*. 1988 Jan 1;259(1):81-2 http://optimalhealthresearch.com/archives/wilk.html

[3] Carter JP. <u>Racketeering in Medicine: The Suppression of Alternatives</u>. Norfolk: Hampton Roads Pub; 1993

[4] Morley J, Rosner AL, Redwood D. A case study of misrepresentation of the scientific literature: recent reviews of chiropractic. *J Altern Complement Med*. 2001 Feb;7:65-78

[5] Terrett AG. Misuse of the literature by medical authors in discussing spinal manipulative therapy injury. *J Manipulative Physiol Ther*. 1995;18(4):203-10

[6] National Alliance of Professional Psychology Providers. AMA Seeks To Control and Restrict Psychologist's Scope of Practice. www.nappp.org/scope.pdf Accessed Nov 2006

[7] "In an effort to marshal the medical community's resources against the growing threat of expanding scope of practice for allied health professionals, the AMA has formed a national partnership to confront such initiatives nationwide... The committee will use $25,000..." Daly R, American Psychiatric Association. AMA Forms Coalition to Thwart Non-M.D. Practice Expansion. *Psychiatric News* 2006 March; 41: 17 http://pn.psychiatryonline.org/cgi/content/full/41/5/17-a?eaf Accessed November 25, 2006

[8] Spivak JL. <u>The Medical Trust Unmasked</u>. Louis S. Siegfried Publishers; New York: 1961

[9] Trever W. <u>In the Public Interest</u>. Los Angeles; Scriptures Unlimited; 1972. This is probably the most authoritative documentation of the illegal actions of the AMA up to 1972; contains numerous photocopies of actual AMA documents and minutes of official meetings with overt intentionality of destroying Americans' healthcare options so that the AMA and related organizations would have a monopoly in national healthcare.

[10] Wenban AB. Inappropriate use of the title 'chiropractor' and term 'chiropractic manipulation' in the peer-reviewed biomedical literature. *Chiropr Osteopat*. 2006;14:16 http://chiroandosteo.com/content/14/1/16

[11] Orme-Johnson DW, Herron RE. An innovative approach to reducing medical care utilization and expenditures. *Am J Manag Care*. 1997 Jan;3:135-44 http://www.ajmc.com/Article.cfm?Menu=1&ID=2154

[12] van der Steen WJ, Ho VK. Drugs versus diets: disillusions with Dutch health care. *Acta Biotheor*. 2001;49(2):125-40

[13] Texas Medical Association. Physicians Ask Court to Protect Patients From Illegal Chiropractic Activities. http://www.texmed.org/Template.aspx?id=5259 Accessed Feb 2007

[14] Starfield B. Is US health really the best in the world? *JAMA*. 2000 Jul 26;284(4):483-5

[15] "Recent estimates suggest that each year more than 1 million patients are injured while in the hospital and approximately 180,000 die because of these injuries. Furthermore, drug-related morbidity and mortality are common and are estimated to cost more than $136 billion a year." Holland EG, Degruy FV. Drug-induced disorders. *Am Fam Physician*. 1997;56(7):1781-8, 1791-2

[16] Freedman KB, Bernstein J. The adequacy of medical school education in musculoskeletal medicine. *J Bone Joint Surg Am*. 1998;80(10):1421-7

[17] Freedman KB, Bernstein J. Educational deficiencies in musculoskeletal medicine. *J Bone Joint Surg Am*. 2002;84-A(4):604-8

[18] Matzkin E, Smith ME, Freccero CD, Richardson AB. Adequacy of education in musculoskeletal medicine. *J Bone Joint Surg Am*. 2005;87-A(2):310-4

[19] Schmale GA. More evidence of educational inadequacies in musculoskeletal medicine. *Clin Orthop Relat Res*. 2005 Aug;(437):251-9

[20] "...Americans made an estimated 425 million visits to providers of unconventional therapy. This number exceeds the number of visits to all U.S. primary care physicians (388 million)." Eisenberg DM, Kessler RC, Foster C, Norlock FE, Calkins DR, Delbanco TL. Unconventional medicine in the United States. Prevalence, costs, and patterns of use. *N Engl J Med*. 1993 Jan 28;328(4):246-52

[21] "Estimated expenditures for alternative medicine professional services increased 45.2% between 1990 and 1997 and were conservatively estimated at $21.2 billion in 1997, with at least $12.2 billion paid out-of-pocket. This exceeds the 1997 out-of-pocket expenditures for all US hospitalizations." Eisenberg DM, Davis RB, Ettner SL, Appel S, Wilkey S, Van Rompay M, Kessler RC. Trends in alternative medicine use in the United States, 1990-1997: results of a follow-up national survey. *JAMA* 1998 Nov 11;280(18):1569-75

of pathophysiologic phenomena is a huge step forward in creating improved health and preventing future illness in the patients who seek our professional assistance. However, even complete multidimensional treatment plans still fall short of the goal of creating wellness, if for no other reasons than 1) they are still disease- and problem-oriented, rather than health-oriented, 2) they are prescribed from outside ("The doctor told me to do it.") rather than originating internally and spontaneously by the patient's own direction and affirmation ("I *do* this because I *am* this."), and, finally and most

difficult to relay, 3) they are mechanistic rather than organic, they can do no better than the sum of their parts, they flow exclusively from the mind ("do") and not also from the body-soul ("am"). The art of creating wellness takes time to understand, longer to implement clinically, and even longer to apply to one's own life. Wellness is a state of being rather than a checklist of activities in a "preventive health program." The subtle differences that distinguish "wellness" from any "program" or "prescription" are the differences between *leading* versus *following* and *flowing* versus *performing*. **Wellness is multidimensional self-actualization, full integration of one's life — present, past, and future; physical, mental, emotional, spiritual, biochemical — one's shadow[22], work[23], feelings, thoughts, and goals into a cohesive living whole – "a wheel rolling from its own center."[24]**

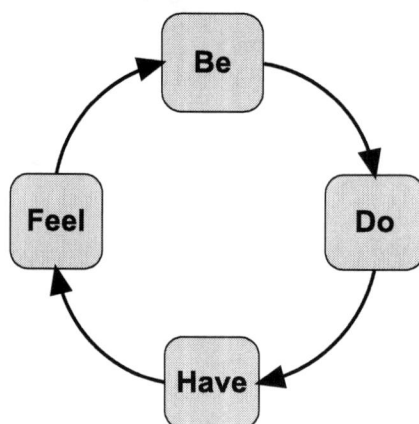

---

[22] Robert Bly. The Human Shadow. Sound Horizons 1991 [ISBN: 1879323001] and Bly R. A Little Book on the Human Shadow. [ISBN: 0062548476]
[23] Rick Jarow. Creating the Work You Love: Courage, Commitment and Career; Inner Traditions Intl Ltd; (December 1995) [ISBN: 0892815426]
[24] Walter Kaufmann (Translator), Friedrich Wilhelm Nietzsche. Thus Spoke Zarathustra: A Book for None and All. Penguin USA; 1978, page 27

Acute Care and Musculoskeletal Care: Opportunities for Health Optimization

Clinicians should appreciate that every patient encounter is an opportunity for comprehensive care, disease prevention, and health optimization. This is true whether the presenting complaint is acne, psoriasis, a respiratory infection, or musculoskeletal pain. Given the relatively high frequency of musculoskeletal complaints in clinical practice in general and chiropractic and osteopathic practices in particular, the following section will emphasize the clinical presentation of musculoskeletal complaints as an underappreciated opportunity for wellness care.

Since **approximately 1 of every 7 (14% of total) visits to a primary healthcare provider is for the treatment of musculoskeletal pain or dysfunction**[25], every healthcare provider needs to have 1) knowledge of important concepts related to musculoskeletal medicine, 2) the ability to recognize urgent and emergency conditions, 3) the ability to competently perform orthopedic examination procedures and interpret laboratory assessments, and 4) the knowledge and ability to design and implement effective treatment plans and to coordinate patient management.

In pharmacosurgical allopathic medicine, the goal of musculoskeletal treatment is to address the patient's injury or disorder by alleviating pain with the use of drugs, preventing further injury, and returning the patient to his/her previous status and activities. The most commonly employed interventions are 1) rest and "watchful waiting", 2) non-steroidal anti-inflammatory drugs (NSAIDS) and cyclooxygenase-2-inhibitors (COX-2 inhibitors, or "coxibs"), and 3) surgery. The more action-oriented approaches used by many chiropractic, naturopathic, and osteopathic physicians differs from the allopathic approach because, although avoidance of and "rest" from damaging activities is reasonable and valuable, too much rest without an emphasis on active preventive rehabilitation ❶ encourages patient passivity and ❷ the assumption of the sick role, and it ❸ fails to actively promote tissue healing and ❹ fails to address the underlying proprioceptive deficits that are common in patients with chronic musculoskeletal pain and recurrent injuries.[26,27,28] **NSAIDs are considered "first line" therapy for musculoskeletal disorders by allopaths** despite the data showing that "**There is no evidence that widely used NSAIDs have any long-term benefit on osteoarthritis.**"[29] What is worse than this lack of efficacy is the evidence showing that NSAIDs *exacerbate* musculoskeletal disease (rather than *cure* it). **NSAIDs are known to inhibit cartilage formation and to promote bone necrosis and joint degradation with long-term use**[30,31,32,33] and **NSAIDs are responsible for more than 16,000 gastrohemorrhagic deaths and 100,000 hospitalizations each year.**[34] The "coxibs" were supposed to provide anti-inflammatory benefits with an enhanced safety profile, but the gastrocentric focus of the drug developers failed to appreciate

> **Allopathic medicine has been sold to the public under the banner of "scientific" from a time when this was not the case**
>
> "…only about 15% of medical interventions are supported by solid scientific evidence…"
>
> Smith R. Where is the wisdom…? The poverty of medical evidence. *BMJ*. 1991 Oct 5;303:798-9

that COX-2 is necessary for the formation of prostacyclin, a prostaglandin created from arachidonic acid via COX-2 that plays an important role in vasodilation and antithrombosis; not surprisingly therefore, use of COX-2-inhibiting drugs has consistently been associated with increased risk for adverse cardiovascular effects including

---

[25] American College of Rheumatology Ad Hoc Committee on Clinical Guidelines. Guidelines for the initial evaluation of the adult patient with acute musculoskeletal symptoms. *Arthritis Rheum*. 1996 Jan;39(1):1-8 See also: **Vasquez A**. Musculoskeletal disorders and iron overload disease: comment on the American College of Rheumatology guidelines. *Arthritis Rheum* 1996;39: 1767-8

[26] McPartland JM, Brodeur RR, Hallgren RC. Chronic neck pain, standing balance, and suboccipital muscle atrophy--a pilot study. *J Manipulative Physiol Ther*. 1997;20:24-9

[27] Bullock-Saxton JE, Janda V, Bullock MI. Reflex activation of gluteal muscles in walking. An approach to restoration of muscle function for patients with low-back pain. *Spine* 1993 May;18(6):704-8

[28] Sinaki M, Brey RH, Hughes CA, Larson DR, Kaufman KR. Significant reduction in risk of falls and back pain in osteoporotic-kyphotic women through a Spinal Proprioceptive Extension Exercise Dynamic (SPEED) program. *Mayo Clin Proc*. 2005 Jul;80(7):849-55

[29] Beers MH, Berkow R (eds). *The Merck Manual. 17th Edition*. Whitehouse Station; Merck Research Laboratories 1999 page 451

[30] "At…concentrations comparable to those… in the synovial fluid of patients treated with the drug, several NSAIDs suppress proteoglycan synthesis… These NSAID-related effects on chondrocyte metabolism … much more profound in osteoarthritic cartilage than in normal cartilage, due to enhanced uptake of NSAIDs by the osteoarthritic cartilage." Brandt KD. Effects of nonsteroidal anti-inflammatory drugs on chondrocyte metabolism in vitro and in vivo. *Am J Med*. 1987 Nov 20; 83(5A): 29-34

[31] "The case of a young healthy man, who developed avascular necrosis of head of femur after prolonged administration of indomethacin, is reported here." Prathapkumar KR, Smith I, Attara GA. Indomethacin induced avascular necrosis of head of femur. *Postgrad Med J*. 2000 Sep; 76(899): 574-5

[32] "This highly significant association between NSAID use and acetabular destruction gives cause for concern, not least because of the difficulty in achieving satisfactory hip replacements in patients with severely damaged acetabula." Newman NM, Ling RS. Acetabular bone destruction related to non-steroidal anti-inflammatory drugs. *Lancet*. 1985 Jul 6; 2(8445): 11-4

[33] Vidal y Plana RR, Bizzarri D, Rovati AL. Articular cartilage pharmacology: I. In vitro studies on glucosamine and non steroidal antiinflammatory drugs. *Pharmacol Res Commun*. 1978 Jun;10(6):557-69

[34] Singh G. Recent considerations in nonsteroidal anti-inflammatory drug gastropathy. *Am J Med*. 1998;105(1B):31S-38S

myocardial infarction, unstable angina, cardiac thrombus, resuscitated cardiac arrest, sudden or unexplained death, ischemic stroke, and transient ischemic attacks.[35] Additionally, the use of a COX-2 inhibiting treatment in patients who overconsume arachidonic acid (i.e., most people in America and other industrialized nations[36]) would be expected to shunt bioavailable arachidonate into the formation of leukotrienes, a group of inflammatory mediators now known to contribute directly to atherogenesis.[37] Thus, the outcome was entirely predictable: overuse of COX-2 inhibitors should have been expected to create a catastrophe of iatrogenic cardiovascular death, and this is exactly what was allowed to occur—clearly indicating independent but synergistic failures on the part of pharmaceutical companies, the FDA, and the medical profession.[38,39,40,41] According to statements by David J. Graham, MD, MPH, (Associate Director for Science, Office of Drug Safety, FDA) in 2005, an estimated 139,000 Americans who took Vioxx suffered serious complications including stroke or myocardial infarction; between 26,000 and 55,000 Americans died as a result of their doctors' prescribing Vioxx.[42] Additionally, the surgical procedures employed by allopaths for the treatment of musculoskeletal pain do not consistently show evidence of efficacy, safety, or cost-effectiveness. Arthroscopic surgery for osteoarthritis of the knee, for example, costs thousands of dollars to each individual and billions of dollars to the American healthcare system but is no more effective than placebo.[43,44,45] In a review which also noted that only 15% of medical procedures are supported by literature references and that only 1% of such references are deemed scientifically valid, Rosner[46] showed that the risks of serious injury (i.e., cauda equina syndrome or vertebral artery dissection) associated with spinal manipulation are "*400 times lower* than the death rates observed from gastrointestinal bleeding due to the use of nonsteroidal anti-inflammatory drugs and *700 times lower* than the overall mortality rate for spinal surgery."

In chiropractic, osteopathic, and naturopathic medicine, the goal and means of musculoskeletal treatment is to address the patient's injury or disorder by simultaneously alleviating pain with the use of natural, noninvasive, low-cost, and low-risk interventions while improving the patient's overall health, preventing future health problems, and "upgrading" the patient's overall paradigm of health maintenance and disease prevention from one that is passive and reactive to one that is empowered and pro-active. Commonly employed therapeutics include spinal manipulation[47,48,49], exercise[50] and the use of nutritional supplements and botanical medicines[51,52] which have been demonstrated in peer-reviewed clinical trials to be safe and effective for the alleviation of musculoskeletal pain. More specifically, chiropractic and naturopathic physicians are particularly well-versed in the clinical utilization of such treatments as niacinamide[53], glucosamine and chondroitin sulfates[54], vitamin D[55], vitamin B-12[56], balanced and complete fatty acid therapy[57,58], anti-inflammatory diets[59,60,61], proteolytic/pancreatic

[35] Mukherjee D, Nissen SE, Topol EJ. Risk of cardiovascular events associated with selective COX-2 inhibitors. *JAMA*. 2001 Aug 22-29;286(8):954-9

[36] Seaman DR. The diet-induced proinflammatory state: a cause of chronic pain and other degenerative diseases? *J Manipulative Physiol Ther*. 2002;25(3):168-79

[37] Dwyer JH, Allayee H, Dwyer KM, Fan J, Wu H, Mar R, Lusis AJ, Mehrabian M. Arachidonate 5-lipoxygenase promoter genotype, dietary arachidonic acid, and atherosclerosis. *N Engl J Med*. 2004 Jan 1;350(1):29-37

[38] Topol EJ. Arthritis medicines and cardiovascular events--"house of coxibs". *JAMA*. 2005 Jan 19;293(3):366-8. Epub 2004 Dec 28

[39] Ray WA, Griffin MR, Stein CM. Cardiovascular toxicity of valdecoxib. *N Engl J Med*. 2004 Dec 23;351(26):2767. Epub 2004 Dec 17

[40] Topol EJ. Failing the public health--rofecoxib, Merck, and the FDA. *N Engl J Med*. 2004 Oct 21;351(17):1707-9

[41] Horton R. Vioxx, the implosion of Merck, and aftershocks at the FDA. *Lancet*. 2004 Dec 4-10;364(9450):1995-6

[42] David J. Graham, MD, MPH, (Associate Director for Science, Office of Drug Safety, US FDA) estimated that 139,000 Americans who took Vioxx suffered serious side effects; he estimated that the drug killed between 26,000 and 55,000 people. http://www.commondreams.org/views05/0223-35.htm http://www.fda.gov/cder/drug/infopage/vioxx/vioxxgraham.pdf Accessed November 25, 2006

[43] Gina Kolata. A Knee Surgery for Arthritis Is Called Sham. *The New York Times*, July 11, 2002

[44] Moseley JB, O'Malley K, Petersen NJ, Menke TJ, Brody BA, Kuykendall DH, Hollingsworth JC, Ashton CM, Wray NP. A controlled trial of arthroscopic surgery for osteoarthritis of the knee. *N Engl J Med*. 2002;347:81-8

[45] Bernstein J, Quach T. A perspective on the study of Moseley: questioning the value of arthroscopic knee surgery for osteoarthritis. *Cleve Clin J Med* 2003;70:401, 405-6, 408-10

[46] Rosner AL. Evidence-based clinical guidelines for the management of acute low-back pain: response to the guidelines prepared for the Australian Medical Health and Research Council. *J Manipulative Physiol Ther*. 2001;24(3):214-20

[47] Manga P, Angus D, Papadopoulos C, et al. *The Effectiveness and Cost-Effectiveness of Chiropractic Management of Low-Back Pain*. Richmond Hill, Ontario: Kenilworth Publishing; 1993

[48] Meade TW, Dyer S, Browne W, Townsend J, Frank AO. Low-back pain of mechanical origin: randomised comparison of chiropractic and hospital outpatient treatment. *BMJ*. 1990;300(6737):1431-7

[49] Meade TW, Dyer S, Browne W, Frank AO. Randomised comparison of chiropractic and hospital outpatient management for low-back pain: results from extended follow up. *BMJ*. 1995;311(7001):349-5

[50] Harold Elrick, MD. Exercise is Medicine. *The Physician and Sportsmedicine* - Volume 24 - No. 2 - February 1996

[51] **Vasquez A**. Revisiting the Five-Part Nutritional Wellness Protocol: The Supplemented Paleo-Mediterranean Diet. *Nutritional Perspectives* 2011 January http://optimalhealthresearch.com/part8.html

[52] **Vasquez A**. Reducing pain and inflammation naturally - Part 3: Improving overall health while safely and effectively treating musculoskeletal pain. *Nutritional Perspectives* 2005; 28: 34-38, 40-42 http://optimalhealthresearch.com/part3.html

[53] Kaufman W. Niacinamide therapy for joint mobility. Therapeutic reversal of a common clinical manifestation of the "normal" aging process. *Conn State Med J* 1953;17:584-591

[54] Reginster JY, Deroisy R, Rovati LC, Lee RL, Lejeune E, Bruyere O, Giacovelli G, Henrotin Y, Dacre JE, Gossett C. Long-term effects of glucosamine sulphate on osteoarthritis progression: a randomised, placebo-controlled clinical trial. *Lancet*. 2001;357(9252):251-6

[55] **Vasquez A**, Manso G, Cannell J. The clinical importance of vitamin D: a paradigm shift with implications for all healthcare providers. *Altern Ther Health Med* 2004;10:28-36 http://optimalhealthresearch.com/monograph04.html

[56] Mauro GL, Martorana U, Cataldo P, Brancato G, Letizia G. Vitamin B12 in low back pain: a randomised, double-blind, placebo-controlled study. *Eur Rev Med Pharmacol Sci*. 2000 May-Jun;4(3):53-8

enzymes[62], and botanical medicines such as *Boswellia*[63], *Harpagophytum*[64], *Uncaria*, and willow bark[65,66] —each of these interventions has been validated in peer-reviewed research for safety and effectiveness.[67] Furthermore, from the perspective of integrative chiropractic and naturopathic medicine, aiming for such a limited accomplishment as mere "returning the patient to previous status and activities" would be considered substandard, since the patient's overall health was neither addressed nor improved and since returning the patient to his/her previous status and activities would be a direct invitation for the problem to recur indefinitely. Chiropractic and naturopathic physicians appreciate that, especially regarding chronic health problems, any treatment plan that allows the patient to resume his/her previous lifestyle is by definition doomed to fail because a return to the patient's previous lifestyle and activities that allowed the onset of the disease/disorder in the first place will most certainly result in the perpetuation and recurrence of the illness or disorder. **Stated more directly: for** *healing* **to truly be effective, the comprehensive treatment plan must generally result in a permanent and profound change in the patient's lifestyle and emotional climate, which are the primary modifiable determinants of either health or disease.**

[57] **Vasquez A**. Reducing Pain and Inflammation Naturally. Part 1: New Insights into Fatty Acid Biochemistry and the Influence of Diet. *Nutritional Perspectives* 2004; Oct: 5, 7-10,12,14 http://optimalhealthresearch.com/part1.html

[58] **Vasquez A**. Reducing Pain and Inflammation Naturally. Part 2: New Insights into Fatty Acid Supplementation and Its Effect on Eicosanoid Production and Genetic Expression. *Nutritional Perspectives* 2005; January: 5-16 http://optimalhealthresearch.com/part2.html

[59] Seaman DR. The diet-induced proinflammatory state: a cause of chronic pain and other degenerative diseases? *J Manipulative Physiol Ther*. 2002 Mar-Apr;25(3):168-7

[60] **Vasquez A**. *Integrative Orthopedics*. http://optimalhealthresearch.com/orthopedics.html

[61] **Vasquez A**. Reducing Pain and Inflammation Naturally. Part 1: New Insights into Fatty Acid Biochemistry and the Influence of Diet. *Nutritional Perspectives* 2004; October: 5, 7-10, 12, 14 http://optimalhealthresearch.com/part1.html

[62] Trickett P. Proteolytic enzymes in treatment of athletic injuries. *Appl Ther*. 1964;30:647-52

[63] Kimmatkar N, Thawani V, Hingorani L, Khiyani R. Efficacy and tolerability of Boswellia serrata extract in treatment of osteoarthritis of knee--a randomized double blind placebo controlled trial. *Phytomedicine*. 2003 Jan;10(1):3-7

[64] Chrubasik S, Junck H, Breitschwerdt H, Conradt C, Zappe H. Effectiveness of Harpagophytum extract WS 1531 in the treatment of exacerbation of low-back pain: a randomized, placebo-controlled, double-blind study. *Eur J Anaesthesiol* 1999 Feb;16(2):118-29

[65] Chrubasik S, Eisenberg E, Balan E, Weinberger T, Luzzati R, Conradt C. Treatment of low-back pain exacerbations with willow bark extract: a randomized double-blind study. *Am J Med*. 2000;109:9-14

[66] **Vasquez A**, Muanza DN. Comment: Evaluation of Presence of Aspirin-Related Warnings with Willow Bark. *Ann Pharmacotherapy* 2005 Oct;39(10):1763

[67] **Vasquez A**. Reducing pain and inflammation naturally. Part 3: Improving overall health while safely and effectively treating musculoskeletal pain. *Nutritional Perspectives* 2005;28:34-42 http://optimalhealthresearch.com/part3.html

Clinical Assessments

The clinical assessments reviewed in the following sections are history-taking, orthopedic/musculoskeletal, and neurologic examinations, and commonly used laboratory tests. **History taking is the art of conducting an *informative* and *collaborative* patient interview.**

The role of the doctor during the interview process is not merely that of a data-collecting machine, spewing out questions and receiving responses. Patient interviews can be a creative, enjoyable, comforting opportunity to build rapport and to establish meaningful connection with another human being. Patients are not simply people with health problems – they are first and foremost our fellow human beings, not so dissimilar from ourselves perhaps, and always full of complexity. Our task is not to fully understand their complexity nor to solve all of their mysteries, but rather to help orchestrate these dynamics into a coordinated if not unified direction that promotes health and healing.

Beyond its diagnostic value, the interview process also provides a key opportunity to gain insight into the patient's psychoepistimology—the patient's operating system for interacting with data and the world and internalizing and metabolizing external inputs in such a way as to merge these with internal experiences (i.e., emotions, feelings, preferences, responses). Epistemology is the branch of philosophy concerned with the nature and scope of knowledge. Per Rand[68], psychoepistimology is a person's "method of awareness"; a person's psychoepistimology creates a "corollary view of existence" and in turn, "A man's method of using his consciousness determines his method of survival." By understanding how the patient views him/herself in the world, understanding his/her goals, and—in essence—what "drives" the patient and what "makes him/her tick", clinicians can shape the nuances of the conversation and the treatment plan to promote the desired cognitive-conceptual-behavioral changes in behavior that are prerequisite for the attainment of optimized health outcomes.

History & Assessment

History of the primary complaint: "D.O.P.P. Q.R.S.T."
- Description/location
- Onset
- Provocation: exacerbates
- Palliation: alleviates
- Quality
- Radiation of pain
- Severity
- Timing

Associated complaints
- Additional manifestations
- Concomitant diseases

Review of systems
- Head-to-toe inventory of health status, associated health problems, and complications

Past health history
- Surgeries
- Hospitalizations
- Traumas
- Vaccinations and medications
- Successful and failed treatments for the current complaint(s)

Family health history
- Genotropic illnesses and predispositions
- Lifestyle patterns
- Emotional expectations

Social history
- Hobbies, work, exposures
- Relationships and emotional experiences
- Interpersonal support
- Malpractice litigation

Health Habits
- Diet: appropriate intake of protein, fruits, vegetables, fats, sugars
- Sleep
- Stress management
- Exercise / Sedentary Lifestyle
- Spirituality / Centeredness
- Caffeine and tobacco
- Ethanol and recreational drugs

Medication and supplements
- Reason, doses, duration, cost
- Side-effects
- Interactions

Responsibility and Compliance
- Ability and willingness to comply with prescribed treatment plan and to incorporate the necessary diet-exercise-relationship-emotional-lifestyle modifications
- *Internal* versus *external* locus of control

---

[68] Rand A. For the New Intellectual. New York; Signet:1961, 16

```
┌──────────────────┐         ╔═══════════════╗
│  Patient History │ ──────▶ ║  Establish a  ║
└──────────────────┘         ║ relationship of║
         │                   ║ trust, empathy,║
         ▼                   ║  and mutual   ║
   ╔═══════════╗             ║   respect     ║
   ║  Obtain   ║             ╚═══════════════╝
   ║information║
   ║ about the ║
   ║  illness  ║
   ║and the patient║
   ╚═══════════╝
   ╱    │    │    ╲
  ▼     ▼    ▼     ▼
┌─────┐┌──────┐┌──────┐┌──────┐
│History││Physical││Imaging││ Lab │
│      ││ exam  ││studies││tests │
└─────┘└──────┘└──────┘└──────┘
    ╲     │    │    ╱
     ▼    ▼    ▼   ▼
   ┌──────────────────┐
   │  Assessment of   │
   │   the patient    │
   │        &         │
   │   Diagnosis of   │
   │  health disorder │
   └──────────────────┘
            │
            ▼
   ╭──────────────────╮
   │ Determine course(s) of │
   │ action for each problem │
   ╰──────────────────╯
      │      │      │      │
   ┌─────┐┌────────┐┌──────┐┌──────────────┐
   │Refer││Co-manage││Treat &││Follow-up, reevaluate,│
   │     ││        ││Educate││update treatment plan │
   └─────┘└────────┘└──────┘└──────────────┘
```

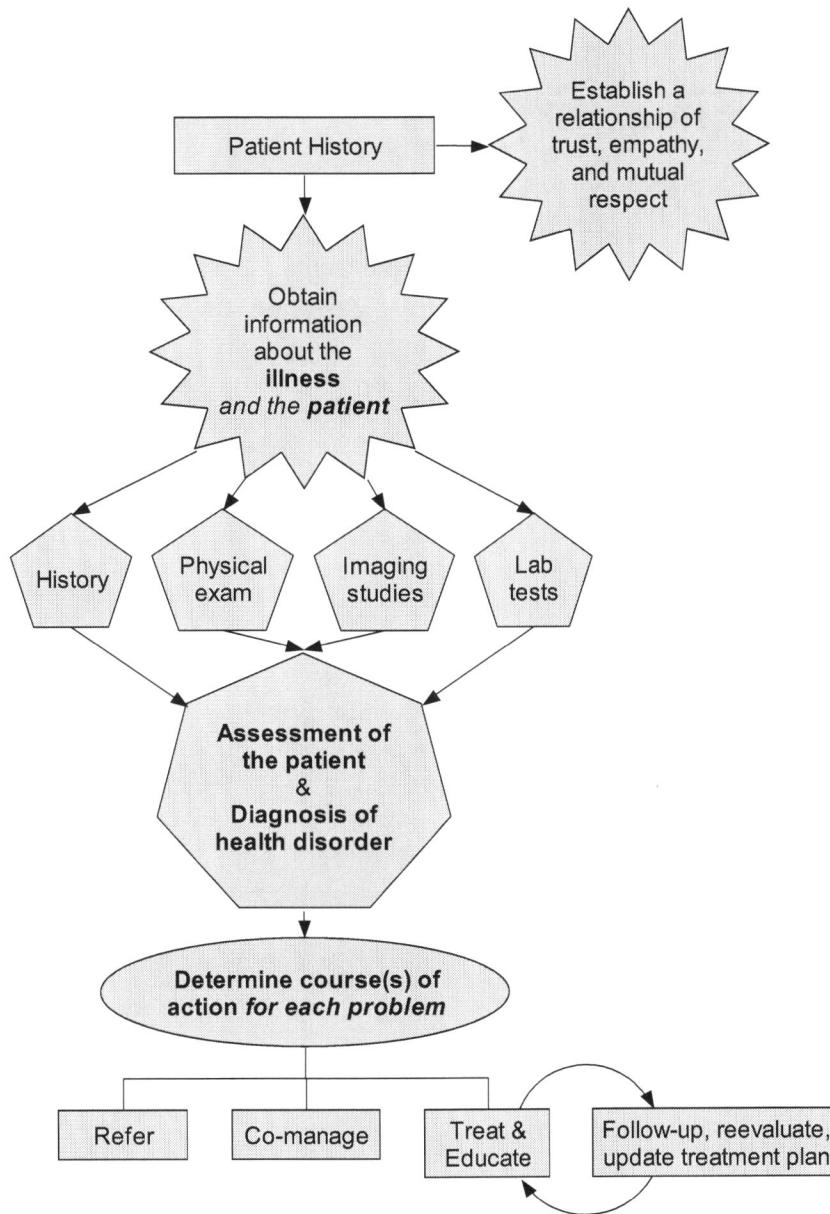

Key components of patient assessment and management: Patient assessment and management is an on-going process that begins with the initial history taken at the first clinical encounter and continues through the physical examination and laboratory assessments and thereafter by monitoring the patient's implementation of and response to the treatment plan. The plan is complete when the desired outcome of health optimization is achieved and sustained.

Components of a Complete Patient History: "D.O.P.P. Q.R.S.T."

Category	Patient history questions and implications
Description, Location: Always start with open-ended questions	• *What is it like for you?* • *What do you experience?* • *What are you feeling?* • *Where is the pain/sensation/problem)?* • Ask about specifics: **Pain, numbness, weakness, tingling**, fatigue, recent or chronic infections, burning, aching, dull, sharp, cramping, stretching, pins and needles, weakness, changes in function (i.e., bowel and bladder continence).
Onset	• *When did it begin? Have you ever had anything like this before?* • *Was there a specific event associated with the onset of the problem, such as an injury or an illness, or did the problem start gradually or insidiously?* • *How has it changed over time?* • *Prior injuries to site?* • *Why are you seeking care for this now (rather than last week or last month)?* • *What has changed? How is the pain/problem developing over time—getting worse or getting better?*
Palliation	• *How have you tried treating it? Does anything make it go away?* • *What makes it better? What relieves the pain?* • Ask about prior and current treatments, radiographs, medications, supplements (herbs, vitamins, minerals), injections, surgery, massage, manipulation, counseling. • Knowing response/resistance to previous treatments can provide clinical insight.
Provocation	• *Are your symptoms constant, or does the problem come and go?* • *What makes it worse? What makes the pain worse?* • *When during the day/week/month/year are your symptoms the worst?*
Quality	• *Can you describe the pain to me?* • *What does it feel like?* • *What do you experience?* • Get a clear understanding of the type of sensation(s): stabbing, shooting pain, pins and needles, sharp pain, electric sensation, numbness, burning, aching, throbbing, weakness, tingling, gel phenomenon (stiffness worsened by inactivity), dizziness, confusion, fatigue, shortness of breath.
Radiation	• *Does the pain stay localized or does it move to your arm/leg/head/face?* • *Do you feel pain in other areas of your body?*
Severity	• *How bad is it? How would you rate it on a scale of one to ten if one were almost no pain and ten was the worst pain you could imagine?* Use the validated VAS—visual analog scale—to quantify the level of pain and impairment. • *Does this problem prevent you from engaging in your daily activities, such as work, exercise, or hobbies?* This is a very important question for determining functional impairment and internal consistency; if the patient is "too injured to work" yet is still able to fully participate in recreational activities that are physically challenging, then malingering is likely.
Timing	• *When do you notice this problem?* • *Is it constant, or does it come and go? Where are you when you notice it the most?* • *Is it worse in the morning, or worse in the evening?* • *Does anyone else in your [home/office/worksite] have this same problem?* • *What times of the day or what days of the week is it the worst?*

Components of a Complete Patient History: "D.O.P.P. Q.R.S.T." —*continued*

Category	Patient history questions and implications
Associated manifestations and constitutional symptoms	• *Have you noticed any other problems associated with this problem?* • **Fatigue?** • **Fever?** • **Weight loss?** *Weight gain?* • *Night* **sweats?** • **Diarrhea? Constipation?** • **Weakness?** • *Nausea?* • *Bowel or bladder difficulties or changes? Difficulty with sexual function?* These could be related to hormonal imbalances, drug side-effects, relationship problems, nutritional deficiencies, nerve compression, and/or depression. • *Change in sensation near your anus/genitals?* Cauda equina syndrome is an important consideration in patients with low-back pain. • *Loss of appetite?* • *Difficulty sleeping?* • *Skin rash or change in pigmentation?*
ROS: review of systems	• <u>General constitution</u>: fatigue, malaise, fever, chills, weight gain/loss… • *"Now we are going to conduct a head-to-toe inventory just to make sure that we have covered everything."* • <u>Head</u>: headaches, head pain, pressure inside head, difficulty concentrating, difficulty remembering, mental function • <u>Ears</u>: ringing in ears, dizziness, hearing loss, hypersensitivity to noise, ear pain, discharge from ear, pressure in ears • <u>Eyes</u>: eye pain, loss of vision or decreased vision or ability to focus, redness or irritation, seeing flashing lights or spots, double vision • <u>Nose</u>: sinus problems, chronically stuffy nose, difficulty smelling things, nose bleeds, change or decrease in sense of smell or taste • <u>Mouth</u>, teeth, TMJ, pain or sores in mouth, difficulty chewing, sensitive teeth, bleeding gums, pain in jaw joint, change or decrease in sense of taste • <u>Neck</u>: pain at the base of skull, pain in neck, stiffness • <u>Throat</u>: difficulty swallowing, pain in throat, feeling like things get stuck in throat, change in voice, difficulty getting air or food in or out • <u>Chest and breasts</u>: any chest pain, difficult breathing, wheezing, coughing, pain, lumps, or discharge from nipple • <u>Shoulders</u>: pain or aching in your shoulders, restricted motion or stiffness • <u>Arms, elbows, hands</u>: pain or problems with your arms, elbows, hands, …in the joints or the muscles…, numbness, tingling, weakness, swelling, changes in fingernails, cold hands? • <u>Stomach, abdomen, pelvis, genitals, urinary tract, rectum,</u> : pain in stomach or abdomen, difficulty with digestion, gas, bloating, regurgitation, ulcer, any problems lower down in your abdomen—near your lower intestines? Pain, lumps, swelling, difficulty passing stool, pain or itching near your anus, genitalia; any genital pain, burning, discharge, redness, irritation, sexual dysfunction or impotence, loss of bowel or bladder control? Diarrhea or constipation? How often do you have a bowel movement? • <u>Hips, legs, knees, ankles, feet</u>: numbness, weakness, pain or tingling in the hips, knees, ankles, or feet; pain in calves with walking, swelling of ankles, cold feet • *Is there anything else that you think I should know in order to help you?*

Components of a Complete Patient History: "D.O.P.P. Q.R.S.T." —*continued*

Category	Patient history questions and implications

Medical history	• *Are you taking any* **medications**? *What medications have you taken in the past few years?* Finding out that your new patient recently discontinued his 20-year regimen of valproic acid, lithium, and risperidone may significantly change your interpretation of the clinical interview
	• *Have you been* **treated for any medical conditions** *or health problems?*
	• *Have you ever been* **hospitalized**?
	• *Have you ever had* **surgery**?
	• *Have you ever been* **diagnosed with any health problems** *such as high blood pressure or diabetes?*
	• Investigate for specific problems in the past health history that would be a major oversight to miss:
	   ○ Current or past diseases: Cancer, Diabetes, Mental illness
	   ○ Hypertension or high cholesterol
	   ○ Medications, especially corticosteroids
	   ○ Surgeries & Hospitalizations
	   ○ Infections, Immune disorders
	   ○ Trauma or previous injuries

Social history	• **Work**—*What do you do for work? Are you exposed to chemicals or fumes at your workplace?* • **Hobbies**—*What do you do for recreation or hobbies? Are you exposed to chemicals or fumes at home or with your hobbies (e.g., painting, gardening)?* • **Eat**—*Tell me about your breakfast, lunch, dinner, snacks… Do you consume foods or drinks that contain aspartame* (linked to increased incidence of brain tumors[69]) *or carrageenan* (possibly linked to increased risk of breast cancer and inflammatory bowel disease[70,71])? • **Exercise**—*What do you do for exercise or physical activity?* • **Drink**—*Do you* **drink alcohol**? *Coffee/caffeine? Water?* • **Drugs**—*Do you use recreational* **drugs**? **Now or in the past?** • **Smoke**—*Do you* **smoke**? • **Sex**—*Are you* **sexually** *active? If so, do you practice safer sex practices?* For all women: *Is there any chance you could be pregnant right now? A "yes" reply may contraindicate radiographic assessment and the use of certain nutrients, botanicals, and/or drugs.* • **Emotional support** • **Family contact and relationships**
Family health history	• *Does anyone in your family have any health problems, especially your parents and siblings?* • *Do you have any children? Do they have any health problems?* • *Do any diseases "run in the family" such as cancer, diabetes, arthritis, heart disease?*
Additional questions	• *Do you have any other information for me? Is there anything that I did not ask?* • *What is your opinion as to why you are having this health problem?* • *Are you in litigation for your illness or injuries?*

---

[69] "In the past two decades brain tumor rates have risen in several industrialized countries, including the United States... Compared to other environmental factors putatively linked to brain tumors, the artificial sweetener aspartame is a promising candidate to explain the recent increase in incidence and degree of malignancy of brain tumors." Olney JW, Farber NB, Spitznagel E, Robins LN. Increasing brain tumor rates: is there a link to aspartame? *J Neuropathol Exp Neurol* 1996 Nov;55(11):1115-23

[70] Tobacman JK. Review of harmful gastrointestinal effects of carrageenan in animal experiments. *Environ Health Perspect.* 2001 Oct;109(10):983-94

[71] "However, the gum carrageenan which is comprised of linked, sulfated galactose residues has potent biological activity and undergoes acid hydrolysis to poligeenan, an acknowledged carcinogen." Tobacman JK, Wallace RB, Zimmerman MB. Consumption of carrageenan and other water-soluble polymers used as food additives and incidence of mammary carcinoma. *Med Hypotheses.* 2001 May;56(5):589-98

Physical Examination

Goals and purpose of the orthopedic/musculoskeletal examination:

1. **To establish an accurate diagnosis (or diagnoses),**
2. **To assess the patient's functional status and current condition,**
3. **To assess for concomitant and/or underlying and preexisting problems,**
4. **To rule out emergency situations**

- *Example*: If your patient presents with low back and leg pain, and you determine that his fall off a horse resulted in ischial bursitis, have you also excluded a lumbar compression fracture? You can send the patient home with anti-inflammatory treatments and icepacks for the bursitis; but if you missed the spinal fracture, your patient could suffer neurologic injury resultant from your "failure to diagnose." **Don't assume that the patient has only one problem until you have proven with your history and examination that other likely problems do not exist.**

Functional assessment: When working with patients with acute injuries and systemic diseases, **take a wider view of the patient than simply diagnosing the problem.**

- *Will she be able to return to work?*
- *Will he be able to drive home safely?*
- *Will she need help with activities of daily living?*
- *Is there an occult disease, infection, malignancy, or toxic exposure that is causing these problems?*
- *Is this an acute presentation of a new problem, or an acute exacerbation of a chronic problem?*

Neurologic examination: One of the most important areas to assess when a patient presents with a musculoskeletal complaint is the neurologic system, especially if the complaint is related to a recent traumatic injury. Blood circulation is essential for life; but lack of circulation is only a major consideration in a small number of injuries, and it is usually readily apparent when severe because the problem will become acute quickly. Nerve injuries, however, can be subtle. All patients with spine (neck, thoracic, low back) pain must be questioned thoroughly for evidence of neurologic compromise. **Neurologic insults—such as cauda equina syndrome and transverse myelitis—can be painless**, can progress rapidly, and can lead to permanent functional disability from muscle weakness or paralysis. **Every patient with pain, weakness, or recent trauma must be evaluated for neurologic deficits before the patient is treated and released from care.** Neurologic examinations are briefly reviewed in the pages that follow; citations can be used for sources of additional information.

Resources for students on neurologic assessment:

- Goldberg S. <u>The Four-Minute Neurologic Exam</u>. Medmaster http://www.medmaster.net/
- http://www.neuroexam.com/neuroexam/ Information and free videos of a neurologic exam.
- http://rad.usuhs.mil/rad/eye_simulator/eyesimulator.html Excellent interactive simulation of assessment of extraocular muscles in a neurologic examination.
- http://emedicine.medscape.com/article/1147993-overview Excellent review, noteworthy for its description of a "+5" level of reflex grading denoting sustained clonus.

Orthopedic Musculoskeletal Examination: Concepts and Goals

Orthopedic tests are detailed or reviewed in each respective chapter of *Integrative Orthopedics*[72] (i.e., shoulder exams are in the chapter on shoulders, knee exams in the chapter on knees). This section reviews the concepts and goals that provide the rationale for performing these tests. **Orthopedic tests are designed to place particular types of stress on specific body tissues.** Types of stress include tension/distraction, compression/pressure, shear force, vibration, friction, and percussion. Each type of stress is applied to elicit specific information about the exact tissue or structure that is being tested. *If you understand the reason for the type of stress that you are applying, and you are aware of the tissue/structure that you are testing, then you will find it much easier to perform the dozens of tests that are required in clinical practice. If you understand the "how" and the "why" then you won't be overwhelmed with named tests that otherwise appear illogical or superfluous.*

> **Types of stress applied during the physical examination for specific purposes**
>
> - **Tension, traction**: To provoke pain from injured/compromised tissues: tendons, muscles, ligaments, and nerves
> - **Compression, pressure**: To provoke pain from inflamed tissues; also used to assess for swelling and fluid accumulation in subcutaneous tissue, bursa, and joint spaces such as the knee
> - **Shearing force**: To test the integrity of ligaments and intervertebral discs
> - **Vibration (using ultrasound or 128 Hz tuning fork)**: To assess vibration sense (neurologic: peripheral nerves and dorsal columns) and screen for broken bones (orthopedic)
> - **Friction, grinding**: To elicit pain from injured tissues (cross-fiber friction) and articular surfaces (grinding tests)
> - **Percussion, over bone and discs**: To assess for bone fractures, bone infections, and acute disc injuries
> - **Percussion, over peripheral nerves**: To assess hypesthesia/tingling suggesting reduced threshold for depolarization secondary to nerve irritation or compression, i.e., Tinel's sign
> - **Fulcrum tests**: To assess for bone fractures: commonly the doctor's arm or a firm object is placed centrally under the bone in question and increasingly firm downward stress is applied to both ends of the bone to test for occult fracture
> - **Torque, twisting**: To test joint integrity (restriction or laxity) or for occult bone fracture (particularly of the digits)

The tests that are described in *Integrative Orthopedics* meet at least one of the following two criteria: 1) it is a common test that all doctors know and which is needed for the sake of communication and for passing academic and licensing examinations, or 2) it is going to be a useful test in clinical practice.

Always remember that abnormalities found during the physical examination—particularly the neurologic examination—are often indicative of an underlying *nonmusculoskeletal* problem that must be identified or—at the very least—considered and then excluded by additional testing. For example, a patient **shoulder pain** and neurologic deficits found during the neuromusculoskeletal portion of your examination could have a **herniated cervical disc** as the underlying cause; but the cause could also be **syringomyelia**, or an **apical lung tumor** that is invading local bone and destroying the nerves of the brachial plexus.[73] As a clinician, the successful management and treatment of your patients depends in large part on the following: ❶ **knowledge**: your ability to conceptualize broadly and to consider many *functional* and *pathologic* causes of your patient's complaints, ❷ **tact**: the efficiency and accuracy with which you assess, accept, and exclude the various differential diagnoses into your final working diagnosis from which your treatment, management, referral, and co-management decisions are made, ❸ **art**: your ability to create the changes in your patient's outlook, lifestyle, biochemistry, biomechanics/anatomy, and physiology to effect the desired outcome.

Neurologic Assessment

Clinical neurology is a complex area of study. However, for most doctors, knowledge of clinical neurology hinges on answering three questions:

- **Is this patient's presentation normal or abnormal?**
- **If it is abnormal, does it indicate a specific disease or lesion?**
- **Does this condition require referral to a specialist or emergency care?**

---

[72] **Vasquez A**. <u>Integrative Orthopedics: Concepts, Algorithms, and Therapeutics</u>. www.OptimalHealthResearch.com
[73] "Pancoast tumor has long been implicated as a cause of brachial plexopathy...The possibility of Pancoast lesion should be considered not only in the presence of brachial plexopathy, but also when C8 or T1 radiculopathy is found." Vargo MM, Flood KM. Pancoast tumor presenting as cervical radiculopathy. *Arch Phys Med Rehabil*. 1990 Jul;71(8):606-9

Every clinician needs thorough training in anatomy and clinical neurology to be competent in the management of patients, because even common problems such as "pain" and "fatigue" and "headache" may herald devastating neurologic illness that must be assessed accurately and managed skillfully. While a complete review of clinical neurology is beyond the scope of this text, the following section provides a basic review of the clinical essentials. Clinicians needing an refresher course in clinical neurology are encouraged to read the concise reviews by Goldberg.[74,75]

Reliable indicators of organic neurologic disease: These cannot be feigned and must be assumed to reveal organic neurologic illness that **must be evaluated by a neurologist**:
- **Significant asymmetry of pupillary light reflex,**
- **Ocular divergence,**
- **Papilledema,**
- **Marked nystagmus,**
- **Muscle atrophy and fasciculation,**
- **Muscle weakness with neurologic deficit**; upper motor neuron lesions (UMNL) indicate a central nervous system (CNS) lesion and need to be fully evaluated by a specialist; the need for referral is less necessary in cases of peripheral neuropathy of known cause.

Purpose of Neurologic Examination and *Principle of Neurologic Localization*:
The purpose of the neurologic examination is to qualify ("yes" or "no") the presence of a neurologic deficit, and —if present—to localize the lesion so that it can be further assessed with the proper laboratory, imaging, electrodiagnostic, or biopsy techniques. The following 9-point summary of localized lesions does not supplant independent studies of neurology and neuroanatomy but is useful for a quick clinically-relevant review:
1. **Cerebral cortex and internal capsule**: Neurologic deficit depends on location of lesion but is typically a combination of sensory/motor deficit and impaired higher neurologic function such as comprehension (superior temporal gyrus) or socially appropriate behavior (frontal lobe, ventral frontal gyri).
2. **Basal ganglia and striatal system**: Athetosis (lentiform nucleus: putamen and globus pallidus), (hemi)ballism (subthalamic nucleus), chorea (putamen), akinesia, bradykinesia, hypokinesia (lack of nigrostriatal dopamine).
3. **Cerebellum**: Ataxia, awkward clumsy execution of *intentional* motions; may have nystagmus, hypotonia.
4. **Brainstem**: Cranial nerve deficit(s) with contralateral distal sensory and/or UMN motor deficits.
5. **Spinal cord**: Cranial nerves and higher cortical functions are intact; lesion can be a combination of sensory and motor (UMN and LMN) deficits and the pattern distal to lesion may be a complete or incomplete pattern of sensory and motor deficits on one or both sides of body depending on area of spinal cord affected.
6. **Nerve root**: Segmental unilateral motor deficit; dermatomal distribution pain or sensory disturbance.
7. **Peripheral nerve**: Localized combination of sensory and motor deficits; may be bilateral or unilateral.
8. **Neuromuscular junction**: Painless weakness and "fatigable weakness": weakness that *worsens* with repeated testing; typically involves cranial nerves first in myasthenia gravis; also consider Lambert-Eaton Syndrome (LES: autoimmune neuromuscular junction disorder associated with occult malignancy; contrasts with myasthenia gravis in that in LES strength *increases* with repeated testing).
9. **Muscle disease**: Painless weakness, typically involving proximal hip/shoulder muscles first; test for elevated serum aldolase and (phospho)creatine kinase.

---

[74] Goldberg S. Clinical Neuroanatomy Made Ridiculously Simple. Miami, Medimaster, Inc, 1990. Now in a third edition with interactive CD.
[75] Goldberg S. The Four-Minute Neurologic Exam. Miami, Medimaster, Inc, 1992

Clinical assessments of neurologic function and structures

Cortex	Cerebellum
• <u>Orientation</u>: Person, place, time, situation. • <u>Mood and cooperation</u> • <u>Level of consciousness</u>: Alert, lethargic, stupor, coma (indirect assessment of reticular system in brainstem) • <u>Memory</u>: Remember objects or numbers; *recent* memory is most commonly affected by brain lesions: *What day of the month is it? How did you get here?* • <u>Mentation</u>: *Count backward from 100 by 7's.* • <u>Spelling</u>: *Spell the word "hand" backwards.* • <u>Stereognosis</u>: Identify by touch a familiar object such as a key or coin. • <u>Hoffman's reflex</u>: Doctor rapidly extends distal joint of patient's middle finger and watches for patient's hand to perform grasp reflex; this test is performed for motor tract lesions involving the cerebral cortex, cerebellum, and upper motor neurons of the spinal cord. • <u>Pronator drift</u>: Supinated hands and arms outstretched forward for 30 seconds; doctor taps on palms; falling of hands and arms into pronation suggests UMNL. • <u>Babinski reflex</u>: Scraping the bottom of the foot results in splaying and flexing of the toes and extension (dorsiflexion) of the big toe; normal in infants.	• <u>Gait</u> (lesion: ataxia) • <u>Heel-to-toe walk</u> • <u>Tandem gait</u> • <u>Hand flip</u>, <u>foot tap</u> (lesion: dysdiadochokinesia) • <u>Finger-to-nose</u>: Patient reaches out to doctor's finger, then patient touches patient nose, then back to new location of doctor's finger. • <u>Heel-to-shin</u>: Slide heel along shin. • <u>Walk in circle around chair</u> • <u>Move eyes in a rapid "figure 8"</u>: Technique for provoking latent nystagmus • <u>Rhomberg's test</u>: Patient stands with feet close together and eyes closed; tests proprioception (peripheral nerves, dorsal columns, spinocerebellar tracts); vision (eyes open tests optic righting reflex) and coordinated motor activity (cerebellum).

Several of the above '"cerebral" deficits may also result from intoxicative, nutritional, or metabolic disorders rather than an organic irreversible physical lesion. Likewise "cerebellar" deficits may also result from lesion of the brainstem tracts/nuclei and cerebellar peduncles, rather than the cerebellum itself.

Brainstem and Cranial Nerves	Spinal Cord, Roots, Nerves

1. Olfactory: **smell**
  • Smell: Test with strong and common odors such as coffee; do not use ammonia or other irritants which are perceived via trigeminal nerve (cranial nerve 5)
  • This is a worthwhile test in patients with recent head trauma (direct or indirect) such as from motor vehicle accidents (MVA); any violent motion of the head may result in injury to the olfactory fibers passing through the cribiform plate; patients may have associated anosmia or altered sense of flavor; frontal lobe disorders such as altered social behavior may be noted in lesioned patients
2. Ophthalmic: **reading, peripheral vision, fundoscopic**
  • Snellen chart for far vision, Rosenbaum card for near vision
  • Peripheral vision
  • Fundoscopic examination
3. Oculomotor: **move eyes and constrict pupils**
  • Eye motion in cardinal fields of gaze
  • Pupil contraction to light
  • Pupil contraction to accommodation
4. Trochlear: **motor to superior oblique**
  • Look "down and in" toward nose
5. Trigeminal: **bite, sensory to face and eyes**
  • Bite (motor to muscles of mastication)
  • Feel (sensory to face, eyes, and tongue)
6. Abducens: **motor to lateral rectus**
  • Looks laterally to the ear
7. Facial: **face muscles and taste to anterior tongue**
  • Furrow forehead, close eyes forcefully, smile and frown
  • Taste to anterior tongue
8. Vestibulocochlear: **hearing and balance**
  • Hearing, Rinne-Weber tests[76]
  • Balance: observe gait and Romberg test
9. Glossopharyngeal: **swallowing, and gag reflex**
  • Swallow
  • Gag reflex (sensory component)
10. Vagus: **motor to palate**
  • Say "ahh" to raise uvula
  • Gag reflex (motor component)
11. Spinal accessory: **motor to SCM and trapezius**
  • Raise your shoulders (against resistance)
  • Turn your head (against resistance)
12. Hypoglossal: **motor to tongue**
  • Stick out tongue to front
	Motor and reflex
	  • Strength: Specific muscles are tested and rated 0-5
	  • Plantar (Babinski) reflex: Signifies UMNL
	  • Abdominal reflexes: "Present" or "absent" (not rated 0-4); superficial reflexes are lost (rather than hyperactive) with UMNL
	    ○ Upper abdominal: T8-10
	    ○ Lower abdominal: T10-12
	  • Anal reflex: Cauda equina and sacral nerve roots
	  • Reflexes: Rate 0-4; asymmetric reflexes are more significant than finding absent or hyperactive (+3) reflexes; +4 reflex with sustained clonus is almost always pathologic and requires neurologist referral. Deep tendon reflexes with main spinal root levels are as follows:
	    ○ Biceps: C5
	    ○ Brachioradialis: C6
	    ○ Triceps: C7
	    ○ Patellar: L3-L4
	    ○ Hamstring: L5
	    ○ Achilles: S1
	Sensory
	  • Light touch
	  • Two-point discrimination
	  • Vibration (use 128 Hz tuning fork)
	  • Joint position sense and proprioception (eyes closed, locate position of joint)
	  • Sharp and dull
	  • Hot and cold
	  • Sensory loss mapping (if deficits are found)
	  • Romberg (peripheral nerves, dorsal columns, vestibular, cerebellar)
	  • Nerve root tension tests such as straight leg raising
	  • **Subjective pain and discomfort can be indicated on pain diagrams and VAS (visual analog scale) as shown on the following page**

---

[76] "The Rinne and Weber tuning fork tests are the most important tools in distinguishing between conductive and sensorineural hearing loss." Ruckenstein MJ. Hearing loss. A plan for individualized management. *Postgrad Med.* 1995 Oct;98(4):197-200, 203, 206

Deep tendon reflexes are summarized below and on the following page. Hyperreflexia is noted with upper motor neuron lesions (UMNL) in the cortex, subcortical nuclei, brainstem, or corticospinal tracts of the spinal cord, whereas hyporeflexia can result from lesions of lower motor neurons (LMNL) in spinal cord, peripheral nerves, as well as from sensory/afferent defects including diabetic neuropathy, vitamin B-12 deficiency, and Guillain-Barre disorder. Muscle strength should always be "five over five" to be considered normal, whereas in the testing of reflexes, symmetry/asymmetry is generally more important than the grade of response (except with sustained clonus). **Asymmetry of reflex or strength (especially when seen together) is never normal and requires clinical correlation and investigation.** Reflexes and strength are evaluated as follows in the following table.

Deep tendon reflexes	Muscle strength
+5 Hyperreflexia with sustained clonus: Sustained clonus strongly suggests UMNL and requires investigation; most textbooks use a 0-4 scale, yet this 0-5 scale facilitates clear communication of observed lesions.[77]	5/5 Normal: Full strength: able to withstand gravity and full resistance.
+4 Marked hyperreflexia: Up to 4 beats of unsustained clonus may be normal[78]; suggests UMNL but may be caused by medications, electrolyte disturbances, etc.	4/5 Partial strength: Able to withstand gravity and partial resistance.
+3 Hyperreflexia: More than normal.	3/5 Partial strength: Only able to resist gravity.
+2 Normal: Neither hyporeflexia nor hyperreflexia.	2/5 Partial strength: Able to contract muscle but unable to resist gravity.
+1 Hyporeflexia: Less than normal	1/5 Slight flicker of muscle contraction: Does not result in joint movement.
0 No reflex: Requires clinical correlation for lesion of sensory receptors, peripheral nerve, spinal cord, anterior horn, or neuromuscular junction; this is a common finding in normal individuals.	0/5 No clinically detectable contraction: Correlate with lesion of peripheral nerve, cord, cerebrum, anterior horn, or neuromuscular junction.

---

[77] Oommen K, edited by Berman SA, et al. Neurological History and Physical Examination. Last Updated: October 4, 2006. *eMedicine* http://www.emedicine.com/neuro/topic632.htm
[78] "…three to four beats of clonus can be elicited at the ankles in some normal individuals." Waxman SG. Clinical Neuroanatomy 25th Edition. McGraw Hill Medical, New York, 2003, p 325

Patients can be asked to <u>localize</u> and <u>describe</u> their pain/discomfort on drawings such as these.
Examples of descriptions:

- Numb
- Hypersensitive
- Tingling

- Shooting pain
- Electrical pain
- Stabbing pain

- Burning pain
- Dull ache
- Muscle weakness

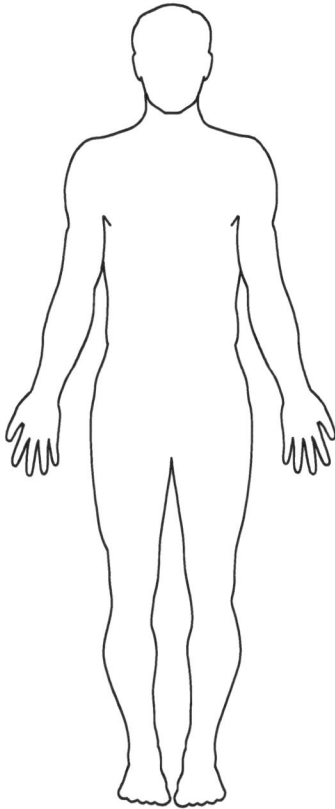

FRONT OF BODY

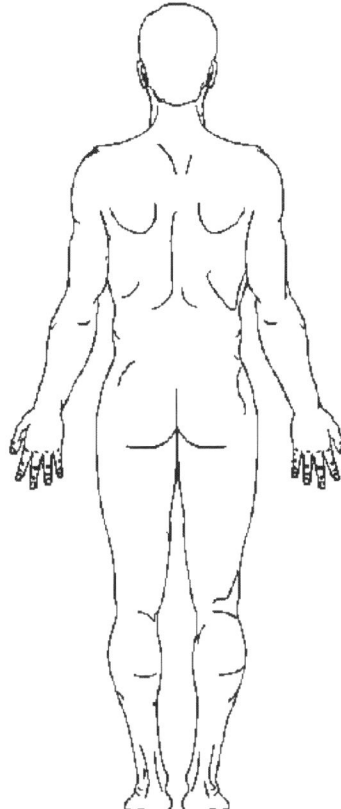

BACK OF BODY

On the lines below, indicate which pain/discomfort you are referring to and then quantify it by placing an "X" on the line.

Location of pain:_____

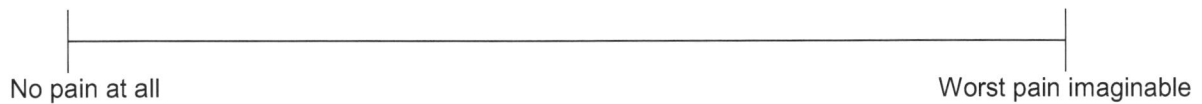

No pain at all   Worst pain imaginable

Location of pain:_____

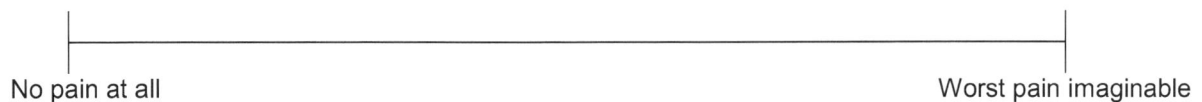

No pain at all   Worst pain imaginable

Laboratory Assessments: General Considerations of Commonly Used Tests

"The laboratory evaluation of patients with rheumatic disease is often informative but rarely definitive."[79]

Laboratory tests are immensely important in evaluating patients with musculoskeletal pain, as these tests allow the clinician to 1) assess for infection (e.g., subacute osteomyelitis), 2) quantify the degree of inflammation (i.e., with CRP or ESR), 3) assess or exclude other disease processes that may be the cause of pain or dysfunction, and 4) assess for concomitant diseases (e.g., septic arthritis complicating rheumatoid arthritis). Additionally, 5) these tests open the door to more complete patient care and holistic management of the whole person because they allow for a more comprehensive and complete understanding of the patient's underlying physiology. **The recommended routine is to use the following panel of tests when assessing patients with musculoskeletal pain: 1) CBC, 2) CRP, 3) chemistry/metabolic panel, and preferably also 4) ferritin, 5) 25(OH)-vitamin D, and 6) thyroid assessment, minimally including TSH** and optimally including free T4, total T3, reverse T3 and anti-thyroid antibodies. The use of a screening evaluation on a routine basis helps identify patients with occult diseases and also allows for more comprehensive management of the patient's overall health. Other tests are indicated in specific situations. *Orthopedics* relies heavily upon physical examination and imaging, whereas *Rheumatology* relies more heavily upon laboratory analysis. In Orthopedics, laboratory tests are used mainly for the purposes of discovering or excluding rheumatic and systemic diseases. In Rheumatology, lab tests are used to specifically identify the type of illness, quantify the severity of the condition, and to assess for concomitant illnesses and complications.

Essential Tests: These Tests are Required for Basic Patient Assessment

Test	Purpose	Clinical application
CRP (or ESR)	Screening for **infection**, **inflammation**, and possibly **cancer**; if inflammation is present, then these tests allow for a generalized quantification of severity.	**Useful in all new patients** for helping to differentiate systemic/inflammatory disorders from those which are noninflammatory and mechanical. Also very helpful as a general "barometer" of health since higher values correlate with increased risk for diabetes mellitus and cardiovascular disease; thus this test helps bridge the gap between acute care and wellness promotion.
CBC	Screening for **anemia**, **infection**, certain cancers (namely **leukemia**).	Useful in any patient with **nontraumatic musculoskeletal pain** or **systemic manifestations**, especially **fever or weight loss;** occasionally detects occult B-12 and folate deficiencies.
Chemistry panel	Screening for **diabetes**, **liver disease, kidney failure**, bone lesions (alkaline phosphatase), **electrolyte disturbances,** adrenal insufficiency (hyponatremia with hyperkalemia), **hyperparathyroidism, hypercalcemia.**	Use this panel in any patient with **nontraumatic musculoskeletal pain** or **systemic manifestations**; all patients with **hypertension, diabetes**, or who use **medications** that cause **hepatotoxicity, nephrotoxicity,** etc.
Thyroid assessments	Hypothyroidism is a common problem and is an often overlooked cause of musculoskeletal pain.[80]	This is a reasonable test panel for any patient with fatigue, cold extremities, depression, "arthritis", muscle pain, hypercholesterolemia, or other manifestations of hypothyroidism.

---

[79] Klippel JH (ed). Primer on the Rheumatic Diseases. 11th Edition. Atlanta: Arthritis Foundation. 1997 page 94
[80] "Hypothyroidism is frequently accompanied by musculoskeletal manifestations ranging from myalgias and arthralgias to true myopathy and arthritis." McLean RM, Podell DN. Bone and joint manifestations of hypothyroidism. *Semin Arthritis Rheum*. 1995 Feb;24(4):282-90

Overview of Important Tests: Common Components of Routine Evaluation

Test	Purpose	Clinical Application
Ferritin *For more details on the treatment of iron overload and iron deficiency, see the guidelines on the website.[81]*	Important for assessing for **iron overload** (e.g., hemochromatoic polyarthropathy), and **iron deficiency** (e.g., low back pain due to colon cancer metastasis). Ferritin values less than 20 in adults (e.g., iron deficiency) or greater than 200 in women and 300 in men (e.g., iron overload) necessitate evaluation and effective treatment.	*Ferritin is the ideal test for both iron overload and iron deficiency.* All patients should be screened for hemochromatosis and other hereditary forms of iron overload regardless of age, gender, or ethnicity.[82] Iron deficiency—particularly in adults—may be the first clue to gastric/colon cancer and generally necessitates referral to gastroenterologist.
Serum 25-hydroxy-vitamin D, 25(OH)D	**Vitamin D deficiency is a common cause of musculoskeletal pain and inflammation**[83,84], and vitamin D deficiency is a significant risk factor for cancer and other serious health problems.[85,86,87]	Measurement of serum 25(OH) vitamin D (or empiric treatment with 2,000 – 4,000 IU vitamin D3 per day for adults) is indicated in patients with chronic musculoskeletal pain.[88,89] Optimal vitamin D status correlates with serum 25(OH)D levels of 50 – 100 ng/mL.[90]
Antinuclear antibodies (ANA)	Sensitive (but not specific) for the detection of several autoimmune diseases, especially systemic lupus erythematosus (SLE).	This test is particularly valuable for assessing patients with polyarthropathy, facial rash, and/or fatigue.
Rheumatoid factor (RF)	The primary value of this test is in supporting a diagnosis of rheumatoid arthritis; specificity is low.	RF may be positive in normal health, iron overload, chronic infections, hepatitis, sarcoidosis, and bacterial endocarditis.
Cyclic citrullinated protein (CCP) antibodies	Cyclic citrullinated protein (CCP) antibodies are currently the single best laboratory test for rheumatoid arthritis (RA) and have largely replaced RF.	Citrullinated protein antibodies are rapidly becoming *the test* for diagnosing and confirming RA; used with RF for highly specific "conjugate seropositivity."
Lactulose-mannitol assay	Assesses for malabsorption and excess intestinal permeability—"leaky gut."	Diagnostic test for intestinal damage; excellent nonspecific screening test for pathology or pathophysiology such as celiac and Crohns.
Comprehensive parasitology, stool analysis	Identification and quantification of intestinal yeast, bacteria, and other microbes.	Extremely valuable test when working with patients with chronic fatigue syndromes, fibromyalgia, or autoimmunity; see chapter 4 of *Integrative Rheumatology*.

---

[81] Excerpt from **Vasquez A**. Integrative Rheumatology on iron overload http://optimalhealthresearch.com/hemochromatosis.html

[82] **Vasquez A**. Musculoskeletal disorders and iron overload disease: comment on the American College of Rheumatology guidelines for the initial evaluation of the adult patient with acute musculoskeletal symptoms. *Arthritis Rheum* 1996;39: 1767-8 http://optimalhealthresearch.com/hemochromatosis.html

[83] Masood H, Narang AP, Bhat IA, Shah GN. Persistent limb pain and raised serum alkaline phosphatase the earliest markers of subclinical hypovitaminosis D in Kashmir. *Indian J Physiol Pharmacol.* 1989 Oct-Dec;33(4):259-61

[84] Al Faraj S, Al Mutairi K. Vitamin D deficiency and chronic low back pain in Saudi Arabia. *Spine.* 2003 Jan 15;28(2):177-9

[85] Grant WB. An estimate of premature cancer mortality in the U.S. due to inadequate doses of solar ultraviolet-B radiation. *Cancer.* 2002;94(6):1867-75

[86] Zittermannn A. Vitamin D in preventive medicine: are we ignoring the evidence? *Br J Nutr.* 2003 May;89(5):552-72

[87] Holick MF. Vitamin D: importance in the prevention of cancers, type 1 diabetes, heart disease, and osteoporosis. *Am J Clin Nutr.* 2004;79(3):362-71

[88] Plotnikoff GA, Quigley JM. Prevalence of severe hypovitaminosis D in patients with persistent, nonspecific musculoskeletal pain. *Mayo Clin Proc.* 2003 Dec;78(12):1463-70

[89] Al Faraj S, Al Mutairi K. Vitamin D deficiency and chronic low back pain in Saudi Arabia. *Spine.* 2003 Jan 15;28(2):177-9

[90] **Vasquez A**, Manso G, Cannell J. The Clinical Importance of Vitamin D (Cholecalciferol): A Paradigm Shift with Implications for All Healthcare Providers. *Alternative Therapies in Health and Medicine* 2004;10:28-37 and *Integrative Medicine* 2004;3:44-54 http://optimalhealthresearch.com/cholecalciferol.html

Chemistry/metabolic panel	
Overview and interpretation:	<ul><li>Accurate interpretation requires knowledge and pattern-recognition by the doctor to translate numbers into differential diagnoses that are correlated with the clinical presentation, examination, and imaging findings to arrive at probable diagnoses.</li><li>Variation exists in the components and ranges offered by different laboratories.</li></ul>
Advantages:	<ul><li>Inexpensive and easy to perform—venipuncture + serum separator tube.</li><li>Provides a quick screen for diabetes, hepatitis, renal insufficiency, suggestions of alcohol abuse, hyperparathyroidism, electrolyte imbalances, etc.</li></ul>
Limitation and considerations:	<ul><li>Individual tests and the most common clinical considerations for low and high values are listed in the following section. These values and considerations are provided with the routine adult outpatient in mind and are not inclusive of every possible differential diagnosis and therapeutic consideration. Consult your laboratory texts and reference manuals as needed per patient.</li><li>Abnormal laboratory results are always due to one of four problems:<ol><li>Technical error: Error with the laboratory analysis, improper patient identification correlating with the sample, alteration of the sample before delivery to the laboratory (e.g., too much time, too much heat, lysis of cells). Given the importance of laboratory accuracy and the life-and-death decisions that are based upon such reports, this type of error is inexcusable, however, it does occur, occasionally producing results that defy physiologic possibility or which contradict the clinical picture. Repeating the test is appropriate. *Example*: Hypercalcemia (elevated serum calcium) may be reported in error by the laboratory due to problems with the analyzing machinery.</li><li>Drug effect: An otherwise healthy patient may develop a laboratory abnormality due to a drug effect. *Example*: Hypercalcemia can be secondary to the effect of a calcium-sparing diuretic, such as hydrochlorothiazide (HCTZ).</li><li>Pathology: The patient has a diagnosable disease causing the laboratory abnormality. *Example*: Hypercalcemia can be secondary to a parathyroid adenoma which secretes abnormally high amounts of parathyroid hormone; hypercalcemia can also be a presentation of malignancy such as breast cancer or prostate cancer, or from a granulomatous disease such as sarcoidosis.</li><li>Physiologic abnormality: The patient has a physiologic abnormality causing the laboratory abnormality. *Example*: Hypercalcemia can be secondary to excess intake of vitamin D. In practice, hypercalcemia from hypervitaminosis D is very rare because vitamin D has a wide safety margin; but for the sake of this discussion, vitamin D toxicity will be listed as a possible cause of hypercalcemia.</li></ol></li></ul>
Comments:	<ul><li>All abnormalities require follow-up—repeat test within 2-4 weeks as part of routine follow-up along with additional investigation and clinical re-assessment. Extraordinary abnormalities and those with life-threatening implications should of course be retested immediately; often, the laboratory will hold the blood sample for 7 days and the repeat analysis can be performed on the same blood sample to exclude technical error.</li><li>Many ill patients (such as those with chronic fatigue syndrome, fibromyalgia, etc) will have normal results with the metabolic panel and other basic routine laboratory assessments. Therefore, normal results do not ensure that the patient is healthy nor without life-threatening illness.</li><li>Generally, laboratory tests are performed in the morning under fasting conditions; such is the standard but is not necessarily required depending on the nature of the test, convenience, and the clinical situation.</li></ul>

Practical overview of common abnormalities on the chemistry/metabolic panel—*continued*

Low values—considerations	Analyte[91]	High values—considerations
Technical error due to faulty processing of sample (i.e., hemolysis); insulinoma, exogenous insulin administration (test serum C-peptide), overdose of anti-hyperglycemic drugs, hypopituitarism and adrenal insufficiency.	**Glucose**: 65-99 mg/dL *Clinical pearl: Fasting glucose levels can miss mild type-2 diabetes mellitus; a better test for long-term glucose status is hemoglobin A1c.*	Postprandial sample, diabetes mellitus type-1 or type-2, Cushing disease or syndrome, acromegally, pheochromocytoma, glucagonoma, hyperthyroidism. If glucose is >300 mg/dL and patient is unstable (e.g., tachypnic or stuporous), evaluate for diabetic ketoacidosis or hyperosmolar state. Optimal fasting serum glucose is in the range of 70-75 up to 85 mg/dL, since levels >85 mg/dL have been associated with increased mortality.
Hyponatremia is potentially fatal and is also a cause of permanent neurologic injury (e.g., pontine myelinolysis). Clinicians should be particularly concerned when the sodium level drops below 125 mmol/L. Symptomatic hyponatremia is worthy of treatment in hospital setting; mild cases due to a recent event such as excess diaphoresis (e.g., prolonged sweating and exercise) or excess fluid intake (e.g., beer potomania [i.e., binge drinking], overhydration with unmineralized water) might be managed with sodium replacement and water restriction. Older patients, patients with pulmonary disease, and patients taking certain drugs such as serotonin-reuptake inhibitors may develop a chronic and relatively benign mild hyponatremia associated with "reset osmostat syndrome." Sodium levels can be altered downward by conditions that introduce osmotically active substances into the serum, such as immunoglobulins (e.g., multiple myeloma), hyperglycemia, and hypertriglyceridemia; corrective equations are available for such situations. For additional information see on-line reviews by Goh[92] and Decaux and Musch.[93]	**Sodium**: 136 to 144 mEq/L (mmol/L)	Hypernatremia in outpatients is rare; assess for drug effect and dehydration with hemoconcentration. Some clinicians will determine the free water deficit, while others will treat with oral or IV hydration with plain water or half-normal saline, respectively. Electrolyte abnormalities—particularly involving sodium—should generally be corrected slowly and with close supervision.

[91] The reference range for this table and some provisional information was derived from Medline Plus provided by the U.S. Department of Health and Human Services and National Institutes of Health. http://www.nlm.nih.gov/medlineplus/ency/article/003468.htm Accessed June 28, 2011. However, the majority of the information in this table comes from the author's (Dr Vasquez's) clinical training and experience. Editorial and peer reviews were provided by colleagues Barry Morgan MD (emergency medicine), Holly Furlong DC, Kris Young DC, Erika Mennerick DC, and Bill Beakey DOM of Professional Co-op Services, Inc. professionalco-op.com.
[92] Goh KP. Management of hyponatremia. *Am Fam Physician*. 2004;69:2387-94 http://www.aafp.org/afp/2004/0515/p2387.html Accessed June 2011.
[93] Decaux G, Musch W. Clinical laboratory evaluation of the syndrome of inappropriate secretion of antidiuretic hormone. *Clin J Am Soc Nephrol*. 2008 Jul;3(4):1175-84 http://cjasn.asnjournals.org/content/3/4/1175.full.pdf Accessed June 29, 2011.

Practical overview of common abnormalities on the chemistry/metabolic panel—*continued*

Low values—considerations	Analyte	High values—considerations
Hypokalemia can cause fatal cardiac arrhythmias and needs to be taken seriously. Replacement is generally via oral administration of potassium-rich foods, juices, or supplements such as potassium citrate (best option) or potassium chloride (KCl, inexpensive and therefore commonly used in medical settings even though KCl is clearly not optimal therapy due to the acidifying effect of the chloride anion). Recalcitrant hypokalemia is often a sign of magnesium depletion.[94] Causes of hypokalemia include diarrhea, vomiting, diuretics, Cushing disease/syndrome, dietary insufficiency, overhydration with mineral-free fluids, hyperaldosteronism and renal artery stenosis. Acute metabolic acidosis should cause relative or absolute elevations in serum K; the finding of normal or low serum K in a patient with acidosis (e.g., diabetic ketoacidosis) indicates (severe) potassium depletion.	<u>Potassium</u>: 3.6 to 5.2 mEq/L (mmol/L)	**Hyperkalemia is defined as a potassium level greater than 5.5 mmol/L. Severe hyperkalemia (>7 mmol/L) can be fatal and needs to be taken seriously.** In severe hyperkalemia, treatment and emergency management should be implemented before a complete evaluation and differential diagnosis are performed.[95] ❶ Ensure that blood sample was not hemolyzed. Repeat test if patient is stable and time allows. ❷ If hyperkalemia is severe or patient is symptomatic or has electrocardiographic changes, treat hyperkalemia with intravenous calcium, beta-adrenergic agonists (e.g., albuterol), bicarbonate, insulin and glucose; magnesium sulfate may also help alleviate arrhythmias; oral sodium polystyrene sulfonate (SPS, also known as Kayexalate) is a frequently used potassium-binding agent. ❸ DDX includes adrenal insufficiency, potassium-sparing diuretics, ACE-inhibitors and ARBs, NSAIDs, rhabdomyolysis, renal failure, massive cell necrosis such as with tumor lysis syndrome.
Evaluate hypocalcemia clinically with Chvostek's sign (~30% sensitive) and Trousseau sign (~90% sensitive) which may also be present in hypomagnesemia; evaluate clinically for arrhythmia, muscle spasm/hypertonicity, and hyperreflexia. Measure serum albumin and perform equation for "corrected calcium" if albumin is low. DDX includes renal failure, hypoparathyroidism, malabsorption, and drug effect (e.g., rarely a loop diuretic such as furosemide). Chronic mild hypocalcemia is treated with oral vitamin D and calcium supplementation; subacute symptomatic hypocalcemia can be treated with intravenous calcium gluconate especially if cardiac arrhythmias are present.	<u>Calcium</u>: 8.6 to 10.2 mg/dL	Outpatient hypercalcemia is potentially serious and needs to be evaluated in a stepwise manner: ❶ repeat the test to rule out lab error unless you are confident in the performance of the laboratory and stability of the submitted sample, ❷ review drug list for adverse effect, such as from hydrochlorothiazide (HCTZ) or rarely from excess cholecalciferol intake, ❸ test intact parathyroid hormone (iPTH) to evaluate for hyperparathyroidism, ❹ evaluate for possible granulomatous disease such as sarcoidosis, tuberculosis, Crohns disease, and possible leukemia or lymphoma, ❺ consider metabolic bone disease such as Paget disease of bone or metastatic bone disease, ❻ evaluate for cancer, ❼ test urine calcium for familial hypocalciuric hypercalcemia, ❽ refer to specialist such as internist or endocrinologist if hypercalcemia persists and answer is not forthcoming.

Corrected calcium (cCa) equations: Used when both serum calcium and albumin are low
<u>American units</u>: cCa (mg/dL) = serum Ca (mg/dL) + 0.8 (4.0 - serum albumin [g/dL])
<u>International units</u>: cCa (mmol/L) = measured total Ca (mmol/L) + 0.02 (40 - serum albumin [g/L])

---

[94] "Herein is reviewed literature suggesting that magnesium deficiency exacerbates potassium wasting by increasing distal potassium secretion." Huang CL, Kuo E. Mechanism of hypokalemia in magnesium deficiency. *J Am Soc Nephrol*. 2007;18:2649-52 jasn.asnjournals.org/content/18/10/2649

[95] "If the hyperkalemia is severe (potassium >7.0 mEq/L) or if the patient is symptomatic, begin treatment before diagnostic investigation of the underlying cause." Garth D. Hyperkalemia in emergency medicine treatment and management. *Medscape Reference* http://emedicine.medscape.com/article/766479-treatment#a1126 Accessed June 2011

Practical overview of common abnormalities on the chemistry/metabolic panel—*continued*

Low values—considerations	Analyte	High values—considerations
Clinically meaningful hypochloremia is rare among outpatients. Hypochloremic metabolic alkalosis is commonly seen after persistent vomiting. Consider syndrome of inappropriate diuretic hormone (SIADH) secretion, cardiopulmonary disease, and adrenal insufficiency.	**Chloride**: 97 to 111 mmol/L	Hyperchloremia in outpatients is rare; assess for drug effect and dehydration with hemoconcentration; assess for acid-base disturbance, especially acidosis.
Reduced CO_2 correlates with hyperventilation; consider acid-base disturbance, salicylate overdose, asthma. Slight decrements in healthy outpatients are probably due to anxious hyperventilation at time of venipuncture.	**CO_2 (carbon dioxide)**: 20 - 30 mmol/L	Elevated CO_2 can suggest cardiopulmonary compromise and/or acid-base disturbance; assess clinically. Slight elevations in otherwise healthy outpatients are probably due to breath-holding at time of venipuncture.
Reduced total protein with normal albumin suggests hypogammaglobulinemia; evaluate for nephrotic syndrome, liver disease, protein deficiency and malabsorption/enteropathy, immunosuppressive syndromes and consider intravenous gammaglobulin therapy.	**Total protein (albumin + globulins)**: 6.3 - 8.0 g/dL	Elevated total protein with normal albumin suggests hypergammaglobulinemia, such as due to infection or plasma cell dyscrasia (e.g., multiple myeloma and Waldenstrom's disease). Evaluate within the clinical context; order serum protein electrophoresis if cause remains elusive, especially if patient has immune complex disease, neuropathy, or nephropathy.
Assess for liver disease, nephrotic syndrome, protein deficiency, malabsorption (consider celiac disease).	**Albumin**: 3.9 - 5.0 g/dL	Assess for dehydration/hemoconcentration.
Loss of hepatic mass due to cirrhosis, possible pyridoxine deficiency.	**ALT (alanine aminotransferase)**: 10 - 40 IU/L	Hepatocellular liver injury due to chemical toxicity, viral hepatitis, hemochromatosis, metastatic or infectious disease, muscle injury. ALT is preferentially elevated over AST in viral hepatitis.
Loss of hepatic mass due to cirrhosis, possible pyridoxine deficiency.	**AST (aspartate aminotransferase)**: 10 - 40 IU/L	Hepatocellular liver injury due to chemical toxicity, viral hepatitis, hemochromatosis, metastatic or infectious liver disease, myocardial infarct, muscle injury. AST is preferentially elevated over ALT in alcoholic hepatitis and rhabdomyolysis.
Consider zinc deficiency, malnutrition.	**Alkaline phosphatase**: 44 - 147 IU/L	Metabolic bone disease, metastatic bone disease, vitamin D deficiency, congestive liver disease. Test isoenzymes to differentiate bone versus hepatic origin if cause of elevation remains unclear.

Low values—considerations	*Analyte*	*High values—considerations*
Low values are rare but might be noted with severe chronic anemia.	**Total bilirubin**: 0.2 to 1.5 mg/dL **Direct (conjugated) bilirubin**: 0 to 0.3 mg/dL **Indirect (unconjugated) bilirubin**: Determined by subtracting the *direct* from the *total* bilirubin.	Indirect/unconjugated bilirubin is elevated with hemolysis (e.g., hemolytic anemia) and impaired enzymatic conjugation (e.g., Gilbert's syndrome) or both (e.g., neonates). Direct/conjugated bilirubin has been enzymatically conjugated with glucuronic acid but is blocked from hepatobiliary excretion; consider performing liver and gall bladder sonogram (or CT or MRI) to evaluate for causes of biliary obstruction in addition to a careful abdominal exam. In patients with advanced liver disease, perform the Model for End-Stage Liver Disease (MELD) score and/or the MELD-Na score to predict 3-month mortality.[96] Fluoridated water inhibits glucuronidation in some patients with Gilbert's syndrome; biochemical improvement follows avoidance of fluoridated water.[97]

Low values—considerations	*Analyte*	*High values—considerations*
Liver disease, nephrotic syndrome, protein deficiency and malabsorption. **BUN-to-creatinine ratio (normal = 10)** ≥10-20: Renal underperfusion, post-renal obstruction ≤10: Suggests intrinsic renal disease	**BUN (blood urea nitrogen)**: 7 to 20 mg/dL	Consider renal underperfusion (e.g., due to heart failure, GI bleeding, renal artery stenosis, dehydration), intrinsic renal failure, post-renal urinary tract obstruction. When renal disease is initially considered, order a urinalysis with microscopic analysis—see following section on urinalysis (UA).

Low values—considerations	*Analyte*	*High values—considerations*
Sarcopenia (insufficient muscle mass), protein deficiency and malabsorption. **Methods for estimating creatinine clearance, glomerular filtration rate (GFR)** 1. Modification of Diet in Renal Disease (MDRD) equation*, 2. 24-hour urine creatinine measurement, 3. Serum cystatin-C measurement, 4. Cockcroft-Gault equation (below): $$GFR = \frac{(140 - age\ years) \times wt\ kg \times (0.85\ if\ female)}{72 \times serum\ creatinine\ in\ mg/dL}$$ Clinical pearls for managing the chronic kidney disease (CKD) patient with declining renal function: • When the GFR ≤ 60 (CKD stage 3): Modify dosages or withdraw certain drugs. Treat the causative problem and/or begin specialist co-management. • When the GFR ≤ 30 (CKD stage 4): The patient needs to consult a nephrologist. • When the GFR ≤ 15 (CKD stage 5): The patient needs a transplant or dialysis. *National Institute of Diabetes and Digestive and Kidney Diseases (NIDDK). GFR MDRD Calculator for Adults (Conventional units). Accessed June 2011 nkdep.nih.gov/professionals/gfr_calculators/idms_con.htm	**Creatinine**: 0.8 to 1.3 mg/dL	Excess dietary protein, creatine supplementation, renal hypoperfusion; the most important consideration is intrinsic renal failure. Creatinine production (from arginine and creatine) is proportional to muscle mass. A rise in creatinine does not become evident until renal function (measured by glomerular filtration rate [GFR]) has fallen by approximately 50%. Creatinine levels indicative of impaired renal function to such an extent that modifications in diet, medications, and co-management become relevant are 1.4 mg/dL in women and 1.5 mg/dL in men. In the evaluation of renal function, the patient's age is a crucial determinant of how the serum creatinine is interpreted for the estimation of renal function (via GFR—see the Cockcroft-Gault equation). Cystatin C is more sensitive than are singular or conjugate interpretations of BUN and creatinine. If drug-induced nephritis is suspected, test urine eosinophils.

---

[96] MELD calculations are best performed electronically, such as with http://www.mayoclinic.org/meld/mayomodel8.html or other medical calculator.
[97] Lee J. Gilbert's disease and fluoride intake. *Fluoride* 1983; 16: 139-45

Cystatin C	
Overview and interpretation:	<ul><li>Cystatin C is gaining acceptance as studies confirm and define its usefulness, especially as an early, sensitive marker for chronic kidney disease. Concentrations of cystatin C are not affected by gender, age, or race, and cystatin C is not affected by most drugs (prednisone increases; cyclosporine decreases), infections, diet, or inflammation.[98]</li><li>Produced at a constant rate by all nucleated cells.</li><li>Freely filtered by the glomerulus.</li><li>Elevated in: renal disorders.<ul><li>Cystatin C rises more rapidly than creatinine (Cr) in early renal impairment.</li><li>Good predictor of the severity of ATN (acute tubular necrosis).</li><li>The cystatin C concentration is an independent risk factor for heart failure, mortality, CVD and non-CVD outcomes in older adults and appears to provide a better measure of risk assessment than the serum Cr concentration.</li></ul></li></ul>
Advantages:	<ul><li>More accurate assessment of renal function than creatinine-based assessments.</li><li>Can be used to accurately assess renal function when creatinine-based assessments suggest impending renal impairment inconsistent with clinical presentation.</li></ul>
Limitations:	<ul><li>Cost is approximately US $80.</li><li>False "non-renal" elevations may occur with cancer and/or rheumatic disease.</li></ul>

Presentation: 40yo male presenting for follow-up on abnormal renal function assessment—use of cystatin C to confirm normal kidney function: This apperantly healthy and athletic 40yo man displays consistently elevated creatinine and an estimated glomerular filtration rate (eGFR) that is close enough at 62 to warrant concern. Clinicians must appreciate that eGFR <60 is consistent with stage 3 chronic kidney disease (CKD) which warrants monitoring and which often necessitates changes in drug dosing (e.g., to avoid metformin-induced lactic acidosis) and diet (e.g., to avoid hyperkalemia).

Date and Time Collected	Date Entered	Date and Time Reported	Physician Name	NPI	Physician ID
12/07/11 11:10	12/08/11	12/13/11 04:07ET	VASQUEZ , A		

Tests Ordered
Comp. Metabolic Panel (14); FSH+TestT+LH+DHEA S+Prog+E2...; Chlamydia pneumoniae(IgG/M); Venipuncture

TESTS	RESULT	FLAG	UNITS	REFERENCE INTERVAL	LAB
Comp. Metabolic Panel (14)					
Glucose, Serum	89		mg/dL	65 - 99	01
BUN	18		mg/dL	6 - 24	01
Creatinine, Serum	**1.41**	**High**	mg/dL	0.76 - 1.27	01
eGFR If NonAfricn Am	62		mL/min/1.73	>59	
eGFR If Africn Am	72		mL/min/1.73	>59	

    Note: A persistent eGFR <60 mL/min/1.73 m2 (3 months or more) may indicate chronic kidney disease. An eGFR >59 mL/min/1.73 m2 with an elevated urine protein also may indicate chronic kidney disease. Calculated using CKD-EPI formula.

BUN/Creatinine Ratio	13			9 - 20	

In this situation, cystatin C was performed and confirmed normal renal function despite persistently elevated creatinine, which is probably attributable to this patient's athleticism and muscle mass.[99]

Date and Time Collected	Date Entered	Date and Time Reported	Physician Name	NPI	Physician ID
12/07/11 11:10	12/12/11	12/15/11 07:14ET	VASQUEZ , A		

Tests Ordered
Cystatin C; Written Authorization

TESTS	RESULT	FLAG	UNITS	REFERENCE INTERVAL	LAB
Cystatin C	0.71		mg/L	0.53 - 0.95	01

---

[98] http://labtestsonline.org/understanding/analytes/cystatin-c/tab/test Accessed April 2012
[99] Thank you, Bill Beakey DOM of Professional Co-op Services, Inc. professionalco-op.com for provision of these laboratory services.

Presentation: 69yo female presenting for routine outpatient health assessment with no acute complaints: Review the following labs and outline your treatment plan before reading the discussion below.

PATIENT NAME	PATIENT ID	ROOM NUMBER	AGE	SEX	PHYSICIAN
			69 Y 1941	F	Vasquez

REQUISITION NO	ACCESSION NO	ID.NO.	COLLECTION DATE & TIME	LOG-IN-DATE	REPORT DATE & TIME
			09/22/10 08:00 AM	09/22/10 06:37 PM	09/23/10 03:36AM

NOTES:
PT FASTING

TEST	RESULTS OUT OF RANGE	RESULTS WITHIN RANGE	UNITS	EXPECTED RANGE	LAB
BASIC METABOLIC PROFILE					
GLUCOSE		98	MG/DL	65-100	
BUN		19	MG/DL	8-25	
CREATININE		1.2	MG/DL	0.6-1.3	
EGFR AFRICAN AMER.	54		ML/MIN/1.73	>60	
EGFR NON-AFRICAN AMER.	45		ML/MIN/1.73	>60	
SODIUM		136	MEQ/L	133-146	
POTASSIUM	8.5		MEQ/L	3.5-5.3	

RESULTS RECHECKED AND VERIFIED
NOTE: NO VISIBLE HEMOLYSIS OBSERVED.

TEST	OUT OF RANGE	WITHIN RANGE	UNITS	EXPECTED RANGE	
CHLORIDE		100	MEQ/L	97-110	
CARBON DIOXIDE		27	MEQ/L	18-30	
CALCIUM		10.0	MG/DL	8.5-10.5	
LIPID PANEL					
CHOLESTEROL		193	MG/DL	<200	
TRIGLYCERIDES		129	MG/DL	<150	
HDL CHOLESTEROL		52	MG/DL	>39	
CALCULATED LDL CHOL	115		MG/DL	<100	
RISK RATIO LDL/HDL		2.22	RATIO	<3.22	
HEMOGLOBIN A1C	7.0		%	4.0-5.6	

AMERICAN DIABETES ASSOCIATION GUIDELINES FOR HGB A1C:
GLYCEMIC GOAL IN DIABETES . . . . . . <7.0%
DIAGNOSIS OF DIABETES . . . . >/=6.5%
CONFIRMED ON REPEAT ANALYSIS OR
WITH APPROPRIATE SYMPTOMS.
INCREASED RISK FOR DIABETES 5.7-6.4%

| TSH | 10.6 | | UIU/ML | 0.3-5.1 | |

PERFORMING LAB(S) LEGEND:

> **Chemistry/metabolic panels should be performed on all new patients prior to the initiation of treatment and periodically on all established patients to monitor for disease emergence, disease progression, and response to treatment**
>
> Treating this diabetic patient with a potassium-rich diet emphasizing low-carbohydrate fruits and vegetables would exacerbate her already life-threatening hyperkalemia. Note also that her hypothyroidism would be expected to contribute to her obesity which is exacerbating her diabetes and that (somewhat theoretically since we don't have her vital signs here) hypothyroid bradycardia could also reduce renal perfusion and contribute to her low GFR and hyperkalemia.

Assessments and plan: ❶ Life-threatening hyperkalemia: The clinician must focus on the emergency issue(s). Many books quote a potassium of 6 mEq/L as a panic value; note that the laboratory already excluded technical error and checked for hemolysis, which are the two most common causes of spurious hyperkalemia. This patient should be called at home and advised to immediately seek transportation by a secondary driver (e.g., taxi, ambulance, friend, neighbor, or relative) to the nearest hospital. If the patient is demented or otherwise incompetent, the clinician should contact the patient's caretaker or call directly for an ambulance. Attention must be given to the reliability of the driver, the urgency of the situation, and the speed by which the driver can get the patient to the hospital; failure by the clinician to ensure proper patient care—which in this case and most situations is best ensured by enrolling the ambulance service—could easily result in medicolegal complications. Hospital treatment for hyperkalemia will include assessment for electrocardiographic changes and treatment of hyperkalemia with intravenous calcium to stabilize cardioelectroconductivity, beta-adrenergic agonists, bicarbonate, diuretics, insulin and glucose; magnesium may also help alleviate arrhythmias; oral sodium polystyrene sulfonate (Kayexalate) is a potassium-binding agent. ❷ Diabetes mellitus: Notice that this patient's fasting glucose level is "normal" and yet the patient is clearly diabetic per the hemoglobin A1c value >6.5%. This patient needs a comprehensive nutritional plan for diabetes management. Promoting dependence on drugs at this early point should be considered inappropriate. ❸ Hypothyroidism: The TSH >10 indicates primary hypothyroidism by any standard; in all probability, unless major contraindications exist (of which very few exist), this patient should be started on a thyroid hormone combination as discussed in the section on thyroid assessment. ❹ Renal insufficiency: This patient has stage-3 chronic kidney disease and should begin a renoprotective and renorestorative program—beyond the basics of hypertension and hyperglycemia control—as discussed in *Chiropractic and Naturopathic Mastery of Common Clinical Disorders*. Use of ACE-inhibitor or ARB is contraindicated due to hyperkalemia. ❺ Dyslipidemia: The elevated LDL cholesterol and triglycerides should both be below 100 mg/dL. Diet is key, followed by fatty acid therapy, niacin, berberine.

Lipid panel:	
Overview and interpretation:	• "High cholesterol" was a buzz phrase many years ago indicating an unfavorable lipid profile causally associated with accelerated atherogenesis and the resultant CVD in its myriad forms. The next step was to identify low-density lipoprotein (LDL) cholesterol as the most obvious kingpin of vascular villains. Advances over the past decade include: 1. Appreciation that other non-lipid molecules such as homocysteine and c-reactive protein (CRP) are important contributors to the atherogenic process, 2. Renewed interest in the beneficial effects of high-density lipoprotein (HDL) cholesterol in mediating vasculoprotection, 3. "Non-standard" CVD risk factors such as very-low-density lipoprotein (VLDL), β-VLDL, intermediate-density lipoprotein (IDL) cholesterol, and lipoprotein-a (Lp-a) are also clinically important. For the sake of this introductory section on the basics of laboratory interpretation, the discussion will be limited to the components of the standard lipid panel; additional tests and details are provided in disease-specific chapters on metabolic/inflammatory disorders.

Lipids: Goals	*Clinical notes*:
Total cholesterol: < 200 mg/dL	• Higher cholesterol levels correlate with increased risk for CVD. Except in very rare cases of genotropic disease, the vast majority of humans should be able to achieve a total cholesterol <200 mg/dL via nutritional optimization, exercise, and proper endocrine (especially thyroid) status. The so-called "statin" drugs which block HMG-CoA reductase (3-hydroxy-3-methyl-glutaryl-CoA reductase, the rate-limiting enzyme for the endogenous production of cholesterol) would and should be *orphan drugs*. Reducing serum levels of insulin—the primary inducer of HMG-CoA reductase—is the most rational means by which to reduce total cholesterol levels. Thyroid hormone downregulates HMG-CoA reductase; this explains the well-established association of hypothyroidism with dyslipidemia and hypercholesterolemia.
LDL: <100 mg/dL	• O'Keefe and Cordain and colleagues[100] have noted that optimal LDL is 50-70 mg/dl and that lower is better and is physiologically normal for humans who eat appropriate diets and who are physically active.
HDL: >50-60 mg/dL	• Per the American Heart Association[101], "An HDL of 60 mg/dL and above is considered protective against heart disease." Of note, a recent report linked accumulation of persistent organic pollutants (POP) with elevated HDL levels.[102]
Triglycerides: <100 mg/dL	• Elevated serum triglycerides—except in rare cases of genotropic disease—are indicators of dietary carbohydrate excess and/or alcohol excess and/or insulin resistance. Hypertriglyceridemia is associated with increased CVD risk, higher body mass index (BMI), vitamin D deficiency, and increased risks of breast cancer and prostate cancer. Extreme hypertriglyceridemia (500 mg/dL or more) can cause pancreatitis; administration of omega-3 fatty acids from fish oil is protective.
Advantages	• Allows for the monitoring of established cardiovascular risk factors and a surrogate marker for dietary compliance and lifestyle optimization.
Limitations:	• Other non-lipid risk factors should also be monitored and optimized.
Comments:	• Important panel for overall patient management and disease prevention.

---

[100] O'Keefe JH Jr, Cordain L, Harris WH, Moe RM, Vogel R. Optimal low-density lipoprotein is 50 to 70 mg/dl: lower is better and physiologically normal. *J Am Coll Cardiol.* 2004 Jun 2;43(11):2142-6

[101] American Heart Association. heart.org/HEARTORG/Conditions/What-Your-Cholesterol-Levels-Mean_UCM_305562_Article.jsp Accessed June 2011

[102] "However, unlike the findings with p,p'-DDE, after the initial decrease of HDL-cholesterol from the 1st to 2nd quartile, HDL-cholesterol increased from the 2nd to 4th quartile of these PCBs." Lee DH, Steffes MW, Sjödin A, Jones RS, Needham LL, Jacobs DR Jr. Low dose organochlorine pesticides and polychlorinated biphenyls predict obesity, dyslipidemia, and insulin resistance among people free of diabetes. *PLoS One.* 2011 Jan 26;6(1):e15977

CBC: complete blood count

Overview and interpretation:	This test measures numbers and indices of white and red blood cells and platelets. A routine "CBC with differential" is affordable, practical, and thus preferred for the vast majority of situations (step 1); the next step when the clinical picture remains unclear is—generally—to order a peripheral blood smear (step 2) before proceeding to a hematologist referral (step 3). Additional tests—more components of step 2—are listed below per topic. If all three blood cell populations are reduced (pancytopenia) consider nutritional anemia, hypersplenism (especially secondary to hepatic cirrhosis), autoimmunity (especially systemic lupus erythematosus), or bone marrow disorder such as myelofibrosis or aplastic anemia.

- WBC (white blood cells): The three most commonly encountered disorders that cause an abnormal WBC count are ❶ bone marrow suppression (causing low WBC count) and conditions associated with elevated WBC count including ❷ leukemia/lymphoma and ❸ response to infection. An elevated WBC count suggests the possibility of infection (especially bacterial infection) or leukemia/lymphoma and therefore requires the clinician's attention. However, relying on the WBC count for the assessment of serious infection is potentially misleading, particularly since, for example, it is elevated in less than 50% of patients with acute and chronic musculoskeletal infections; per Shaw et al[103] "Therefore, it [the WBC count] is helpful when it is high, but potentially misleading when it is normal." Clinicians can gain additional information by assessing percentage and quantitative indices of neutrophils, lymphocytes, and eosinophils, elevations of which may suggest bacterial infections, viral infections, or allergic or parasitic conditions, respectively. Primary care clinicians may also choose to perform lymphocyte immunophenotyping by flow cytometry in patients with unexplained lymphocytosis prior to hematologist consult.

  - Neutropenia: Severe suppression of WBC count resulting in neutropenia can occur in liver disease, viral infections (including but not limited to HIV), autoimmune disorders, bone marrow infiltration/failure, and toxin/alcohol exposure. For severe neutropenia, hospitalization, isolation precautions, prophylactic antibiotics, and marrow-stimulating agents are often indicated. Neutropenia is defined by an absolute neutrophil count (ANC) less than

    > **Absolute neutrophil count (ANC) = Total WBC x (% "Segs" + % "Bands")**
    > - <u>Normal value</u>: ≥ 1500 cells/mm3,
    > - <u>Mild neutropenia</u>: 1000-1500/mm3,
    > - <u>Moderate neutropenia</u>: 500-1000/mm3,
    > - <u>Severe neutropenia</u>: ≤ 500/mm3; hospitalization is generally advised

    1500 neutrophilic cells per mm3. Neutropenia is most commonly due to use of anti-cancer cytotoxic agents; other drugs that can cause neutropenia include anticonvulsants (e.g., carbamazepine, valproic acid, diphenylhydantoin), thyroid inhibitors (carbimazole, methimazole, propylthiouracil), antibacterial drugs (penicillins, cephalosporins, sulfonamides, chloramphenicol, vancomycin, trimethoprim-sulfamethoxazole), antipsychotic drugs (clozapine), antiarrhythmics (procainamide), antirheumatic drugs (penicillamine, gold salts, hydroxychloroquine), and NSAIDs.[104] The ANC is calculated with "segs" (segmented neutrophils) and "bands" (band neutrophils) reported on CBC with differential: ANC = Total WBC x (% Segs + % Bands).

---

[103] Shaw BA, Gerardi JA, Hennrikus WL. How to avoid orthopedic pitfalls in children. *Patient Care* 1999; Feb 28: 95-116
[104] Tefferi A, Hanson CA, Inwards DJ. How to interpret and pursue an abnormal complete blood cell count in adults. *Mayo Clin Proc*. 2005 Jul;80(7):923-36 www.mayoclinicproceedings.com/content/80/7/923.long This article serves as the main review for this section on CBC interpretation.

CBC: complete blood count—*continued*

<table>
<tr>
<td>Overview and interpretation —continued:</td>
<td>

- <u>RBC (red blood cells and associated indices)</u>: Since polycythemia is relatively rare, in most situations the clinician is looking for anemia, most often related to the categories in the subsections that follow this paragraph. The first step is to classify the anemia based on the mean corpuscular volume (MCV) as microcytic (MCV, <80 fL), normocytic (MCV, 80-95 fL), or macrocytic (MCV, >95 fL)—details on following page.
- <u>Clinical notes on the most common anemias</u>:
  - <u>Nutritional deficiency of B-12 or folate</u>: My approach is to critique the mean corpuscular volume (MCV) and to interpret MCV values greater than 90 with an increased suspicion for folate and/or B-12 deficiency. Clinical experience has shown that MCV values greater than 95 correlate with increased homocysteine levels, and a clinical response (improvement in mood, energy, and a reduction in MCV) is commonly seen following three months of nutritional supplementation. Deficiency of vitamin B-12 can easily be treated with oral administration of 2,000 mcg per day of vitamin B-12.[105] I generally use 5 mg (rarely up to 20 mg) per day of oral folate for the treatment of probable or documented folic acid deficiency; this is safe for most patients, excluding those on antiepileptic drugs.[106] Vitamin B-12 and folic acid *function together* and should be *administered together*. Cyanocobalamin should be avoided due to the cyanide.
  - <u>Iron deficiency (confirmed with assessment of serum ferritin)</u>: While inadequate intake, malabsorption, or menstrual bleeding may cause iron deficiency, **adult patients with iron deficiency are at higher probability for gastrointestinal pathology and should therefore be evaluated with endoscopy or other comprehensive assessment** *beyond fecal occult-blood testing* **to rule out gastrointestinal disease.**[107,108] **The standard of care for all healthcare professionals is that adult patients with inexplicable iron deficiency are referred for gastroenterscopic evaluation to assess for occult gastrointestinal pathology; the major concerns are gastric/colon carcinoma, but malabsorptive conditions and bleeding noncancerous polyps are also worthy of diagnosis.** Iron supplementation should be administered and can reasonably be withheld during acute viral and bacterial infections as it promotes bacterial and viral replication and pathogenicity.
  - <u>The anemia of chronic disease</u>: Generally associated with a corresponding disease history such as long-term RA or renal insufficiency and often associated with increased ESR, CRP, and ferritin. **Do not assume that an anemic patient has iron deficiency until proven with measurement of serum ferritin.** Anemia of chronic kidney disease (CKD) is associated with reduced renal production of erythropoietin, thereby resulting in understimulation of bone marrow.
  - <u>Anemia caused by hemolysis or splenic sequestration</u>: Autoimmune hemolytic anemia most commonly occurs in patients with systemic lupus erythematosus (SLE). Pancytopenia—reduced numbers of RBC, WBC, and platelets—is seen with chronic liver disease that has progressed to cirrhosis and has resulted in hemolysis and splenic sequestration of blood cells; such patients are at risk for esophageal varicies, encephalopathy, and ascites with spontaneous bacterial peritonitis and should be screened and treated appropriately.

</td>
</tr>
</table>

---

[105] Kuzminski AM, et al. Effective treatment of cobalamin deficiency with oral cobalamin. *Blood* 1998 Aug 15;92(4):1191-8

[106] "PGA administered in doses up to 1,000 mg orally a day... The folate was well absorbed, as reflected by marked increases in the serum and erythrocyte folate concentrations... There was no evidence of clinical or laboratory toxicity at these high doses of folate." Boss GR, Ragsdale RA, Zettner A, Seegmiller JE. Failure of folic acid (pteroylglutamic acid) to affect hyperuricemia. *J Lab Clin Med* 1980 Nov;96(5):783-9

[107] Rockey DC, Cello JP. Evaluation of the gastrointestinal tract in patients with iron-deficiency anemia. *N Engl J Med*. 1993;329(23):1691-5

[108] "Endoscopy revealed a clinically important lesion in 23 (12%) of 186 patients. ... CONCLUSIONS: Endoscopy yields important findings in premenopausal women with iron deficiency anemia, which should not be attributed solely to menstrual blood loss." Bini EJ, Micale PL, Weinshel EH. Evaluation of the gastrointestinal tract in premenopausal women with iron deficiency anemia. *Am J Med*. 1998 Oct;105(4):281-6

Anemia—the most common considerations in outpatient practice: Always assess patient for tachycardia, hypovolemia, orthostasis, and adequate perfusion; always test serum ferritin during the initial evaluation then perform peripheral blood smear (PBS) if diagnosis remains unclear

- Microcytic anemia:
  - Iron deficiency anemia (IDA)—Test serum ferritin. The confirmation of iron deficiency in adults generally requires gastroenterologic consultation to assess for occult gastrointestinal blood loss; this is especially true for all men and post-menopausal women but also applies to premenopausal women.* Testing for celiac disease and hematuria is advised.**
  - Thalassemia—Check for polycythemia, test Hgb electrophoresis; because the diagnosis of the various thalassemias can be complex, consider consulting a hematologist,
  - Anemia of chronic disease (ACD)—Assess patient, inflammatory markers, and renal function. The most common causes of ACD are temporal (giant cell) arteritis and polymyalgia rheumatica, rheumatoid arthritis, chronic infection, Hodgkin lymphoma, renal cell carcinoma, myelofibrosis, and Castleman disease (a noncancerous lymphoproliferative disorder).
- Normocytic anemia:
  - Nutritional anemia: Iron deficiency and vitamin B-12 deficiency can both cause normocytic anemia.
  - Bleeding—Assess patient for tachycardia, hypovolemia, and shock; consider transfusion and/or volume repletion as needed. Assess serum ferritin and the reticulocyte count.
  - Chronic renal failure (CRF): Anemia associated with elevated BUN and creatinine.
  - Hypersplenism: Assess for chronic hepatitis and cirrhosis. Cirrhotic patients are at increased risk for gastroesophageal hemorrhage and ascites with spontaneous bacterial peritonitis.
  - Hemolysis: Expect to see elevated reticulocytes (chronic) and lactate dehydrogenase (acute); expect high indirect bilirubin and low serum haptoglobin with intravascular hemolysis; assess for autoimmunity (ANA, direct Coombs test [direct antiglobulin test]), glucose-6-phosphate dehydrogenase (G6PD) deficiency, drug-induced hemolysis, and other causes as case warrants.
  - Bone marrow disorder: Correlate lab findings with patient presentation; consult hematologist if solution is not forthcoming.
- Macrocytosis:
  - Induced by toxins, drugs, alcohol—Assess per patient history and other findings; the most notorious offenders are hydroxyurea, zidovudine, and alcohol.
  - Vitamin B-12 and/or folate deficiency: Consider testing serum methylmalonate and homocysteine followed by empiric supplementation with B-12 at 2,000 or more micrograms per day and folate at 1-5 milligrams per day; determine cause of problem and strongly consider autoimmune gastritis, bacterial overgrowth, celiac disease. Test serum ferritin because nutritional deficiencies commonly occur together. Administration of vitamin B-12 is advised in all patients suspected of having B-12 deficiency.*** Regarding the clinical presentation of vitamin B-12 deficiency, clinicians should remember the adage that one-third of patients will present with anemia, one-third with peripheral neuropathy, and one-third with central neurologic problems such as depression, psychosis, and/or other disturbances of mood, memory, or personality. Failure to diagnose and treat vitamin B-12 deficiency in a timely manner will result in permanent neurologic damage.
  - Hypothyroidism: Measure TSH and free T4 at a minimum; assess basal body temperature, and speed of Achilles reflex return.

* "A gastrointestinal source of chronic blood loss was identified in a substantial proportion of premenopausal women with iron deficiency anemia." Green BT, Rockey DC. Gastrointestinal endoscopic evaluation of premenopausal women with iron deficiency anemia. *J Clin Gastroenterol.* 2004 Feb;38(2):104-9
** Goddard AF, James MW, McIntyre AS, Scott BB; on behalf of the British Society of Gastroenterology. Guidelines for the management of iron deficiency anaemia. *Gut.* 2011 Jun http://www.epocrates.com/dacc/1106/irondefbmj1106.pdf
*** "Thus, therapeutic trials of Cbl are warranted when clinical findings consistent with Cbl deficiency are present..." Solomon LR. Cobalamin-responsive disorders in the ambulatory care setting: unreliability of cobalamin, methylmalonic acid, and homocysteine testing. *Blood* 2005 Feb:978-85 bloodjournal.hematologylibrary.org/content/105/3/978.full.pdf

CBC: complete blood count—*continued*	
Overview and interpretation —continued:	▪ <u>Platelets</u>: Elevated platelet count (thrombocytosis) can be due to malignant primary thrombocytosis, iron-deficiency anemia, hemolysis, asplenia, and reactive thrombocytosis due to cancer, infection, or chronic inflammation. Low platelet count (thrombocytopenia, fewer than 150,000 platelets per microliter) increases risk for spontaneous bleeding and can—rarely but importantly—be associated with serious and potentially life-threatening disorders such as thrombotic thrombocytopenic purpura/hemolytic uremic syndrome (TTP/HUS) and disseminated intravascular coagulation (DIC). In relatively asymptomatic and nonacute outpatients, the most common causes of thrombocytopenia are hypersplenism due to liver cirrhosis, idiopathic thrombocytopenic purpura (ITP), and drug reaction, most notoriously secondary to trimethoprim-sulfamethoxazole ("Bactrim"), cardiac medications (e.g., quinidine, procainamide, thiazide diuretics), antirheumatic drugs (gold salts [rarely used these days]), and heparin. Heparin-induced thrombocytopenia (HIT, type-2) is potentially fatal and requires immediate cessation of heparin administration. Patients with unexplained persistent thrombocytopenia should be tested for HIV, autoimmunity (ANA), and lymphoproliferative disorders (PBS, immunophenotyping, serum protein electrophoresis, and serum immunofixation). Isolated mild to moderate thrombocytopenia (75,000 – 150,000 platelets per microliter) during pregnancy generally is considered nonpathologic.
Advantages:	▪ The **CBC with differential** is inexpensive and easy to perform and is appropriate for asymptomatic patients. The "CBC with diff" is an appropriate first test for patients who are symptomatic (e.g., fatigue, fever) or have an ongoing history of health problems. In certain healthcare settings where cost containment is a major priority, CBC *without* differential is commonly ordered; however, in outpatient private practice, the additional expenditure of $2 for the CBC *with* differential is the preferred evaluation. It provides a quick screen for anemia, leukemia, infection, and for provisional evidence of B-12/folate and iron deficiencies. The CBC can also identify more complex conditions such as pancytopenia and thereby promote comprehensive patient management; for example, pancytopenia may unmask hepatic cirrhosis which may necessitate use of nadolol for prophylaxis against gastroesophageal variceal hemorrhage as well as use of prophylactic antibiotics against spontaneous bacterial peritonitis. ▪ The **peripheral blood smear (PBS)** is used to further evaluate leukocytosis, anemias, and other abnormalities. In the investigation of persistent leukocytosis, the PBS is of limited value and therefore, while the PBS should certainly be performed, it is generally followed by **immunophenotyping by flow cytometry** if not a direct referral to a hematologist. An excellent review by Tefferi et al[109] concluded, "In general, it is prudent to perform a PBS in most instances of abnormal CBC, along with basic tests that are dictated by the type of CBC abnormalities. The latter may include, for example, serum ferritin in patients with microcytic anemia or lymphocyte immunophenotyping by flow cytometry in patients with lymphocytosis..."
Limitations:	▪ WBC count may be normal even in patients with serious infections. ▪ RBC indices may be normal in people with severe iron deficiency. ○ **Dr Vasquez's experience**—*Many outpatients with no evidence of anemia on the CBC will be grossly iron deficient with ferritin values less than 6 mcg/L, clearly indicating iron deficiency. Nonanemic iron deficiency contributes to fatigue, depression, and attention deficit.*
Comments:	▪ The **CBC** is a foundational part of the assessment for all new patients. Generally, "CBC *with* differential" should be ordered.

---

[109] Tefferi A, Hanson CA, Inwards DJ. How to interpret and pursue an abnormal complete blood cell count in adults. *Mayo Clin Proc* 2005;80(7):923-3

Presentation: Classic iron insufficiency in a healthy 32yo athletic female: This limited laboratory report is from a 32yo athletic female whose primary complaint is that of "less endurance than expected" given her healthy lifestyle and frequent participation in physical exercise of various types such as running, biking, hiking, and kayaking. Her TSH is on the low end of normal consistent with her taking 17 mcg daily of liothyroinine (T3); note however that the total T3 level remains on the low end of the normal range, suggesting that she may benefit from additional T3 supplementation. The RBC parameters Hgb and Hct are on the low end of the normal range consistent with recent menstruation; the response of the bone marrow to recent blood loss is noted with the RDW being toward the high end of normal, refecting increased marrow production of reticulocytes. Ferritin is suboptimal at 25 ng/mL, given that the optimal range is approximately 40-70 ng/mL.[110] Altough various iron supplements are available on the market and high-iron foods such as beef and blackstrap molasis can be used, typical treatment is with iron 18 mg per day often provided as ferrous sulfate 90 mg; note that 5 mg ferrous sulfate = 1 mg elemental iron. Other forms of iron such as ferrous aspartate may be better tolerated. Daily iron supplementation for 2-3 months should elevate the ferritin level and improve the feeling of energy not simply by ❶ improving oxygen delivery to tissues but also by ❷ improving function of the electron transport chain where iron is a required cofactor, ❸ improving the conversion of thyroid hormone (T4) into the active form of T3, and by ❹ improving the production of dopamine and norepinephrine, since iron is a required cofactor for the enzyme tyrosine hydroxylase which converts the amino acid tyrosine into L-DOPA which is converted to dopamine and then partially to norepinephrine. Given that this patient menstruates monthly and has no significant medical history and—specifically—no gastrointestinal complaints; the probability is high that her state of iron insufficiency is due to physiologic blood loss; however, a case could be made for endoscopic evaluation[111], and in the event that the patient suffered from an diagnosed intestinal lesion such as colon cancer, the practitioner who did not refer for gastroenterologic evaluation would be challenged to produce effective medicolegal defense. Guidelines[112] published in 2011 support testing for celiac disease, *H. pylori* infection, and hematuria while reserving endoscopy in premenopausal women to those aged 50 years or older, or with symptoms of gastrointestinal disease, or those with a strong family history of colorectal cancer.

Reported: 07/07/2011 / 06:02 CDT

Test Name	In Range	Out Of Range	Reference Range
TSH, 3RD GENERATION	0.54		mIU/L
Reference Range			

> or = 20 Years   0.40-4.50

Pregnancy Ranges
First trimester   0.20-4.70
Second trimester   0.30-4.10
Third trimester   0.40-2.70

Test Name	In Range	Out Of Range	Reference Range
T3, TOTAL	97		76-181 ng/dL
CBC (INCLUDES DIFF/PLT)			
WHITE BLOOD CELL COUNT	7.1		3.8-10.8 Thousand/uL
RED BLOOD CELL COUNT	4.28		3.80-5.10 Million/uL
HEMOGLOBIN	12.1		11.7-15.5 g/dL
HEMATOCRIT	36.2		35.0-45.0 %
MCV	84.5		80.0-100.0 fL
MCH	28.4		27.0-33.0 pg
MCHC	33.6		32.0-36.0 g/dL
RDW	14.8		11.0-15.0 %
PLATELET COUNT	248		140-400 Thousand/uL
ABSOLUTE NEUTROPHILS	3586		1500-7800 cells/uL
ABSOLUTE LYMPHOCYTES	2854		850-3900 cells/uL
ABSOLUTE MONOCYTES	525		200-950 cells/uL
ABSOLUTE EOSINOPHILS	107		15-500 cells/uL
ABSOLUTE BASOPHILS	28		0-200 cells/uL
NEUTROPHILS	50.5		%
LYMPHOCYTES	40.2		%
MONOCYTES	7.4		%
EOSINOPHILS	1.5		%
BASOPHILS	0.4		%
FERRITIN	25		10-154 ng/mL

---

[110] See excerpt from Vasquez A. *Integrative Rheumatology*. http://optimalhealthresearch.com/hemochromatosis.html

[111] "A gastrointestinal source of chronic blood loss was identified in a substantial proportion of premenopausal women with iron deficiency anemia." Green BT, Rockey DC. Gastrointestinal endoscopic evaluation of premenopausal women with iron deficiency anemia. *J Clin Gastroenterol*. 2004 Feb;38(2):104-9

[112] Goddard AF, James MW, McIntyre AS, Scott BB; on behalf of the British Society of Gastroenterology. Guidelines for the management of iron deficiency anaemia. *Gut*. 2011 Jun 6. [Epub ahead of print] http://www.epocrates.com/dacc/1106/irondefbmj1106.pdf

Presentation: Vitamin B-12 deficiency without hematologic abnormality—report and discussion: This elderly patient shows no signs of anemia; note also that the MCV is perfectly normal. Given that the psychiatric literature supports a minimal serum vitamin B-12 level of 600 pg/ml, the advocation by medical reference laboratories of a lower "normal" limit of 200 pg/ml is scientifically absurd and ethically indefensible; this is yet another example of the importance of clinicians' knowledge of the literature overriding the laboratory's reference range. The consistent documentation of the rapid reversibility of severe neuropsychiatric illness with vitamin B-12 therapy as the only intervention[113,114] provides additional justification for empiric vitamin B-12 administration in patients with clinical symptoms consistent with vitamin B-12 deficiency regardless of hematologic and serologic findings.[115] Vitamin B-12 deficiency is very serious because it can lead to permanent brain damage, resulting in personality changes, memory impairment, and overt psychotic disorders, including catatonia; mechanisms of neurologic injury may include homocysteine toxicity, autoimmune neuronal demyelinization, and axonal degeneration and nerve-sheath demyelination especially in the median forebrain bundle area.[116]

HEMATOLOGY

----- CBC - WBC STUDIES -----

Procedure:	WBC 10E3
Reference:	[4.50-11.00]
Units:	/CMM
07DEC06 0926 THU	7.32

----- CBC - RBC STUDIES -----

	RBC 10E6	HEMOGLOBIN	HEMATOCRIT	MCV	MCH	MCHC	RDW-CV
Procedure:	RBC 10E6	HEMOGLOBIN	HEMATOCRIT	MCV	MCH	MCHC	RDW-CV
Reference:	[4.50-5.90]	[13.5-17.5]	[41.0-53.0]	[80.0-94.0]	[27.0-31.0]	[32.0-36.0]	[11.0-16.0]
Units:	/CMM	G/DL	%	FL	PG	%	%
07DEC06 0926 THU	5.16	15.7	46.3	89.7	30.4	33.9	14.1

----- CBC - PLATELET STUDIES -----

	PLATELET 10E3	MPV
Procedure:	PLATELET 10E3	MPV
Reference:	[150-500]	[9.0-13.0]
Units:	/CMM	FL
07DEC06 0926 THU	308	11.2

CHEMISTRY PROFILES

----- ROUTINE CHEMISTRY PROFILES -----

	SODIUM	POTASSIUM	CHLORIDE	CO2	GLUCOSE	BUN	CREATININE	CALCIUM
Procedure:	SODIUM	POTASSIUM	CHLORIDE	CO2	GLUCOSE	BUN	CREATININE	CALCIUM
Reference:	[133-145]	[3.5-5.3]	[100-110]	[22.0-29.0]	[70-110]	[5-25]	[0.5-1.4]	[8.3-10.3]
Units:	MMOL/L	MEQ/L	MMOL/L	MMOL/L	MG/DL	MG/DL	MG/DL	MG/DL
07DEC06 0926 THU	137	4.3	101	27.0	90	16	0.9	9.9

	ANION GAP	OSMOLARITY	BUN/CREAT
Procedure:	ANION GAP	OSMOLARITY	BUN/CREAT
Reference:	[6-14]	[272-305]	
Units:	MEQ/L	MOSM/K	MG/DL
07DEC06 0926 THU	13	275	17.8

SPECIAL CHEMISTRY

----- CHEMISTRY SPECIAL/MISCELLANEOUS -----

	FOLATE	VITAMIN B-12
Procedure:	FOLATE	VITAMIN B-12
Reference:	[2.0-18.0]	[193-982]
Units:	NG/ML	PG/ML
07DEC06 0926 THU	14.7	182 L

[113] Berry N, Sagar R, Tripathi BM. Catatonia and other psychiatric symptoms with vitamin B12 deficiency. *Acta Psychiatr Scand*. 2003 ;108(2):156-9

[114] Newbold HL. Vitamin B-12: placebo or neglected therapeutic tool? *Med Hypotheses*. 1989 Mar;28(3):155-64

[115] Solomon LR. Cobalamin-responsive disorders in the ambulatory care setting: unreliability of cobalamin, methylmalonic acid, and homocysteine testing. *Blood*. 2005 Feb 1;105(3):978-85

[116] Catalano G, Catalano MC, Rosenberg EI, Embi PJ, Embi CS. Catatonia. Another neuropsychiatric presentation of vitamin B12 deficiency? *Psychosomatics*. 1998 Sep-Oct;39(5):456-60 http://psy.psychiatryonline.org/cgi/reprint/39/5/456

Consequences of vitamin B-12 deficiency:

Initially the manifestations are mild and reversible, but over time they become more severe and strongly refractory to treatment to the point that permanent damage (particularly in the CNS) is anticipated:

- "Bipolar disorder"—a condition indistinguishable from a bipolar disorder,
- Organic brain syndrome, delirium, confusion, poor memory, impaired cognition,
- Dementia and erroneous diagnosis of "Alzheimer's disease",
- Mood disorders, depression, catatonia, paranoia, paranoid psychosis, violent behavior,
- Peripheral neuropathy, "combined degeneration" of anterior and posterior columns of the spinal cord,
- As a result of the above problems, patients who are mismanaged by doctors unknowledgeable about basic nutrition often suffer directly from these effects but also suffer from the medical management from these problems. Mood disorders and psychosis may result from B-12 deficiency, and the medical management of mood disorders and psychosis includes medicalization, electroconvulsive therapy (ECT), and institutionalization.

The medical profession's failure to train its students and doctors in nutrition is widely and consistently documented; given that such a profession-wide policy can do nothing other than result in patient harm and/or drug dependency under the guise of "healthcare", it is—borrowing a phrase from Nietzsche—"the highest of all conceivable corruptions."

- Nutritional deficiencies and the medical paradigm (*J Clin Endocrinol Metab* 2003 Nov): "But public health measures in the first half of the 20th century eradicated the most extreme of the vitamin deficiencies in the industrialized nations, and the physician's actual experience of [obvious] deficiency disease dropped to near zero. Perhaps as a result, the medical profession's approach to nutrition today is still dominated by the external agent paradigm, as witnessed in the national campaigns for cholesterol, saturated fat, and salt. Those who think more seriously in terms of the continuing importance of deficiency per se are often derogated or relegated to the quackery fringe. The result, at the very least, is inattention to the real deficiencies that may masquerade as other disorders, or that may simply be ignored altogether."
- Failure of surgical treatment for low-back pain caused by vitamin D deficiency (*J Am Board Fam Med* 2009 Jan): The author of this case series describes six cases of chronic debilitating back pain—three of which "required surgery"—which were greatly relieved or completely cured by correction of vitamin D deficiency. The author notes, "Chronic low back pain and failed back surgery may improve with repletion of vitamin D from a state of deficiency/insufficiency to sufficiency. Vitamin D insufficiency is common; repletion of vitamin D to normal levels in patients who have chronic low back pain or have had failed back surgery may improve quality of life or, in some cases, result in complete resolution of symptoms."

That nutritional deficiencies can cause mood disorders and mental disease is well-known; in contrast to what patients actually need, the general allopathic approach to these clinical presentations is founded upon the administration of drugs, followed by ECT, institutionalization, and psychosurgery and—lately, instead of scalpel-induced brain damage—radiofrequency heating (thermocapsulotomy) or gamma radiation (radiosurgery, gammacapsulotomy) for the destruction of brain structures, and the surgical implantation of brain electrostimulators. Meanwhile, thousands of these psychiatrically-labeled patients simply need nutritional supplementation. Minor exceptions noted, the medical profession as a whole chooses to remain blind to the value of nutrition so that the pharmacosurgical paradigm can remain dominant by continuing to *appear* omnipotent. The dual illusions that are maintained are "Drugs and surgery are the answers to all major health problems" and "If no drug exists for a condition, then it is idiopathic and no curative treatment is available."

As an example, type-2 diabetes mellitus (T2DM) has burgeoned into an epidemic under the dominance of the allopathic disease model, and patients are told that the condition is genetic, progressive and incurable; a review published in the May 2011 issue of *Journal of the American Osteopathic Association* admonished physicians to (mis)educate their patients as follows, with Dr Vasquez's comments in brackets: "Be absolutely clear that T2DM is a lifelong disease [false statement] that will require lifelong treatment [false statement fostering dependency]. Success in controlling the disease and preventing future complications will depend on the patient and physician working together [creation of dependency under the guise of "working together"]. There is often a fatalistic attitude in patients with T2DM [perhaps because they have been lied to and disempowered], so it is important to establish a relationship that on one hand offers hope [creating the illusion of hope while enforcing drug dependency] and on the other does not suggest that the disease will be cured [although the diseases is generally curable with appropriate nutritional intervention]. Be up front with the patient from the first visit and make it clear that T2DM is a chronic illness [enforce drug dependency starting a the first visit]..." This babble

Nutritional deficiency, diet-responsive disorders, and the allopathic medical paradigm: Review and commentary with emphases on diabetes mellitus and vitamins D and B-12

was published in a peer-reviewed medical journal despite clear multi-decade evidence showing that T2DM is reversible with nutritional intervention. Recent examples of the safety and efficacy of diet intervention for T2DM are provided here with many more examples and details in *Nutritional, Integrative and Functional Medicine Mastery of Common Clinical Disorders*.

- T2DM is rapidly reversible with diet (*Diabetologia* 2011 Jun): "Normalization of both beta cell function and hepatic insulin sensitivity in type 2 diabetes was achieved by dietary energy restriction alone. This was associated with decreased pancreatic and liver triacylglycerol stores. **The abnormalities underlying type 2 diabetes are reversible by reducing dietary energy intake.**"
- Diet therapy effective, safe, and is at least as effective as injected insulin for reducing chronic hyperglycemia in T2DM (*Nutr Metab* 2009 May): "The number of patients on sulfonylureas decreased from 7 at baseline to 2 at 6 months. No patient required inpatient care or insulin therapy. In summary, the 30%-carbohydrate diet over 6 months led to a remarkable reduction in HbA1c levels, even among outpatients with severe type 2 diabetes, without any insulin therapy, hospital care or increase in sulfonylureas. **The effectiveness of the [low-carbohydrate] diet may be comparable to that of insulin therapy.**"

Ironically (or not), the first-line drug for T2DM—metformin—causes vitamin B-12 (cobalamin, Cbl) deficiency and exacerbation of the often debilitating peripheral neuropathy of T2DM which is often treated with the drugs gabapentin/Neurontin or pregabalin/Lyrica, which exacerbates obesity and T2DM, thereby promoting a vicious cycle.

- Pregabalin/Lyrica and gabapentin/Neurontin promote fat-weight gain, thereby exacerbating T2DM (*Prescrire Int* 2005 Dec): "Pregabalin, like gabapentin, can lead to weight gain and peripheral edema especially in elderly patients."
- Metformin causes vitamin B-12 deficiency and exacerbates diabetic peripheral neuropathy (*Diabetes Care* 2010 Jan): "Metformin-treated patients had depressed Cbl levels and elevated fasting MMA and Hcy levels. Clinical and electrophysiological measures identified more severe peripheral neuropathy in these patients; the cumulative metformin dose correlated strongly with these clinical and paraclinical group differences. CONCLUSIONS: Metformin exposure may be an iatrogenic cause for exacerbation of peripheral neuropathy in patients with type 2 diabetes."
- Vitamin B-12 deficiency secondary to metformin prescription (*Rev Assoc Med Bras* 2011 Jan): "The present findings suggest a high prevalence of vitamin B12 deficiency in metformin-treated diabetic patients [n=144]. Older patients, patients in long term treatment with metformin and low vitamin B12 intake are probably more prone to this deficiency."
- Metformin-induced vitamin B12 deficiency presenting as a peripheral neuropathy (*South Med J* 2010 Mar): "Chronic metformin use results in vitamin B12 deficiency in 30% of patients. ... **Vitamin B12 deficiency, which may present without anemia and as a peripheral neuropathy, is often misdiagnosed as diabetic neuropathy, although the clinical findings are usually different. Failure to diagnose the cause of the neuropathy will result in progression of central and/or peripheral neuronal damage which can be arrested but not reversed with vitamin B12 replacement.**"
- Low vitamin B-12 status correlates with expedited brain atrophy (*Neurology* 2008 Sep): "The decrease in brain volume was greater among those with lower vitamin B(12) and holoTC levels and higher plasma tHcy and MMA levels at baseline. ... Using the upper (for the vitamins) or lower tertile (for the metabolites) as reference in logistic regression analysis and adjusting for the above covariates, vitamin B(12) in the bottom tertile (<308 pmol/L) was associated with increased rate of brain volume loss (odds ratio 6.17, 95% CI 1.25-30.47)."

Consequences for the clinician:

Given that the evidence in favor of early and empiric treatment for possible vitamin B-12 deficiency is stronger than evidence in favor of allowing vitamin B-12 deficiency or dependency to persist with potentially catastrophic outcomes, no scientific argument can be made in favor of failing to diagnose and treat vitamin B-12 deficiency/dependency. However, since, in general, the allopathic and osteopathic medical professions have failed to educate their students and doctors about nutrition, these professions have established ignorance as their defense and therefore no standard of care exists for the treatment or failure of treatment of chronic nutritional deficiencies. Ethically, the results are failure to achieve beneficence via failure to diagnose and treat, and the widespread implementation of malfeasance via diagnostic/therapeutic failure complicated by the unnecessary expenses and adverse effects of drugs/surgeries/interventions used in place of nutritional supplementation. The enforcement of a standard of care is meaningless when nutritional incompetence is the standard. Fortunately for patients, the biomedical literature uses increasingly strong language in favor of mandating standards for nutritional evaluation and treatment:

- Nutritional deficiencies and the medical paradigm (*J Clin Endocrinol Metab* 2003 Nov): "J. Cannell (submitted for publication) has written that measures such as this editorial will not change the situation, and that only tort litigation will work. One can only hope that he is wrong. Either way, something needs to change"

- Physicians should routinely use vitamin supplementation as treatment for patients (*JAMA* 2002 Jun): "Physicians should make specific efforts to ensure that patients are taking vitamins they should..."

- Testing and treating for vitamin D deficiency among patients with chronic nonspecific musculoskeletal pain should be the standard of care (*Mayo Clin Proc* 2003 Dec): "Because osteomalacia is a known cause of persistent, nonspecific musculoskeletal pain, screening all outpatients with such pain for hypovitaminosis D should be standard practice in clinical care."

- Testing and treating for vitamin D deficiency among patients with chronic low-back pain should be the standard of care (*Spine* 2003 Jan): "Screening for vitamin D deficiency and treatment with supplements should be mandatory in this setting."

Citations for this section:

1. Catalano G, Catalano MC, Rosenberg EI, Embi PJ, Embi CS. Catatonia. Another neuropsychiatric presentation of vitamin B12 deficiency? *Psychosomatics*. 1998 Sep-Oct;39(5):456-60
2. Newbold HL. Vitamin B-12: placebo or neglected therapeutic tool? *Med Hypotheses*. 1989 Mar;28(3):155-64
3. Solomon LR. Cobalamin-responsive disorders in the ambulatory care setting: unreliability of cobalamin, methylmalonic acid, and homocysteine testing. *Blood*. 2005 Feb 1;105(3):978-85
4. Christmas D, Eljamel MS, Butler S, et al. Long term outcome of thermal anterior capsulotomy for chronic, treatment refractory depression. *J Neurol Neurosurg Psychiatry*. 2011 Jun;82(6):594-600
5. Malone DA Jr. Use of deep brain stimulation in treatment-resistant depression. *Cleve Clin J Med*. 2010 Jul;77 Suppl 3:S77-80
6. Heaney RP. Vitamin D, nutritional deficiency, and the medical paradigm. *J Clin Endocrinol Metab*. 2003;88:5107-8
7. Schwalfenberg G. Improvement of chronic back pain or failed back surgery with vitamin D repletion: a case series. *J Am Board Fam Med*. 2009 Jan-Feb;22(1):69-74
8. Gavin JR 3rd, Freeman JS, Shubrook JH Jr, Lavernia F. Type 2 diabetes mellitus: practical approaches for primary care physicians. *J Am Osteopath Assoc*. 2011 May;111(5 Suppl 4):S3-S12
9. Lim EL, Hollingsworth KG, Aribisala BS, et al. Reversal of type 2 diabetes: normalisation of beta cell function in association with decreased pancreas and liver triacylglycerol. *Diabetologia*. 2011 Jun 9. Published on-line.
10. Haimoto H, Sasakabe T, Wakai K, Umegaki H. Effects of a low-carbohydrate diet on glycemic control in outpatients with severe type 2 diabetes. *Nutr Metab* 2009:6;21
11. Gabapentin/Neurontin causes "Gains of up to 15 kg (33lbs) during 3 months of treatment." http://pacmedweightloss.com/docs/medications_that_cause_weight_gain.pdf Accessed July 2011.
12. Vogiatzoglou A, Refsum H, Johnston C, Smith SM, Bradley KM, de Jager C, Budge MM, Smith AD. Vitamin B12 status and rate of brain volume loss in community-dwelling elderly. *Neurology*. 2008 Sep 9;71(11):826-32
13. Wile DJ, Toth C. Association of metformin, elevated homocysteine, and methylmalonic acid levels and clinically worsened diabetic peripheral neuropathy. *Diabetes Care*. 2010 Jan;33(1):156-61
14. Nervo M, Lubini A, Raimundo FV, Faulhaber GA, Leite C, Fischer LM, Furlanetto TW. Vitamin B12 in metformin-treated diabetic patients: a cross-sectional study in Brazil. *Rev Assoc Med Bras*. 2011 Jan-Feb;57(1):46-9
15. Bell DS. Metformin-induced vitamin B12 deficiency presenting as a peripheral neuropathy. *South Med J*. 2010 Mar;103(3):265-7
16. [No authors listed] Pregabalin: new drug. Very similar to gabapentin. *Prescrire Int*. 2005 Dec;14(80):203-6
17. Fletcher RH, Fairfield KM. Harvard Medical School. Vitamins for chronic disease prevention in adults: clinical applications. *JAMA*. 2002;287:3127-9
18. Plotnikoff GA, Quigley JM. Prevalence of severe hypovitaminosis D in patients with persistent, nonspecific musculoskeletal pain. *Mayo Clin Proc*. 2003;78:1463-70
19. Al Faraj S, Al Mutairi K. Vitamin D deficiency and chronic low back pain in Saudi Arabia. *Spine* 2003 ;28:177-9

UA: Urinalysis	
Overview and interpretation:	▪ Collection: Unless catheterized, patients are advised to pass approximately one-third of their available urine into the toilet, then pass approximately the middle-third of their urine into the specimen container. Use of an antiseptic to clean the urethral meatus was once advocated to avoid/reduce specimen contamination, but this step is ineffective and therefore unnecessary because contamination rates remain similar at 32% and 29% whether or not, respectively, urethral meatus cleansing is performed.[117]
	▪ Analysis: Analysis should be performed on fresh urine, preferably within 1-2 hours; in outpatient clinical practice this two-hour timeframe is consistently possible only if the clinician performs in-office dipstick analysis (and perhaps microscopic visualization). Samples that cannot be analyzed within 1-2 hours or those which are destined for a reference laboratory should be refrigerated. Dipstick UA can be performed in office and is simple, inexpensive, and—when performed and interpreted with a modicum of competence— sufficiently accurate. Per Klatt[118], "The color change occurring on each segment of the strip is compared to a color chart to obtain results. However, a careless doctor, nurse, or assistant is entirely capable of misreading or misinterpreting the results." Urine samples can be sent to a reference laboratory for more accurate chemical analysis as well as microscopic analysis, culture and sensitivity. Whether infection is clinically suspected or not, clinicians might chose to order "UA with reflex to microscopy and culture" to ensure that urine samples are appropriately processed if the laboratory finds suspicion of UTI upon dipstick analysis.
	▪ Scope of this review: The purpose of this brief review is to concisely refresh clinicians' appreciation of the components of the routine urinalysis, one that is generally performed in-office with a dipstick reagent stick or that is performed by a reference laboratory. This is not an exhaustive review, and microscopic findings have not been detailed here because most clinicians do not perform microscopy in their offices; additional details on UA and microscopic assessment is available in articles such as the excellent review by Simerville, Maxted, and Pahira published in *American Family Physician* 2005 and available on-line at http://www.aafp.org/afp/2005/0315/p1153.html as of July 2011.
	▪ Components of routine urinalysis:
	○ Visual inspection: Urine should be clear with a color ranging from faint yellow (well hydrated, dilute urine) to bright yellow (especially with B-vitamin supplementation). An amber-brown hue might be due to dehydration or a pathologic process resulting in myoglobinuria (i.e., rhabdomyolysis) or the presence of bile pigments (i.e., biliary tract obstruction). A red color to urine suggests hematuria, recent beet consumption, or use of certain drugs or food dyes; the antibiotic rifampin/rifampicin is notorious for adding a red-orange color to the urine (and to a lesser extent to sweat and tears). The urine of patients with porphyria cutanea tarda will be red-brown in natural light and pink-red in fluorescent light.[119] Cloudy urine is due to pyruia (infection), proteinuria, or precipitated phosphate crystals in alkaline urine.
	○ Strong odor: Odiferous or malodorous urine suggests infection, recent ingestion of foods such as asparagus or nutritional supplements such as lipoic acid, certain medications, concentrated urine due to dehydration or underperfusion of the kidneys.
	○ Specific gravity: Specific gravity is a measure of solute concentration and thus is proportional to urine osmolality; as such it reflects renal perfusion, hydration, and the ability of the kidneys to perform their critical function of concentrating filtrate. Dilute urine has a specific gravity <1.010 and is seen with adequate/excessive hydration, diuretic use, diabetes insipidus, adrenal insufficiency, hyperaldosteronism, and impaired renal

---

[117] Simerville JA, Maxted WC, Pahira JJ. Urinalysis: a comprehensive review. *Am Fam Physician.* 2005 Mar 15;71(6):1153-62 http://www.aafp.org/afp/2005/0315/p1153.html
[118] Klatt EC. WebPath. Savannah, Georgia, USA. http://library.med.utah.edu/WebPath/tutorial/urine/urine.html Accessed July 1, 2011
[119] Rich MW. Porphyria cutanea tarda. Don't forget to look at the urine. *Postgrad Med.* 1999 Apr;105(4):208-10, 213-4

function (i.e., failure of the kidneys to concentrate urine). Concentrated urine has a specific gravity >1.020 and correlates with dehydration, renal artery stenosis, hypoperfusion/shock, glucosuria, and syndrome of inappropriate anti-diuretic hormone secretion (SIADH), which is often associated with hyponatremia.

o pH: Urine pH may range from 4.5 (very acidic) to as high as 8.5 (very alkaline). Urine pH correlates with serum pH except in patients with renal tubular acidosis (RTA type-1, a condition associated with chronically alkaline urine). Therefore, urine pH can be used to screen for various conditions of systemic alkalosis and acidosis. The Western diet—also called the standard American diet or S.A.D.—causes mild diet-induced metabolic acidosis[120] which promotes degenerative diseases; in contrast, a diet rich in fruits and vegetables such as the Paleo-Mediterranean diet[121] promotes mild systemic and urinary alkalinization.[122] From a wellness perspective, urine pH should be 7.5 up to 8.0 because urinary alkalinization facilitates xenobiotic excretion[123], promotes urinary retention of minerals such as potassium, magnesium, and calcium, and causes a reduction in serum cortisol.[124] Urine pH—like urine sodium:potassium ratio—can be used as a marker of compliance for intake of fruits, vegetables, and alkalinizing supplements such as potassium citrate. For some patients (mostly female), urine alkalinization may encourage urinary tract infection, especially if gastrointestinal dysbiosis[125] is present; in such situations, the often causative GI dysbiosis should be treated, and consistent or transient urinary acidification can be achieved with oral ascorbic acid. Urea-splitting bacteria can cause the urine to be alkaline, and such bacteria can also promote development of magnesium-ammonium phosphate crystals and so-called staghorn nephrolithiasis. Acidic urine promotes development of uric acid nephrolithiasis; therapeutic urinary alkalinization such as by use of supplemental potassium citrate or an alkalinizing diet is preventive and therapeutic. On this topic, Cicerello et al[126] wrote, "In conclusion urinary alkalization with maintaining continuously high urinary pH values, could be the treatment of choice for stone dissolution and prevention of uric acid stones."

o Bilirubin in urine: If present, bilirubin in urine is of the direct/conjugated fraction (rather than indirect/unconjugated, which is nonhydrosoluble) and indicates the need to evaluate for biliary tract obstruction.

o Urobilinogen: Urobilinogen is (direct) bilirubin that has been conjugated in the liver, passed through the biliary system into the intestine, partially metabolized by bacteria, then reabsorbed via the portal circulation and filtered by the kidney. Elevated urobilinogen is associated with liver disease and hemolytic diseases.

o Glucose: Glucose is found in the urine when the serum glucose exceeds approximately 190 mg/dL and overwhelms the reabsorptive capacity of the proximal tubule. Glucose in the urine is presumptive evidence supporting the diagnosis of diabetes mellitus. Rare non-diabetic causes of glucosuria/glycosuria include liver disease, pancreatic disease, and Fanconi's syndrome (characterized by a failure of the proximal renal tubules to reabsorb glucose, amino acids, uric acid, phosphate and bicarbonate).

---

[120] "The modern Western-type diet is deficient in fruits and vegetables and contains excessive animal products, generating the accumulation of non-metabolizable anions and a lifespan state of overlooked metabolic acidosis, whose magnitude increases progressively with aging due to the physiological decline in kidney function." Adeva MM, Souto G. Diet-induced metabolic acidosis. *Clin Nutr.* 2011 Aug;30(4):416-21. Epub 2011 Apr 9.

[121] **Vasquez A**. Revisiting the Five-Part Nutritional Wellness Protocol: The Supplemented Paleo-Mediterranean Diet. *Nutritional Perspectives* 2011 January This article is available at http://optimalhealthresearch.com/part8.html and is also included in this textbook.

[122] Cordain L, Eaton SB, Sebastian A, Mann N, Lindeberg S, Watkins BA, O'Keefe JH, Brand-Miller J. Origins and evolution of the Western diet: health implications for the 21st century. *Am J Clin Nutr.* 2005 Feb;81(2):341-54

[123] Proudfoot AT, Krenzelok EP, Vale JA. Position Paper on urine alkalinization. *J Toxicol Clin Toxicol.* 2004;42(1):1-26

[124] Maurer M, Riesen W, Muser J, Hulter HN, Krapf R. Neutralization of Western diet inhibits bone resorption independently of K intake and reduces cortisol secretion in humans. *Am J Physiol Renal Physiol.* 2003 Jan;284(1):F32-40

[125] **Vasquez A**. Reducing Pain and Inflammation Naturally - Part 6: Nutritional and Botanical Treatments Against "Silent Infections" and Gastrointestinal Dysbiosis, Commonly Overlooked Causes of Neuromusculoskeletal Inflammation and Chronic Health Problems. *Nutritional Perspectives* 2006; January. For a more extensive review, see the most recent edition of Integrative Rheumatology: http://optimalhealthresearch.com/rheumatology.html

[126] Cicerello E, Merlo F, Maccatrozzo L. Urinary alkalization for the treatment of uric acid nephrolithiasis. *Arch Ital Urol Androl.* 2010 Sep;82(3):145-8

UA: Urinalysis

- o Ketones: UA dipsticks detect acetic acid; other products of fatty acid metabolism found in urine include acetone and beta-hydroxybutyric acid. Ketonuria indicates either metabolic disturbance such as diabetes mellitus or normal physiology in the fasting or lipolytic state. Many clinicians—particularly medical students and physicians[note 127]—have been taught to view ketonuria as synonymous with ketoacidosis; this is obviously inaccurate since lipolysis and the resulting ketonuria are normal *and quite desirable* physiologic states. Ketonuria can be measured with ketone-specific dipsticks as a marker of weight-loss efficacy and compliance with diet and exercise programs.
- o Protein: Urine should not contain measurable protein on routine urinalysis. Any finding of protein in the urine—even a "trace" amount—requires follow-up; specifically, the test should be repeated within 2-4 weeks and consistently positive results require more detailed testing including serum BUN and creatinine. Urine protein can also be measured in 24-hour urine collections and should not exceed 150 mg/day; greater than this amount is diagnostic of proteinuria, while ≥ 3.5 gm/day is consistent with nephrotic syndrome, mandating a much more comprehensive *and urgent* patient evaluation. Testing for "protein" with a routine urinalysis will not detect all forms of clinically relevant proteinuria; specifically and classically, routine UA is insensitive for the microalbuminuria of diabetes mellitus (detected with the urinary albumin:creatinine ratio) and also the Bence-Jones proteinuria seen with multiple myeloma.

Evaluation of persistent proteinuria
1. Comprehensive evaluation of patient history, physical exam, and overall clinical impression,
2. Measurement of serum BUN, creatinine, albumin, and lipids; consider measuring cystatin c,
3. Microscopic examination of urinary sediment,
4. Assessment for conditions that commonly cause proteinuria, especially hypertension (sphygmomanometry), diabetes (hemoglobin A1c), autoimmune conditions (screen with ANA);
5. Measurement of 24-hour urinary creatinine excretion (or spot urinary albumin-creatinine ratio),
6. Urinary protein electrophoresis,
7. If the above measures are pathoetiologically unfruitful, refer to an internist or nephrologist.

---

[127] One of the arguments most commonly leveled against the ketogenic diet—in particular the Atkins diet—is that the induction of ketosis, as measured by ketonuria, is a potentially problematic state that should be avoided. This is an example of selective medical ignorance since mild ketosis is physiologically normal is clinically advantageous for weight loss and seizure control. In our osteopathic medical school, one lecturer advised our student body of 170 that ketosis was evidence of the "danger from diet therapies." On the contrary, given that most of my medical school professors were obese, they should have more carefully considered the benefits of rational dietary therapy, including low-carbohydrate versions of the Paleo-Mediterranean diet (described in this text) which can produce mild ketosis en route to alleviating diabetes mellitus and hypertension. Examples of selective medical ignorance and bias against low-carbohydrate ketogenic diets abound from allopathic institutions. "One diet that has raised safety concerns among the scientific community is the low-carbohydrate, high-protein diet." Tapper-Gardzina Y, Cotugna N, Vickery CE. Should you recommend a low-carb, high-protein diet? *Nurse Pract.* 2002 Apr;27(4):52-3, 55-6, 58-9. "High Protein / Low Carb (Carbohydrate) Diets. Long term, these fad diets can be harmful. Many of the health claims about these diets are not based on scientific proof. Low carb diets are still just that – a diet. Most people find maintaining a low carb diet difficult if not impossible long term. Even if weight is lost, 90% of fad dieters gain all or most of the weight back in five years." Ohio State University. http://medicalcenter.osu.edu/PatientEd/Materials/PDFDocs/nut-diet/nut-other/high-pro.pdf Accessed July 2011.

Overview and interpretation:	○ <u>Nitrite</u>: Urinary nit<u>ri</u>te is most often the result of bacterial action on excreted urinary nit<u>ra</u>te; students and clinicians can remember this by recalling that nit<u>ra</u>te is consumed in foods via the <u>a</u>limentary tract, while nit<u>ri</u>te in the urine generally indicates urinary tract <u>i</u>nfection (UTI). A small amount of nitrate is naturally present in some foods, including tap water, beer, some cheese products, cured meats and bacon. Additional environmental sources of nitrate include the nitrates that are intentionally added to foods as preservatives, those which are contaminants from nitrate-containing fertilizers, and those which are present in our polluted environment from pesticides and the manufacture of rubber and latex. Not all bacteria can convert nitrate to nitrite; generally, this reaction indicates the presence of Gram-negative rods such as *Escherichia coli*, the causative agent in the vast majority of UTIs in both men and women. Much less commonly, Gram-positive bacteria may also cause nitrite-positive UTI. A negative urine nitrite does not exclude UTI as it may be due to either a low-nitrate diet, diuretic use, or infection with bacteria that are incapable of reducing nitrate to nitrite. **UTI management** Finding evidence of a UTI requires the clinician to determine the nature of that UTI—urethritis, prostatitis/vaginitis, cystitis, pyelonephritis—and to evaluate the severity of the infection in the context of the patient's age and comorbidities. ○ <u>Leukocyte esterase</u>: Leukocyte esterase—as its name suggests—is an enzyme produced by white blood cells and is therefore associated with urinary tract infection. Up to five minutes is required for the enzyme to fully react with the dipstick reagent. Obviously, a positive dipstick leukocyte esterase does not itself distinguish between benign infectious cystitis and life-threatening pyelonephritis. ○ <u>Red blood cells (RBC)</u>: On a dipstick urinalysis (in contrast to a legitimate microscopic exam), "RBC" are reported not because of the presence of cells but because of the peroxidase activity of erythrocytes, which is also noted with myoglobinuria or hemoglobinuria. Thus, a dipstick analysis "positive for RBC" could indicate legitimate hematuria, or the presence of hemoglobin or myoglobin such as from marked intravascular hemolysis or rhabdomyolysis, respectively. Red blood cells in urine are not "normal" per se, but are not necessarily pathologic. Microhematuria can be induced by many benign events, including sexual **Overt hematuria and cancer** "Up to 20 percent of patients with gross hematuria have urinary tract malignancy; a full work-up with cystoscopy and upper-tract imaging is indicated in patients with this condition." Simerville JA, Maxted WC, Pahira JJ. Urinalysis: a comprehensive review. *Am Fam Physician*. 2005 Mar 15;71(6):1153-62 aafp.org/afp/2005/0315/p1153.html intercourse, exercise, and sample contamination from menstruation. Conversely, pathologic causes of hematuria include urinary tract infections, glomerulonephritis, IgA nephropathy, and nephrolithiasis; overt hematuria is often the first sign of renal or bladder carcinoma. Thus, when consistently present over 2-3 samples, overt or microscopic hematuria—just like any degree of proteinuria—always requires the clinician's attention.
Advantages:	▪ Allows point-of-care testing and thereby facilitates assessment and treatment.
Limitations:	▪ Noted above, e.g., insensitivity to microalbuminuria and mild Bence-Jones proteinuria
Comments:	▪ For additional information, please see any of several excellent clinically-oriented reviews such as Simerville JA, Maxted WC, Pahira JJ. Urinalysis: a comprehensive review. *Am Fam Physician* 2005 Mar http://www.aafp.org/afp/2005/0315/p1153.html

Presentation: Routine lab evaluation in an asymptomatic elderly female—part 1: Whereas a healthy young adult might be treated nonpharmacologically such as with fluid loading and cranberry juice for a routine UTI, clinicians should appreciate several nuances of this case that add to the complexity of appropriate management. This female patient presented for a routine annual examination. Note the patient's date of birth and the date of examination in the lower right-hand corner of the report. Because of the patient's advanced age, additional considerations are warranted. This patient was also noted to be vitamin D deficient and diabetic at the time of the exam—how does this change the overall management? Clinicians must appreciate that elderly patients are less likely to mount a symptomatic and febrile response to advanced urinary tract infections; therefore consideration to the possiblity of pyelonephritis (life-threatening) in contrast to a simple cystitis (benign) must be considered. If the patient has dementia or clinically significant forgetfulness (both of which are easily tested during the office visit), compliance with treatment is much less likely, particularly if the patient does not have access to home nursing and/or does not have a spouse, relative, friend or neighbor who can aid with the supervision of care. Urinary tract infections tend to be more aggressive in elderly patients, especially those who are diabetic, especially those with micronutrient deficiencies.

Questions:
1. What additional assessments are warranted?
2. Would fluid-loading and use of cranberry juice be appropriate treatment for this patient's UTI?
3. What follow-up is recommended?

```
URINALYSIS              01/06/10
                        11:21
U COLOR                 YELLOW
U CLARITY               CLOUDY**
U GLUCOSE               NEGATIVE
U BILE                  NEGATIVE
U KETONES               NEGATIVE
U SPEC GRAVITY          1.012
U BLOOD                 NEGATIVE
U PH                    6.0
                        (NOTE06)
U PROTEIN QUAL          20**
U UROBILINOGEN          0.2
U NITRITE               NEGATIVE
U LEUK ESTERASE         MODERATE**
U WBC                   53*H
U WBCC                  RARE**
U RBC                   5*H
U SQUAM EPITH           13
U HYALINE CAST          2
U MUCOUS                RARE
(NOTE06)
URINE SAMPLES SUBMITTED FOR TESTING MORE THAN 2 HOURS AFTER COLLECTION MAY
YIELD UNRELIABLE RESULTS WHICH INCLUDE INCREASED pH, INCREASED CRYSTAL
FORMATION AND BACTERIAL CONTENT, AND DEGRADATION OF CELLULAR ELEMENTS.

                            BDATE: 03/20/1926 SEX: F RACE:
                            13:59 01/29/10
```

Answers:
1. **Assessments**: Clinical examination must include cardiac auscultatory exam, careful pulmonary auscultation for basilar crackles, distal extremity examination for edema and peripheral vascular disease, assessment for tenderness of the flanks, abdomen, and back. Vital signs are assessed: ❶ temperature, ❷ pulse, ❸ blood pressure, ❹ respiratory rate, and ❺ pain. A chemistry panel, CBC with differential, and CRP or ESR should be performed. The urinalysis is sent for microbial culture and sensitivity. Review patient's current drug regimen. If WBC casts were noted on the microscopic exam, then suspected pyelonephritis would warrant hospitalization.
2. **Treatments**: Fluid-loading would not be appropriate in an elderly patient who might have cardiopulmonary failure, renal insufficiency, or plasma electrolyte imbalance. Cranberry juice is not universally effective and is generally used for UTIs in younger patients who have evidence of *E coli* infection as evidenced by positive urinary nitrite; because this patient's nitrite is negative, a more likely probability exists that the UTI is due to Gram-positive bacteria and thus cranberry juice is less likely to be effective. A clinician could reasonably label this a complicated UTI due to the patient's advanced age and diabetes; thus, either an extended course of Bactrim DS (po b.i.d. for 7-10 days), or Ciprofloxacin (250-500 mg po b.i.d. for 3 days), or Nitrofurantoin (50-100 mg po q6h x7 days or 100 mg ER po q12h x7 days; give w/ food) would be considered. Drug choice depends on patient's tolerance, recent exposure, renal status, drugs, and results of culture and sensitivity.
3. **Follow-up**: Review laboratory results as soon as possible; if this visit is occurring at the end of the week, the lab should be alerted to phone the clinician with results over the weekend because concomitant leukocytosis or severe acute phase response (suggesting possible pyelonephritis or urosepsis) would change the management on an urgent basis. Patient should return to the office within 24-48 hours for reassessment and repeat UA. Patient is advised to return to office or go to hospital if symptoms develop— especially fever, chills, dizziness, or persistent nausea.

Presentation: Routine laboratory evaluation in an asymptomatic elderly female—part 2: Readers should review the lab report in the left side of the page before reading the discussion on the right side of the page. *Write the appropriate interpretation and intervention before looking at the answers in the column on the right.* Normal ranges were not provided with the original report.

```
CBC                    01/06/10
                       11:21
WBC 10E3               7.50
NRBC %                 0.0
NRBC 10E3              0.00
RBC 10E6               4.08*L
HGB                    11.7*L
HCT                    35.1*L
MCV                    86.0
MCH                    28.7
MCHC                   33.3
RDW-CV                 13.7
RDW-SD                 43.1
PLATELET 10E3          175
MPV                    12.3
-----------------------------
CHEM PANEL             01/06/10
                       11:21
SODIUM                 140
POTASSIUM              4.2
CHLORIDE               102
CO2 VENOUS             27.0
GLUCOSE                248*H
BUN                    22
SER CREATININE         1.2
CALCIUM                9.5
GLOBULIN               3.2
TOTAL PROTEIN          7.3
ALBUMIN TOT            4.1
BILI TOTAL             0.5
ALKALINE PHOSPHA       63
SGOT (AST)             15
CHOLESTEROL            186
                       (NOTE01)
TRIGLYCERIDES          122
SGPT (ALT)             11
ANION GAP              11
OSMOLRTY CALC          291
BUN/CREAT              18.3
ALB/GLOB RATIO         1.30
HDL                    31
                       (NOTE02)
LDL CALC               131*H
                       (NOTE03)
(NOTE01)
BORDERLINE HIGH RISK = 200-239
HIGH RISK = 240 AND ABOVE.
(NOTE02)
12-16 HR FASTING:
(NOTE03)
NORMAL = LESS THAN 130 MG/DL
130-159 BORDERLINE/HIGH RISK
>/= 160 HIGH RISK
-----------------------------
CHEM SPECIAL           01/06/10
                       11:21
HEMOGLOBIN A1C         7.6*H
                       (NOTE04)
25-OHD TOTAL           29
-----------------------------
BDATE: 03/20/1926 SEX: F
13:59 01/29/10 FROM E585
```

This patient is anemic. The anemia is not of a severity that would be expected to cause cardiopulmonary/perfusion deficits, but the patient should be assessed, particularly if he/she has history of heart failure or lung disease such as emphysema. The MCV is not elevated, nor is it low. This could be due to combined B-12/folate and iron deficiencies; the patient should be tested and treated appropriately. Assuming that the ferritin is low, what is the next mandatory step in the management of this patient? [Answer: Treat the iron deficiency with iron supplementation but be sure to refer the patient for gastrointestinal endoscopy because of the increased probability of intestinal lesion, especially colon cancer.]

This patient is diagnosed with diabetes mellitus because the glucose is above 200. Cardioprotective measures must be implemented, ophthalmologist eye exam initiated, and foot exam performed. An integrative anti-diabetes plan[128] should be implemented.

Clinicians must appreciate the importance of the MDRD equation in this case. The answer is provided below. Perform the Cockcroft-Gault equation on paper (with use of a calculator if necessary), then perform the MDRD equation. Does this change the management of this patient's UTI? Does this change the overall management of this patient? [Answer: This patient has renal insufficiency (GFR 48-55 if African-American and 42-45 if "other race") and therefore some drugs are now contraindicated. Patient is at increased risk of hyperkalemia, especially if taking ACEi or ARB medications. The wise clinician would consider referral to an internist or nephrologist in order to ensure that the patient receives proper monitoring; for example, if the diabetes and renal insufficiency progress, the patient may require dialysis and—possibly—renal transplant, although transplant is unlikely in a patient of this advanced age.][Note 129]

Triglycerides and LDL are higher than optimal. Diet therapy and combination fatty acid supplementation (described later in this text) is indicated. Berberine might be considered as an adjunct.

HgbA1c greater than 6.5% diagnoses diabetes mellitus.

The vitamin D level is low and should be supported with oral administration of 2,000 - 10,000 IU/d and retested at 2-6 months. Serum calcium should be tested after 2-4 weeks of therapy—sooner if the patient is taking a calcium-sparing drug such as hydrochlorothiazide—and again at about 6 and 12 months.

[128] Vasquez A. *Chiropractic and Naturopathic Mastery of Common Clinical Disorders.* http://optimalhealthresearch.com/clinical_mastery.html
[129] Review of this case by Dr Barry Morgan (MD, emergency medicine) is acknowledged and appreciated.

Presentation: 45yo HLA-B27+ woman with recurrent UTIs and a 7-year history of ankylosing spondylitis treated with anti-TNF drugs: Positive urine culture and positive stool culture demonstrating bacteria (*Escherichia coli* and *Klebsiella pneumoniae*) known to share molecular mimicry and cross-reactivity with HLA-B27: The Gram-negative bacterium *E. coli* produces a protein named "hypothetical protein 168" (Protein Identification Resource [PIR] data bank access code #jp0612) which shares the amino acid sequence "**RRYLE**" with HLA-B27, which contains the sequence "EWL**RRYLE**IGKETLQRVDP."[130] Per the same citation, *Klebsiella pneumoniae*'s protein (PIR s01840) nitrogenase (reductase) molybdenum-iron protein NifN contains the sequence "EWLRR." This amino acid homology confers validation to the phenomenon of molecular mimicry and thus that immune system components such as immunoglobulins and activated T-cells can cross-react between microbial peptides and human tissue antigens.[131] This patient was treated with the combination pharmaceutical antibiotic trimethoprim and sulfamethoxazole commonly referred to as "Bactrim DS" in addition to dietary optimization, hormonal optimization, and nutritional supplementation. Antimicrobial treatment with amoxicillin-clavulanate would have been reasonable, too, except for this patient's prior allergic reaction to the drug.

```
Urine Culture, Routine
  Urine Culture, Routine          Final Report
  Result 1
      Escherichia coli
      50,000-100,000 colony forming units per mL
  Antimicrobial Susceptibility
          ***** S = Susceptible; I = Intermediate; R = Resistant *****
                  P = Positive; N = Negative
          MICS are expressed in micrograms per mL
```

Antibiotic	RSLT#1
Amoxicillin/Clavulanic Acid	S
Ampicillin	S
Cefazolin	S
Cefepime	S
Ceftriaxone	S
Cefuroxime	S
Cephalothin	I
Ciprofloxacin	R
ESBL	N
Ertapenem	S
Gentamicin	S
Imipenem	S
Levofloxacin	R
Nitrofurantoin	S
Piperacillin	S
Tetracycline	S
Tobramycin	S
Trimethoprim/Sulfa	S

Comprehensive Stool Analysis / Parasitology x3

BACTERIOLOGY CULTURE		
Expected/Beneficial flora	**Commensal (Imbalanced) flora**	**Dysbiotic flora**
4+ Bacteroides fragilis group	3+ Alpha hemolytic strep	3+ Klebsiella pneumoniae ssp pneumoniae
3+ Bifidobacterium spp.		
4+ Escherichia coli		
3+ Lactobacillus spp.		
NG Enterococcus spp.		
2+ Clostridium spp.		
NG = No Growth		

PRESCRIPTIVE AGENTS				
	Resistant	**Intermediate**	**Susceptible**	
Amoxicillin-Clavulanic Acid			S	Susceptible results imply that an infection due to the bacteria may be appropriately treated when the recommended dosage of the tested antimicrobial agent is used.
Ampicillin	R			**Intermediate** results imply that response rates may be lower than for susceptible bacteria when the tested antimicrobial agent is used.
Cefazolin			S	
Ceftazidime			S	**Resistant** results imply that the bacteria will not be inhibited by normal dosage levels of the tested antimicrobial agent.
Ciprofloxacin			S	
Trimeth-sulfa			S	

---

[130] Scofield RH, Warren WL, Koelsch G, Harley JB. A hypothesis for the HLA-B27 immune dysregulation in spondyloarthropathy: contributions from enteric organisms, B27 structure, peptides bound by B27, and convergent evolution. *Proc Natl Acad Sci U S A.* 1993 Oct 15;90(20):9330-4
[131] Rashid T, Ebringer A. Ankylosing spondylitis is linked to Klebsiella--the evidence. *Clin Rheumatol.* 2007 Jun;26(6):858-64

CRP: C-reactive protein	
Overview and interpretation:	<ul><li>CRP is a protein made by the liver in response to the immunologic activation characteristic of infectious and inflammatory conditions. Generally, any tissue injury or inflammatory process especially that involves the immune system's increased production of IL-6 will result in increased production of CRP.[132] High sensitivity CRP (hsCRP) is preferred over regular CRP due to its greater sensitivity and use in assessing cardiovascular risk.</li><li>Elevated values are seen with:<ul><li>Infections: Bacterial, fungal, parasitic, viral diseases; some patients with dysbiosis[133] will have mildly-moderately elevated CRP,</li><li>Inflammatory bowel disease: Crohn's disease and ulcerative colitis (higher in CD than UC),</li><li>Autoimmune disease: Rheumatoid arthritis, polymyalgia rheumatica, giant cell arteritis, polyarteritis nodosa, (not always SLE),</li><li>Acute myocardial infarction or other tissue ischemia</li><li>Organ transplant rejection: Renal, (not cardiac),</li><li>Trauma: Burns, surgery,</li><li>Obesity: Leads to modest elevations in CRP.</li></ul></li></ul>
Advantages:	<ul><li>This is an excellent screening test for differentiating "serious problems" (e.g., inflammatory and infectious arthropathy) from "benign problems" such as osteoarthritis.</li><li>Since higher values of CRP are a well-recognized risk factor for cardiovascular disease, screening "musculoskeletal patients" with hsCRP provides data for cardiovascular risk assessment and a more comprehensive and holistic treatment approach, thus bridging the gap between acute care and preventive care.</li></ul>
Limitations:	<ul><li>Elevations in CRP are completely nonspecific, requiring clinical investigation to determine the underlying cause of the immune activation.</li><li>CRP may be normal in some patients with severe systemic diseases (such as lupus or cancer), and therefore a normal CRP does not entirely exclude the presence of significant illness.</li></ul>
Comments:	<ul><li>Writing in *The New England Journal of Medicine*, authors Gabay and Kushner[134] note that measurements of plasma or serum **C-reactive protein can help differentiate inflammatory from non-inflammatory conditions and are useful in managing the patient's disease, since "the concentration often reflects the response to and the need for therapeutic intervention."** Additionally, they note, "Most normal subjects have plasma C-reactive protein concentrations of 2 mg per liter or less, but some have concentrations as high as 10 mg per liter." Deodhar[135] noted that **"Any clinical disease characterized by tissue injury and/or inflammation is accompanied by significant elevation of serum CRP…"** and that **CRP should replace ESR as a method of laboratory evaluation.** Deodhar also noted that **some patients with severe SLE will have normal CRP levels.**</li></ul>

---

[132] Deodhar SD. C-reactive protein: the best laboratory indicator available for monitoring disease activity. *Cleve Clin J Med* 1989 Mar-Apr;56(2):126-30

[133] See chapter 4 of *Integrative Rheumatology* and Vasquez A. Reducing Pain and Inflammation Naturally. Part 6: Nutritional and Botanical Treatments Against "Silent Infections" and Gastrointestinal Dysbiosis, Commonly Overlooked Causes of Neuromusculoskeletal Inflammation and Chronic Health Problems. *Nutr Perspect* 2006; Jan http://optimalhealthresearch.com/part6

[134] Gabay C, Kushner I. Acute-phase proteins and other systemic responses to inflammation. *N Engl J Med.* 1999 Feb 11;340(6):448-54

[135] Deodhar SD. C-reactive protein: the best laboratory indicator available for monitoring disease activity. *Cleve Clin J Med* 1989 Mar-Apr;56(2):126-30

Presentation: Elevated hsCRP (high-sensitivity c-reactive protein) in a male patient with metabolic syndrome and rheumatoid arthritis—response to treatment protocol in *Integrative Rheumatology*: This 52-year-old male patient presented with a 4-year history of rheumatoid arthritis which was unresponsive to prednisone and anti-TNF (tumor necrosis factor alpha) drugs, ie, "biologics." As expected, the prednisone exacerbated the patient's insulin resistance and hypertension; the drug failed to produce an anti-inflammatory benefit for this patient. At a cost of several thousand dollars per treatment, the anti-TNF "biologic" drugs failed to provide any benefit. At the intial visit in July 2005, the hsCRP level was 124 mg/L (normal range 0-3 mg/L), as shown in these lab results.

DATE OF SPECIMEN	TIME	DATE RECEIVED	DATE REPORTED	TIME		Houston		TX	77036-0000
7/08/2005	16:19	7/08/2005	7/11/2005	7:38	419	ACCOUNT NUMBER:	42407150		

TEST	RESULT	LIMITS	LAB
C-Reactive Protein, Cardiac			
> C-Reactive Protein, Cardiac	124.00H mg/L	0.00 - 3.00	HD
	Relative Risk for Future Cardiovascular Event		
	Low	<1.00	
	Average	1.00 - 3.00	
	High	>3.00	

The patient was treated with the protocol outlined in Chapter 4 of *Integrative Rheumatology*.[136] Stool testing showed *Citrobacter freundii* (renamed *Citrobacter rodentium*) which was addressed with botanical medicines; the insufficiency dysbiosis was also corrected per the five-part protocol. Slightly low testosterone and slightly elevated estradiol was optimized with a pharmaceutical aromatase inhibitor (Arimidex) given twice weekly. The five-part nutritional wellness protocol (supplemented Paleo-Mediterranean diet [SPMD]) was implemented.[137]

Comprehensive Parasitology, stool, x2

MICROBIOLOGY

Bacteriology Culture

Beneficial flora		Imbalances		Dysbiotic flora	
Bifidobacter	0+	Gamma strep	1+	Citrobacter freundii	1+
E. coli	2+	Enterobacter sp.	1+		
Lactobacillus	0+				

Mycology (Yeast) Culture

Normal flora	Dysbiotic flora
No yeast isolated	

PARASITOLOGY

	Sample 1		Sample 2
No	Ova or Parasites	No	Ova or Parasites

No anti-inflammatory drugs or botanicals were used. Within five weeks of treatment, the patient's hsCRP dropped from 124 mg/L to 7.58 mg/L—a reduction of approximately 95%—far superior to any previoius response to corticosteroid and biologic drugs. Patient experienced significant alleviation of pain and improved mobility.

8/17/2005	11:06	8/18/2005	8/18/2005	12:32	738	ACCOUNT NUMBER:	42407150

TEST	RESULT	LIMITS	LAB
C-Reactive Protein, Cardiac			
C-Reactive Protein, Cardiac	7.58H mg/L	0.00 - 3.00	HD

[136] Vasquez A. *Integrative Rheumatology*. http://optimalhealthresearch.com/textbooks/rheumatology.html
[137] Vasquez A. Revisiting the Five-Part Nutritional Wellness Protocol. *Nutritional Perspectives* 2011 January http://optimalhealthresearch.com/spmd

ESR: erythrocyte sedimentation rate	

Overview and interpretation:	▪ Values may be elevated even when no pathology is present because ESR increases with anemia and with age.
	
	▪ Much more sensitive than WBC count when screening for infection.[138]
	
	▪ May be normal in about 10% of patients who have pathology such as **giant cell arteritis** and **polymyalgia rheumatica** (conditions where it is generally the only lab abnormality, besides anemia); may also be normal in several other diseases.
	
	▪ **May be normal in patients with septic arthritis and patients with crystal-induced arthritis: joint aspiration for synovial fluid analysis is indicated if septic arthritis is suspected.**[139]
	
	▪ Increased with age, anemia, inflammation; higher in women than men. Age-adjusted normal ranges: any value over 25 is considered high in young people, or 40 in elderly women.
	
	▪ Age-related adjustments for men and women are as follows:
	    1. Men: age divided by 2
	    2. Women: (age + 10) divided by 2

Advantages:	▪ Inexpensive and easy to perform—use the same lavender-topped tube that you use for CBC. ▪ Provides a quick screen for infection, inflammation, and multiple myeloma—the most common primary bone tumor in adults. ▪ In patients with elevated levels, ESR can be used to monitor progression of disease and response to treatment.[140] However, a negative/normal test result does not exclude the presence of significant disease; some noteworthy examples include the following: 1) elderly—due to diminished ability to mount an inflammatory response, 2) patients taking anti-inflammatory drugs and immunosuppressants, 3) a significant proportion of patients with lupus will have normal ESR despite aggressive disease, and 4) some cancer patients with clinically significant tumor burden will not show signs of systemic inflammation. ▪ **ESR may be more reliable than CRP for multiple myeloma.**[141]
Limitations:	▪ ESR may be normal in a subset of patients with clinically significant infection or inflammation. ▪ Values are elevated in the elderly and patients with anemia and are thus not necessarily indicative of disease in these populations.
Comments:	▪ **This test is generally considered *outdated* and has been replaced in most circumstances by CRP for the evaluation of inflammation and infection.** ▪ **The only time I use this test clinically is when I am highly suspicious of inflammation and the CRP is normal. Further, this test may be preferred when assessing for temporal arteritis and for multiple myeloma, two conditions which are classically associated with elevated ESR.**

[138] Shaw BA, Gerardi JA, Hennrikus WL. How to avoid orthopedic pitfalls in children. *Patient Care* 1999; Feb 28: 95-116

[139] Klippel JH (ed). Primer on the Rheumatic Diseases. 11th Edition. Atlanta: Arthritis Foundation. 1997 page 94

[140] Shojania K. Rheumatology: 2. What laboratory tests are needed? *CMAJ*. 2000 Apr 18;162(8):1157-63 http://www.cmaj.ca/cgi/content/full/162/8/1157

[141] "We conclude that ESR, a simple and easily performed marker, was found to be an independent prognostic factor for survival in patients with multiple myeloma." Alexandrakis MG, Passam FH, Ganotakis ES, Sfiridaki K, Xilouri I, Perisinakis K, Kyriakou DS. The clinical and prognostic significance of erythrocyte sedimentation rate (ESR), serum interleukin-6 (IL-6) and acute phase protein levels in multiple myeloma. *Clin Lab Haematol*. 2003;25:41-6

Ferritin	
Overview and interpretation:	▪ Ferritin levels are directly proportional to body iron stores, except in patients with inflammation, infection, hepatitis, or cancer. Therefore, measuring ferritin allows assessment for iron deficiency (a cause of fatigue, or early manifestation of GI cancer) and allows for assessment of iron overload (as a cause of joint pain and arthropathy). This test should be performed in all African Americans[142,143], white men over age 30 years[144], diabetics[145], and patients with peripheral arthropathy[146], and exercise-associated joint pain[147,148] The research also justifies testing children[149], women[150], young adults[151] and the general asymptomatic public.[152] ▪ <u>Low ferritin = iron deficiency</u> ▪ <u>High ferritin = iron overload, cancer, inflammation, infection, and/or hepatitis (viral, alcoholic, or toxic)</u>
Advantages:	▪ Reliable screening test for iron overload when used in conjunction with patient assessment and evidence (e.g., normal CRP) of no infection or acute phase response. ▪ This is the blood test of choice for iron deficiency *and* iron overload.
Limitations:	▪ Iron-deficient patients with an acute phase response may have a falsely normal level of ferritin since ferritin is an acute phase reactant and will be elevated *disproportionate to iron status* during inflammation. ▪ Elevations of ferritin (i.e., >200 mcg/L in women and >300 mcg/L in men) need to be retested along with CRP (to rule out false elevation due to excessive inflammation) before making the presumptive diagnosis of iron overload. **In the absence of significant inflammation, ferritin values >200 mcg/L in women and >300 mcg/L in men indicate iron overload and the need for treatment regardless of the absence of symptoms or end-stage complications.**[153]
Comments:	▪ Note that since ferritin is an acute-phase reactant, a high level of serum ferritin by itself does not allow differentiation between iron overload, infection, and the inflammation associated with tissue injury or metastatic disease. Ferritin must be evaluated within the context of the patient's clinical condition and the assessment of at least one other marker for inflammation such as CRP. If the patient is not acutely ill or has not recently suffered tissue injury (e.g., myocardial infarction) and the CRP is normal, then an elevated ferritin value indicates iron overload until proven otherwise with diagnostic phlebotomy, which is safer and less expensive than liver biopsy or MRI. Transferrin saturation can also be measured when the interpretation of ferritin is unclear. By itself, serum iron is unreliable.

[142] Barton JC, Edwards CQ, Bertoli LF, Shroyer TW, Hudson SL. Iron overload in African Americans. *Am J Med*. 1995 Dec;99(6):616-23

[143] Wurapa RK, Gordeuk VR, Brittenham GM, et al. Primary iron overload in African Americans. *Am J Med*. 1996;101(1):9-18

[144] Baer DM, Simons JL, et al. Hemochromatosis screening in asymptomatic ambulatory men 30 years of age and older. *Am J Med*. 1995 May;98:464-8

[145] Phelps G, Chapman I, Hall P, Braund W, Mackinnon M. Prevalence of genetic haemochromatosis among diabetic patients. *Lancet* 1989; 2: 233-4

[146] Olynyk J, Hall P, Ahern M, KwiatekR, MackinnonM. Screening for hemochromatosis in a rheumatology clinic. *Aust NZ J Med* 1994; 24: 22-5

[147] McCurdie I, Perry JD. Haemochromatosis and exercise related joint pains. *BMJ*. 1999 Feb 13;318(7181):449-5

[148] "RESULTS: Our findings indicate a high prevalence of HFE gene mutations in this population (49.2%) compared with sedentary controls (33.5%). No association was detected in the athletes between mutations and blood iron markers. CONCLUSIONS: The findings support the need to assess regularly iron stores in elite endurance athletes." Chicharro JL, Hoyos J, Gomez-Gallego F, et al. Mutations in the hereditary haemochromatosis gene HFE in professional endurance athletes. *Br J Sports Med*. 2004 Aug;38(4):418-21. Erratum in: *Br J Sports Med*. 2004 Dec;38(6):793 http://bjsm.bmjjournals.com/cgi/content/full/38/4/418 Accessed September 12, 2005

[149] Kaikov Y, Wadsworth LD, Hassall E, Dimmick JE, Rogers PCJ. Primary hemochromatosis in children: report of three newly diagnosed cases and review of the pediatric literature. *Pediatrics* 1992; 90: 37-42

[150] Edwards CQ, Kushner JP. Screening for hemochromatosis. *N Engl J Med* 1993; 328: 1616-20

[151] Gushusrt TP, Triest WE. Diagnosis and management of precirrhotic hemochromatosis. *W Virginia Med J* 1990; 86: 91-5

[152] Balan V, et al. Screening for hemochromatosis: a cost-effectiveness study based on 12, 258 patients. *Gastroenterology* 1994; 107: 453-9

[153] **Barton JC, McDonnell SM, Adams PC, Brissot P, Powell LW, Edwards CQ, Cook JD, Kowdley KV. Management of hemochromatosis. Hemochromatosis Management Working Group. *Ann Intern Med*. 1998 Dec 1;129(11):932-9—one of the best papers ever written on this topic.**

Ferritin—*Interpretation of serum levels*

Ferritin	Categorization and management
≥ 800 mcg/L	<u>Practically diagnostic of iron overload</u>[154]: Repeat tests; rule out inflammation or occult pathology. Initiate phlebotomy and consider liver biopsy or MRI.
≥ 300 mcg/L	<u>Probable iron overload</u>[155]: Repeat tests; rule out inflammation or occult pathology. In men, initiate phlebotomy and consider liver biopsy or MRI.[156]
≥ 200 mcg/L	<u>*In women*: Suggestive of iron overload</u>[157]: Repeat tests, rule out inflammation or occult pathology. In women, initiate phlebotomy and consider liver biopsy or MRI.[158] <u>*In men*: High-normal *unhealthy* iron status with increased risk of myocardial infarction</u>[159]: Rule out inflammation or occult pathology. No follow-up is mandated, yet blood donation and/or abstention from dietary iron are recommended preventative healthcare measures.
≥ 160 mcg/L	<u>*In women*: Abnormal iron status</u>[160]: Repeat tests, rule out inflammation or occult pathology. Consider phlebotomy and liver biopsy or MRI.
≥80-120 mcg/L	<u>High-normal unhealthy iron status</u>[161,162]: No follow-up is mandated; blood donation and abstention from dietary iron are suggested preventative healthcare measures. A subset of patients with restless leg syndrome (RLS, a condition also causally associated with intestinal bacterial overgrowth dysbiosis) have impaired transport of iron into the brain and therefore require slightly elevated ferritin/iron levels (up to 120) to enhance cerebral iron uptake.
40-70 mcg/L	**<u>Optimal iron status for most people</u>**[163,164]
< 20 mcg/L	<u>Iron deficiency</u>: Search for occult gastrointestinal blood loss with endoscopy or imaging assessments in adults; refer to gastroenterologist.[165,166]

Ferritin is an acute-phase reactant, which means that its production is increased during the acute phase of inflammatory and/or infectious disorders. Therefore the numeric value and hence its clinical meaning can be interpreted only within a context that also includes assessment of the patient's inflammatory status, which is best assessed with either ESR or CRP. If CRP/ESR is high, then the physician might assume that the ferritin value is "falsely elevated"—disproportionately elevated with respect to body iron stores. *Common clinical examples requiring use and skillful interpretation of ferritin:*

- **Elderly or arthritic patient with iron deficiency despite normal serum ferritin**: An elderly patient with normal ferritin and elevated CRP/ESR is probably iron deficient; retesting of ferritin and measurement of transferrin saturation and CBC should be performed promptly. If iron deficiency is confirmed or cannot be excluded, referral for endoscopic examination must be implemented. In a patient with known inflammatory arthropathy, the ferritin may appear normal even though the patient is iron deficient and in need of supplementation and endoscopy.
- **Non-anemic iron deficiency**: A middle-aged patient (commonly a premenopausal woman) presents with fatigue and during the course of evaluation is found to have a normal CBC. **Do not let a normal CBC prevent you from assessing ferritin; many of these patients are completely iron deficient with ferritin values of 2-6 mcg/L and are in need of iron replacement as well as evaluation for celiac disease,** *H. pylori* **infection, hematuria, and—as is often warranted—gastrointestinal bleeding/lesions.**

[154] Milman N, Albeck MJ. Distinction between homozygous and heterozygous subjects with hemochromatosis using iron status markers and receiver operating characteristic (ROC) analysis. *Eur J Clin Biochem* 1995; 33: 95-8. See also Milman N. Iron status markers in hereditary hemochromatosis: distinction between individuals being homozygous and heterozygous for the hemochromatosis allele. *Eur J Haematol* 1991;47:292-8

[155] Olynyk JK, Bacon BR. Hereditary hemochromatosis: detecting and correcting iron overload. *Postgrad Med* 1994;96: 151-65

[156] "Therapeutic phlebotomy is used to remove excess iron and maintain low normal body iron stores, ... initiated in men with serum ferritin levels of 300 microg/L or more and in women with serum ferritin levels of 200 microg/L or more, regardless of the presence or absence of symptoms." Barton JC, McDonnell SM, Adams PC, Brissot P, Powell LW, Edwards CQ, Cook JD, Kowdley KV. Management of hemochromatosis. Hemochromatosis Management Working Group. *Ann Intern Med.* 1998 Dec 1;129(11):932-9

[157] Barton JC, Edwards CQ, Bertoli LF, Shroyer TW, Hudson SL. Iron overload in African Americans. *Am J Med* 1995; 99: 616-23

[158] Barton JC, McDonnell SM, Adams PC, et al. Management of hemochromatosis. *Ann Intern Med.* 1998 Dec 1;129(11):932-9

[159] Salonen JT, Nyyssonen K, Korpela H,et al. High stored iron levels are associated with excess risk of myocardial infarction in eastern Finnish men. *Circulation* 1992; 86: 803-11

[160] Nicoll D. Therapeutic drug monitoring and laboratory reference ranges. In: Tierney LM, McPhee SJ, Papadakis MA. *Current Medical Diagnosis and Treatment 1996 (35th Edition).* Stamford: Appleton and Lange, 1996: 1442

[161] Lauffer, RB. *Iron and Your Heart.* New York: St. Martin's Press, 1991: 79-8, 83-88, 162

[162] Sullivan JL. Iron and the sex difference in heart disease risk. *Lancet.* 1981 Jun 13;1(8233):1293-4

[163] Lauffer, RB. *Iron and Your Heart.* New York: St. Martin's Press, 1991: 79-8, 83-88, 162

[164] **Vasquez A.** High body iron stores: causes, effects, diagnosis, and treatment. *Nutritional Perspectives* 1994; 17: 13, 15-7, 19, 21, 28 and **Vasquez A.** Men's Health: Iron in men: why men store this nutrient in their bodies and the harm that it does. *MEN Magazine* 1997; Jan:11,21-23 vix.com/menmag/alexiron.htm

[165] Rockey DC, Cello JP. Evaluation of the gastrointestinal tract in patients with iron-deficiency anemia. *N Engl J Med.* 1993;329(23):1691-5

[166] "Endoscopy revealed a clinically important lesion in 23 (12%) of 186 patients. ... CONCLUSIONS: Endoscopy yields important findings in premenopausal women with iron deficiency anemia, which should not be attributed solely to menstrual blood loss." Bini EJ, Micale PL, Weinshel EH. Evaluation of the gastrointestinal tract in premenopausal women with iron deficiency anemia. *Am J Med.* 1998 Oct;105(4):281-6

Arthritis & Rheumatism

Official Journal of the American College of Rheumatology

VOLUME 39   OCTOBER 1996   NO. 10

1767   1768

Musculoskeletal disorders and iron overload disease: comment on the American College of Rheumatology guidelines for the initial evaluation of the adult patient with acute musculoskeletal symptoms

To the Editor:

The recent clinical guidelines for the initial evaluation of the adult patient with acute musculoskeletal symptoms, proposed by the American College of Rheumatology (1), provide useful information and a good review for clinicians. However, there is one important omission in these guidelines. Nowhere in the guidelines is hemochromatosis mentioned. Such a prevalent and potentially life-threatening disease certainly deserves to be considered in the evaluation of patients with musculoskeletal disorders.

Hereditary hemochromatosis is now thought to be the most common genetic disorder in the white population (2). Approximately 1 in 250 persons is homozygous for this disorder and will develop the characteristic clinical manifestations such as diabetes, cardiomyopathy, liver disease, endocrine dysfunction, and, most notable for this discussion, arthropathy or other musculoskeletal disorders (2). Although hereditary iron overload disorders have traditionally been thought of as occurring exclusively in whites, recent research by Barton et al (3) indicates that approximately 1 in 67 African-Americans is affected by an etiologically distinct and severe form of iron overload. Hereditary iron overload disorders have been detected in persons of every ethnic background.

Arthropathy affects up to 80% of iron-overloaded patients and is often the only manifestation of this disease (4). Joint pain is a common and early symptom of iron overload, and "bone pain" has also been described as a common initial complaint (5). Clinically and radiographically, hemochromatoic arthropathy can resemble osteoarthritis, calcium pyrophosphate dihydrate deposition disease, pseudogout, rheumatoid arthritis, ankylosing spondylitis, or generalized osteopenia with osteoporotic fractures (4,6,7). Since iron overload can cause such a wide array of musculoskeletal manifestations and because definitive clinical differentiation of iron overload from other arthropathies is very difficult, patients with peripheral arthropathy should be screened for iron overload. Indeed, recent research by Olynyk et al (8) indicates that the prevalence of iron overload is 5 times higher in patients with peripheral arthropathy than in the general population. Therefore, screening of patients with peripheral arthropathy for the possible presence of iron overload is justified.

Thus, since iron overload affects such a large portion of the population and arthropathy is a common manifestation of this disorder, patients with musculoskeletal symptoms should be screened for iron overload (4,8). The current literature suggests that everyone should be screened for iron overload even if there are no symptoms (8–10).

Alex Vasquez, DC
Seattle, WA

1. American College of Rheumatology Ad Hoc Committee on Clinical Guidelines: Guidelines for the initial evaluation of the adult patient with acute musculoskeletal symptoms. Arthritis Rheum 39:1–8, 1996
2. Olynyk JK, Bacon BR: Hereditary hemochromatosis: detecting and correcting iron overload. Postgrad Med 96:151–165, 1994
3. Barton JC, Edwards CQ, Bertoli LF, Shroyer TW, Hudson SL: Iron overload in African Americans. Am J Med 99:616–623, 1995
4. Faraawi R, Harth M, Kertesz A, Bell D: Arthritis in hemochromatosis. J Rheumatol 20:448–452, 1993
5. Adams PC, Kertesz AE, Valberg LS: Clinical presentation of hemochromatosis: a changing scene. Am J Med 90:445–449, 1991
6. Bywaters EGL, Hamilton EBD, Williams R: The spine in idiopathic hemochromatosis. Ann Rheum Dis 30:453–465, 1971
7. Eyres KS, McCloskey EV, Fern ED, Rogers S, Beneton M, Aaron JE, Kanis JA: Osteoporotic fractures: an unusual presentation of hemochromatosis. Bone 13:431–433, 1992
8. Olynyk J, Hall P, Ahern M, Kwiatek R, Mackinnon M: Screening for hemochromatosis in a rheumatology clinic. Aust N Z J Med 24:22–25, 1994
9. Baer DM, Simmons JL, Staples RL, Runmore GJ, Morton CJ: Hemochromatosis screening in asymptomatic ambulatory men 30 years of age and older. Am J Med 98:464–468, 1995
10. Adams PC, Gregor JC, Kertesz AE, Valberg LS: Screening blood donors for hereditary hemochromatosis: decision analysis model based on a 30-year database. Gastroenterology 109:177–188, 1995

Vasquez A. Musculoskeletal disorders and iron overload disease: comment on the American College of Rheumatology guidelines for the initial evaluation of the adult patient with acute musculoskeletal symptoms. *Arthritis Rheum.* 1996 Oct;39(10):1767-8 http://www.ncbi.nlm.nih.gov/pubmed/8843875

Algorithm flowchart

Screen asymptomatic patients.

Follow-up abnormal laboratory results. (high serum iron, elevated liver enzymes, high blood glucose, etc.)

Screen high-risk and symptomatic patients.

↓

Assess iron status with transferrin saturation and serum ferritin.
Use fasting morning specimen.

IRON-DEFICIENCY
serum ferritin:<10-15 in women, <20 in men, transferrin saturation:<16%

"HEALTHY IRON STATUS"
transferrin saturation:25-30%
serum ferritin: 30-70

"MODERATE IRON OVERLOAD"
transferrin saturation: >33-45%
serum ferritin: 80-160

POSSIBLE SEVERE IRON OVERLOAD
transferrin saturation: >40% and/or
serum ferritin: >160 in women; >200 in men

In adults with no obvious cause of blood loss: Assume pathologic gastrointestinal bleeding until proven otherwise. Simply testing for occult blood in the stool is insufficient. **Refer for complete (endoscopic) evaluation.**

Periodically assess iron status as part of routine health assessment. Consider assessment for impending iron deficiency. Consider periodic blood donation and low-iron diet to maintain healthy iron status.

No treatment is mandatory. Periodically assess iron status as part of routine health assessment. Consider low-iron diet and regular blood donation to reduce risk of cancer and myocardial infarction.

Repeat tests with fasting morning specimen. Consider other causes of elevated transferrin saturation or elevated serum ferritin.*

Second assessment suggests "healthy iron status" or "moderate iron overload": Average results and/or reassess within 1 month, or periodically assess iron status as part of routine health assessment.

PROBABLE SEVERE IRON OVERLOAD
Ferritin >200 in women, or Ferritin >300 in men.
Confirm with diagnostic phlebotomy, or liver biopsy, or MRI.

Refer as needed (usually gastroenterologist, hematologist, or internist) for phlebotomy therapy and/or deferoxamine chelation.

***Factors that alter iron assessment tests**:
False elevations of transferrin saturation: cancer, liver disease, inflammation, infection, excess alcohol consumption, non-fasting specimens.
False elevations of ferritin: inflammation, infection, cancer, excess alcohol consumption, liver disease, early pregnancy, hyperthyroidism, tissue necrosis, hyperferremia-cataract syndrome and other rare genetic/congenital syndromes.

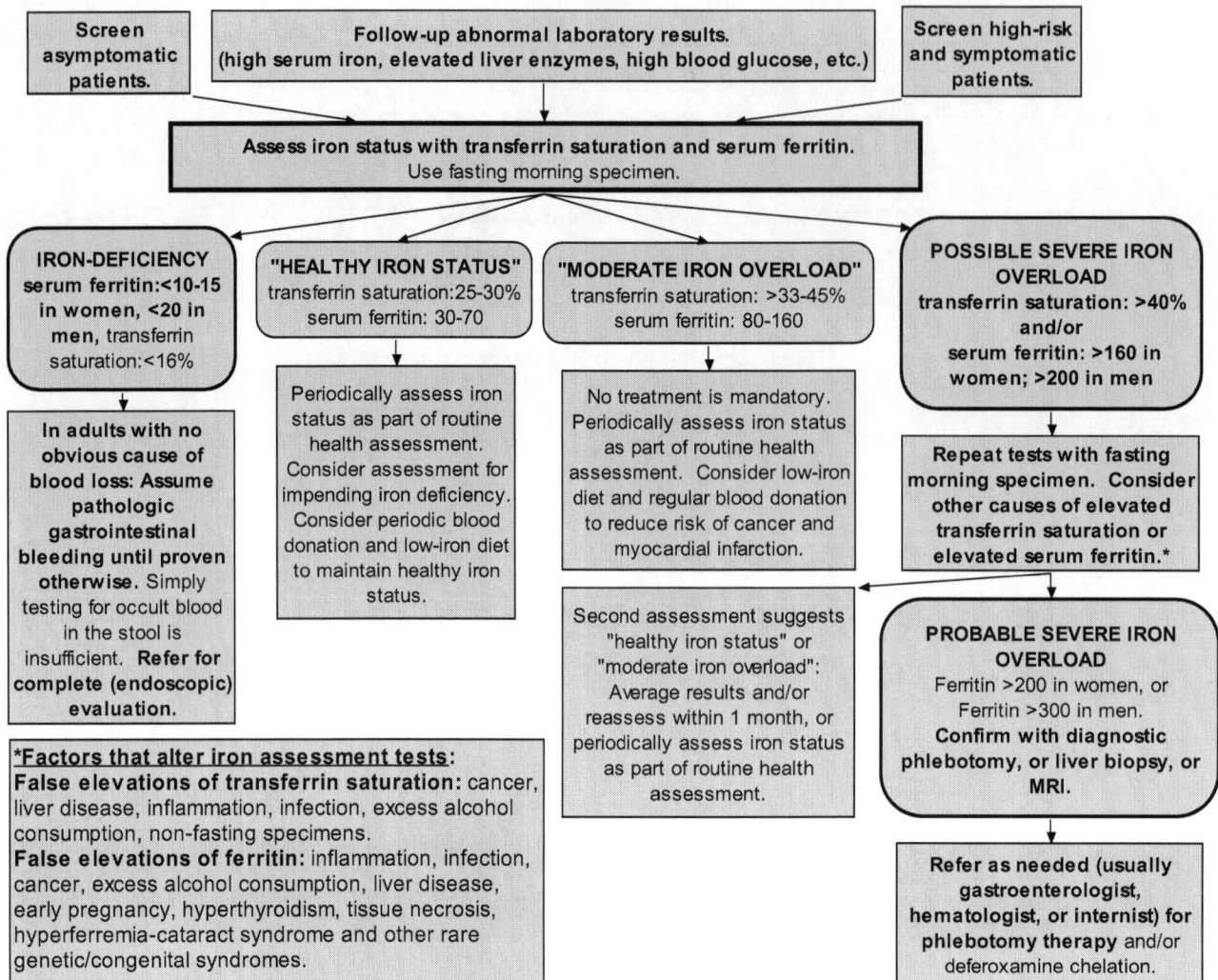

Algorithm for the comprehensive management of iron status: The above flow-chart delineates the management of high-moderate-healthy-low iron status.

Basic treatments for severe iron overload:

- **Iron-removal therapy is mandatory:** Phlebotomy therapy is generally performed weekly or twice-weekly; deferoxamine chelation is reserved for patients who do not withstand phlebotomy (due to cardiomyopathy, severe anemia, or hypoproteinemia) or may be used concurrently with phlebotomy in some patients. Periodically assess hematologic and iron indexes. Continue with weekly iron removal therapy until patient reaches mild iron-deficiency anemia, then decrease frequency and continue phlebotomy as needed (e.g., 4 times per year).
- **Laboratory tests and physical examination:** Assess general physical condition and hepatic, cardiac, endocrine, and general health status.
- **Confirm diagnosis:** Liver biopsy ("gold standard") or diagnostic phlebotomy; perhaps MRI.
- **Assess liver status:** Liver biopsy ("gold standard") or perhaps MRI. Cirrhosis indicates increased risk of hepatocellular carcinoma and reduced life expectancy. Consider liver ultrasound, serum liver enzyme measurement, and serum alpha-fetoprotein to screen for hepatocellular carcinoma every 6 months. Hepatoma surveillance is mandatory in cirrhotic patients.
- **Implement dietary modifications and nutritional therapies:** Avoid iron supplements, multivitamin supplements with iron, iron-fortified foods, liver, beef, pork, alcohol, and excess vitamin C. Ensure adequate protein intake to replace protein lost during phlebotomy. Diet modifications are not substitutes for iron removal therapy. Consider antioxidant therapy.
- **Screen all blood relatives of patients with primary iron overload**. *Mandatory!*
- **Monitor patient condition, and compliance** with lifelong phlebotomy therapy
- **Assess and address psychoemotional issues/concerns**

25(OH)D: serum 25(OH) vitamin D	
Overview and interpretation:	▪ **Vitamin D deficiency is a common cause of musculoskeletal pain**[167,168,169], and vitamin D deficiency is a significant risk factor for cancer and other serious health problems.[170,171,172] ▪ Measurement of serum 25(OH) vitamin D (or empiric treatment with 2,000 – 10,000 IU vitamin D3 per day for adults) is indicated in patients with chronic musculoskeletal pain, particularly low-back pain.[173] Optimal vitamin D status correlates with serum 25(OH)D levels of 50 – 100 ng/mL (125 - 250 nmol/L)—see our review article for more details[174]; levels greater than 100 ng/mL are unnecessary and increase the risk of hypercalcemia. **Excess vitamin D** > 100 ng/mL (250 nmol/L) with hypercalcemia **Optimal range** 50 - 100 ng/mL (125 - 250 nmol/L) **Insufficiency range** < 20- 40 ng/mL (50 - 100 nmol/L) **Deficiency** < 20 ng/mL (50 nmol/L) **Interpretation of serum 25(OH) vitamin D levels**. Modified from Vasquez et al, *Alternative Therapies in Health and Medicine* 2004 and Vasquez A. *Musculoskeletal Pain: Expanded Clinical Strategies* (Institute for Functional Medicine) 2008.
Advantages:	▪ Accurate assessment of vitamin D status.
Limitations:	▪ Patients with certain granulomatous conditions such as sarcoidosis or Crohn's disease and patients taking certain drugs such as thiazide diuretics (hydrochlorothiazide) can develop hypercalcemia due to "vitamin D hypersensitivity" or drug side effects—these patients require frequent monitoring of serum calcium while taking vitamin D supplements.
Comments:	▪ **Routine measurement and/or empiric treatment with vitamin D3 needs to become a routine component of patient care.**[175] ▪ Periodic assessment of 25(OH)D and serum calcium are required to ensure effectiveness and safety of treatment, respectively.

[167] Masood H, Narang AP, Bhat IA, Shah GN. Persistent limb pain and raised serum alkaline phosphatase the earliest markers of subclinical hypovitaminosis D in Kashmir. *Indian J Physiol Pharmacol*. 1989 Oct-Dec;33(4):259-61

[168] Al Faraj S, Al Mutairi K. Vitamin D deficiency and chronic low back pain in Saudi Arabia. *Spine*. 2003 Jan 15;28(2):177-9

[169] Plotnikoff GA, Quigley JM. Prevalence of severe hypovitaminosis D in patients with persistent, nonspecific musculoskeletal pain. *Mayo Clin Proc*. 2003 Dec;78(12):1463-70

[170] Grant WB. An estimate of premature cancer mortality in the U.S. due to inadequate doses of solar ultraviolet-B radiation. *Cancer* 2002;94(6):1867-75

[171] Zittermannn A. Vitamin D in preventive medicine: are we ignoring the evidence? *Br J Nutr*. 2003 May;89(5):552-72

[172] Holick MF. Vitamin D: importance in the prevention of cancers, type 1 diabetes, heart disease, and osteoporosis. *Am J Clin Nutr*. 2004;79(3):362-71

[173] Al Faraj S, Al Mutairi K. Vitamin D deficiency and chronic low back pain in Saudi Arabia. *Spine*. 2003 Jan 15;28(2):177-9

[174] **Vasquez A, Manso G, Cannell J. The Clinical Importance of Vitamin D (Cholecalciferol): A Paradigm Shift with Implications for All Healthcare Providers.** *Alternative Therapies in Health and Medicine* **2004; 10: 28-37** http://optimalhealthresearch.com/cholecalciferol.html

[175] Heaney RP. Vitamin D, nutritional deficiency, and the medical paradigm. *J Clin Endocrinol Metab*. 2003;88:5107-8 http://jcem.endojournals.org/cgi/content/full/88/11/5107

THE LANCET.com

May 6, 2005

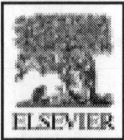

Subphysiologic Doses of Vitamin D are Subtherapeutic: Comment on the Study by The Record Trial Group

Dear Editor,

Based on recently published research, it is clear that the study by The Record Trial Group [1] on vitamin D and calcium in the prevention of fractures suffered from at least four important shortcomings which negatively skewed their results.

First, and most important, the dose of vitamin D used in their study (800 IU/d) is subphysiologic and would therefore not be expected to produce a clinically meaningful effect. The physiologic requirement for vitamin D was determined scientifically in a recent study by Heaney and colleagues [2], who showed that healthy men utilize 3,000 to 5,000 IU of cholecalciferol per day, and several recent clinical trials have been published documenting the safety and effectiveness of administering vitamin D in physiologic doses of at least 4,000 IU per day.[3-5] In fact, studies have shown a dose-response relationship with vitamin D supplementation [6], and low doses (e.g., 600 IU) are clearly less effective than higher doses in the physiologic range (e.g., 4,000 IU).[5] It is important to note that the commonly used dose of vitamin D at 800 IU per day was not determined scientifically; rather this amount was determined arbitrarily before sufficient scientific methodology was available.[2,7] Given that the commonly recommended daily intake of vitamin D in the range of 200-800 IU is not sufficient for maintaining adequate serum levels of vitamin D [8], it is therefore incumbent upon modern researchers and clinicians to use doses of vitamin D that are consistent with the physiologic requirement as established in current research.

Second, the authors recognize that patient compliance in their study population was quite poor. This poor compliance obviously contributed to the purported lack of treatment efficacy.

Third, and consistent with recent data published elsewhere [8], virtually all of their patients were still vitamin D deficient at the end of one year of treatment, thereby affirming the inadequacy of the treatment dose. Vitamin D deficiency is common in industrialized nations, particularly those of northern latitudes [9-11], including the UK, where this study was performed. By modern criteria for serum vitamin D levels [12], virtually all of the patients in this study were vitamin D deficient at the beginning of the study, and the insufficient treatment dose of 800 IU/d failed to correct this deficiency even after 1 year of treatment. Given that vitamin D levels must be raised to approximately 40 ng/mL (100 nmol/L) in order to maximally reduce parathyroid hormone levels and bone resorption [13,14], supplementation that does not accomplish the goal of raising serum vitamin D levels into the optimal physiologic range cannot be considered adequate therapy.[12]

Fourth, and finally, there is reason to question the bioavailability of their vitamin D3 supplement, as the authors note that their dose-response was generally lower than that seen in other studies. Bioavailability is a prerequisite for treatment efficacy, and the elderly have higher likeliness of comorbid conditions that impair digestion and absorption of nutrients. Specifically, it is well documented that vitamin D absorption is decreased in elderly patients compared to younger controls [15,16], and this is complicated by an age-related reduction in renal calcitriol production [17,18] and intestinal vitamin D receptors [19], thereby further impairing vitamin D metabolism and calcium absorption. Since emulsification of fat soluble vitamins is required for their absorption [20], and since pre-emulsification of nutrients has been shown to increase absorption and dose-responsiveness of the fat-soluble nutrient coenzyme Q [21, 22], it seems apparent that attention to the form (not merely the dose) of nutrient supplementation is clinically important, particularly when working with elderly patients.

These shortcomings, when combined, could have lead to an additive or synergistic reduction in treatment potency that skewed their results toward a conclusion of inefficacy. In order to produce more meaningful results in clinical trials, our group published guidelines [12] recommending that future studies 1) ensure patient compliance, 2) use physiologic doses of vitamin D (e.g., 4,000 IU per day), and 3) ensure that serum levels are raised to a minimum of 40 ng/mL (100 nmol/L), since levels below this threshold are associated with increased parathyroid hormone levels, increased bone resorption, and recalcitrance to bone-building interventions.[23,24]

Alex Vasquez
Biotics Research Corporation
Rosenberg, Texas, USA 77471

Competing Interests: Dr. Vasquez is a researcher at Biotics Research Corporation, an FDA-licensed drug manufacturing facility in the USA.

References:
1. Record Trial Group. Oral vitamin D3 and calcium for secondary prevention of low-trauma fractures in elderly people (Randomised Evaluation of Calcium Or vitamin D, RECORD): a randomised placebo-controlled trial. *Lancet* (Early Online Publication), 28 April 2005
2. Heaney RP, Davies KM, Chen TC, Holick MF, Barger-Lux MJ. Human serum 25-hydroxycholecalciferol response to extended oral dosing with cholecalciferol. *Am J Clin Nutr* 2003;77:204-10
3. Vieth R, Chan PC, MacFarlane GD. Efficacy and safety of vitamin D3 intake exceeding the lowest observed adverse effect level. *Am J Clin Nutr.* 2001;73:288-94
4. Al Faraj S, Al Mutairi K. Vitamin D deficiency and chronic low back pain in Saudi Arabia. *Spine.* 2003;28:177-9
5. Vieth R, Kimball S, Hu A, Walfish PG. Randomized comparison of the effects of the vitamin D3 adequate intake versus 100 mcg (4000 IU) per day on biochemical responses and the wellbeing of patients. *Nutr J.* 2004 Jul 19;3(1):8 http://www.nutritionj.com/content/pdf/1475-2891-3-8.pdf
6. Van den Berghe G, Van Roosbroeck D, Vanhove P, Wouters PJ, De Pourcq L, Bouillon R. Bone turnover in prolonged critical illness: effect of vitamin D. *J Clin Endocrinol Metab.* 2003;88:4623-32
7. Vieth R. Vitamin D supplementation, 25-hydroxyvitamin D concentrations, and safety. *Am J Clin Nutr.* 1999;69:842-56 http://www.ajcn.org/cgi/reprint/69/5/842.pdf
8. Glerup H, Mikkelsen K, Poulsen L, Hass E, Overbeck S, Thomsen J, Charles P, Eriksen EF. Commonly recommended daily intake of vitamin D is not sufficient if sunlight exposure is limited. *J Intern Med.* 2000;247:260-8
9. Thomas MK, Lloyd-Jones DM, Thadhani RI, Shaw AC, Deraska DJ, Kitch BT, Vamvakas EC, Dick IM, Prince RL, Finkelstein JS. Hypovitaminosis D in medical inpatients. *N Engl J Med* 1998;338:777-83
10. Dubbelman R, Jonxis JH, Muskiet FA, Saleh AE. Age-dependent vitamin D status and vertebral condition of white women living in Curacao (The Netherlands Antilles) as compared with their counterparts in The Netherlands. *Am J Clin Nutr* 1993;58:106-9
11. Kauppinen-Makelin R, Tahtela R, Loyttyniemi E, Karkkainen J, Valimaki MJ. A high prevalence of hypovitaminosis D in Finnish medical in- and outpatients. *J Intern Med.* 2001;249:559-63
12. Vasquez A, Manso G, Cannell J. The clinical importance of vitamin D (cholecalciferol): a paradigm shift with implications for all healthcare providers. *Altern Ther Health Med.* 2004;10:28-36; quiz 37, 94
13. Kinyamu HK, Gallagher JC, Rafferty KA, Balhorn KE. Dietary calcium and vitamin D intake in elderly women: effect on serum parathyroid hormone and vitamin D metabolites. *Am J Clin Nutr* 1998;67:342-8
14. Dawson-Hughes B, Harris SS, Dallal GE. Plasma calcidiol, season, and serum parathyroid hormone concentrations in healthy elderly men and women. *Am J Clin Nutr* 1997;65:67-71
15. Harris SS, Dawson-Hughes B, Perrone GA. Plasma 25-hydroxyvitamin D responses of younger and older men to three weeks of supplementation with 1800 IU/day of vitamin D. *J Am Coll Nutr.* 1999;18:470-4
16. Barragry JM, France MW, Corless D, Gupta SP, Switala S, Boucher BJ, Cohen RD. Intestinal cholecalciferol absorption in the elderly and in younger adults. *Clin Sci Mol Med.* 1978;55:213-20
17. Tsai KS, Heath H 3rd, Kumar R, Riggs BL. Impaired vitamin D metabolism with aging in women. Possible role in pathogenesis of senile osteoporosis. *J Clin Invest.* 1984;73:1668-72
18. Gallagher JC, Riggs BL, Eisman J, Hamstra A, Arnaud SB, DeLuca HF. Intestinal calcium absorption and serum vitamin D metabolites in normal subjects and osteoporotic patients: effect of age and dietary calcium. *J Clin Invest.* 1979;64:729-36
19. Ebeling PR, Sandgren ME, DiMagno EP, Lane AW, DeLuca HF, Riggs BL. Evidence of an age-related decrease in intestinal responsiveness to vitamin D: relationship between serum 1,25-dihydroxyvitamin D3 and intestinal vitamin D receptor concentrations in normal women. *J Clin Endocrinol Metab.* 1992;75:176-82
20. Gallo-Torres HE. Obligatory role of bile for the intestinal absorption of vitamin E. *Lipids.* 1970;5:379-84
21. Bucci LR, Pillors M, Medlin R, Henderson R, Stiles JC, Robol HJ, Sparks WS. Enhanced uptake in humans of coenzyme Q10 from an emulsified form. *Third International Congress of Biomedical Gerontology*; Acapulco, Mexico: June 1989
22. Bucci LR, Pillors M, Medlin R, Klenda B, Robol H, Stiles JC, Sparks WS. Enhanced blood levels of coenzyme Q-10 from an emulsified oral form. In Faruqui SR and Ansari MS (editors). *Second Symposium on Nutrition and Chiropractic Proceedings.* April 15-16, 1989 in Davenport, Iowa
23. Stepan JJ, Burckhardt P, Hana V. The effects of three-month intravenous ibandronate on bone mineral density and bone remodeling in Klinefelter's syndrome: the influence of vitamin D deficiency and hormonal status. *Bone* 2003;33:589-596
24. Vasquez A. Health care for our bones: a practical nutritional approach to preventing osteoporosis. [letter] *J Manipulative* Physiol Ther. 2005;28:213

Citation: Vasquez A. Subphysiologic Doses of Vitamin D are Subtherapeutic: Comment on the Study by The Record Trial Group. *Lancet* 2005 published online May 6

Internet: Originally posted at http://www.thelancet.com/journals/lancet/article/PIIS0140673605630139/comments and now available at http://optimalhealthresearch.com/cholecalciferol.html

Calcium and vitamin D in preventing fractures

Data are not sufficient to show inefficacy

EDITOR—The study by Porthouse et al had two major design flaws.[1] Firstly, the dose of vitamin D (800 IU per day) is subphysiological and therefore subtherapeutic. Secondly, their use of "self report" as a measure of compliance is unreliable.

The dose of vitamin D at 800 IU daily was not determined scientifically but determined arbitrarily before sufficient scientific methodology was available.[2-4] Heaney et al determined the physiological requirement of vitamin D by showing that healthy men use 4000 IU cholecalciferol daily,[2] an amount that is safely attainable with supplementation[3] and often exceeded with exposure of the total body to equatorial sun.[4]

We provided six guidelines for interventional studies with vitamin D.[5] Dosages of vitamin D must reflect physiological requirements and natural endogenous production and should therefore be in the range of 3000-10 000 IU daily. Vitamin D supplementation must be continued for at least five to nine months. The form of vitamin D should be D_3 rather than D_2. Supplements should be assayed for potency. Effectiveness of supplementation must include measurement of serum 25-hydroxyvitamin D. Serum 25(OH)D concentrations must enter the optimal range, which is 40-65 ng/ml (100-160 nmol/l).

Since the study by Porthouse et al met only the second and third of these six criteria, their data cannot be viewed as reliable for documenting the inefficacy of vitamin D supplementation.

Alex Vasquez, *researcher*

Biotics Research Corporation, 6801 Biotics Research Drive, Rosenberg, TX 77471, USA avasquez@bioticsresearch.com

John Cannell, *president*

Vitamin D Council, 9100 San Gregorio Road, Atascadero, CA 93422, USA

Competing interests: AV is a researcher at Biotics Research Corporation, a drug manufacturing facility in the United States that has approval from the Food and Drug Administration.

References

1. Porthouse J, Cockayne S, King C, Saxon L, Steele E, Aspray T, et al. Randomised controlled trial of calcium and supplementation with cholecalciferol (vitamin D3) for prevention of fractures in primary care. *BMJ* 2005;330: 1003. (30 April.)[Abstract/Free Full Text]
2. Heaney RP, Davies KM, Chen TC, Holick MF, Barger-Lux MJ. Human serum 25-hydroxycholecalciferol response to extended oral dosing with cholecalciferol. *Am J Clin Nutr* 2003;77: 204-10.[Abstract/Free Full Text]
3. Vieth R, Chan PC, MacFarlane GD. Efficacy and safety of vitamin D3 intake exceeding the lowest observed adverse effect level. *Am J Clin Nutr* 2001;73: 288-94.[Abstract/Free Full Text]
4. Vieth R. Vitamin D supplementation, 25-hydroxyvitamin D concentrations, and safety. *Am J Clin Nutr* 1999;69: 842-56.[Abstract/Free Full Text]
5. Vasquez A, Manso G, Cannell J. The clinical importance of vitamin D (cholecalciferol): a paradigm shift with implications for all healthcare providers. *Altern Ther Health Med* 2004;10: 28-36.[ISI][Medline]

Related Article

Randomised controlled trial of calcium and supplementation with cholecalciferol (vitamin D₃) for prevention of fractures in primary care
Jill Porthouse, Sarah Cockayne, Christine King, Lucy Saxon, Elizabeth Steele, Terry Aspray, Mike Baverstock, Yvonne Birks, Jo Dumville, Roger Francis, Cynthia Iglesias, Suezann Puffer, Anne Sutcliffe, Ian Watt, and David J Torgerson
BMJ 2005 330: 1003. [Abstract] [Full Text]

Vasquez A, Cannell J. Calcium and vitamin D in preventing fractures: data are not sufficient to show inefficacy. *BMJ*. 2005 Jul 9;331(7508):108-9 http://www.ncbi.nlm.nih.gov/pubmed/16002891

Thyroid status—laboratory assessments	
Overview and interpretation:	▪ **Context**: Thyroid disorders are common in clinical practice and thus all clinicians need to have a clear understanding of the clinical presentations and laboratory assessments. Although various aspects of thyroid dysfunction, laboratory tests and clinical presentations will be reviewed here, the primary emphasis will be upon hypothyroidism, which is the most common and *unnecessarily* enigmatic of the thyroid disorders. ▪ **Controversy**: In the allopathic medical paradigm, much confusion exists regarding a common but "mysterious" and "enigmatic" condition known as hypothyroidism—low thyroid function. Its converse—**hyper**thyroidism and Graves disease—is well understood, easily diagnosed, and readily treated. Because the medical treatment for **hyper**thyroidism often leaves patients in a **hypo**thyroid state, affected patients thus transition from *clarity* (hyperthyroidism) wherein they feel ill due to the disease process into *"mystery"* (hypothyroidism) wherein they feel ill due to incomplete/inaccurate treatment. The basis for the confusion within the allopathic medical community about hypothyroidism is primarily two-fold: ❶ first, they rely on the wrong test (TSH) as the main basis for laboratory assessment, ❷ second, they use incomplete treatment (T4 without T3) which defies the known physiology of the thyroid gland, which makes at least two hormones rather than one. One might get the impression that perpetual confusion is at times the goal of the medical profession; we certainly see this with the management of hypertension, depression, diabetes mellitus, psoriasis and other inflammatory/autoimmune conditions. For people who seek clarity, it is available. ▪ **Basic physiology**: The hypothalamus produces thyrotropin-releasing hormone (TRH) which stimulates the anterior pituitary gland to make thyroid-stimulating hormone (TSH), which stimulates the thyroid gland to produce thyroxine (T4, approximately 85% of thyroid gland hormone production) and triiodothyronine (T3, approximately 15% of thyroid gland hormone production). In the periphery, the prohormone T4 is converted to active T3 by deiodinase enzymes. Stress, glucagon, and environmental toxins (halogenated phenolics, plastic monomers, flame retardants[176]) impair production of T3 and/or increase production of reverse T3, which is either inert or inhibitory to the action of T3. If the thyroid gland begins to fail, then TSH levels increase as the body attempts to stimulate production of thyroid hormones from a failing gland, which typically fails due to autoimmune attack (Hashimoto's thyroiditis); hence the association of elevated blood TSH levels with "primary hypothyroidism." Thyroid hormones have many different functions in the body, and one of the chief effects is contributing to maintenance of the basal metabolic rate, or the speed of reactions within and the temperature of the body. An insufficiency of thyroid hormone adversely effects numerous biochemical reactions and body/organ functions; hence the myriad of clinical presentations reflecting variations in biochemical and physiologic individuality. Conversely yet similarly, excess thyroid hormone (whether endogenously produced or exogenously administered) also affects numerous body systems. ▪ **Clinical presentation of *hyper*thyroidism**: The clinical pattern of thyroid excess is more narrowly-focused and thus more predictable and consistent than is the presentation of low thyroid function. The clinical manifestations of hyperthyroidism generally fall into three categories: hyper-adrenergic, hypermetabolic, and ophthalmologic/ocular. ❶ hyper-adrenergic: tachycardia, tremor, diaphoresis, insomnia and a feeling of nervousness and psychomotor agitation due to upregulation of adrenergic tone and generally some degree of relative or absolute hyperthermia; increased dopaminergic and noradrenergic tone in the brain accounts for the neuropsychiatric manifestations, such as mania, psychosis, and

[176] "All studied contaminants inhibited DI activity in a dose-response manner... This study suggests that some halogenated phenolics, including current use compounds such as plastic monomers, flame retardants and their metabolites, may disrupt thyroid hormone homeostasis through the inhibition of DI activity in vivo." Butt CM, Wang D, Stapleton HM. Halogenated Phenolic Contaminants Inhibit the In Vitro Activity of the Thyroid Regulating Deiodinases in Human Liver. *Toxicol Sci.* 2011 May 11. [Epub ahead of print]

hypersexuality, ❷ hyper-metabolic: fecal frequency often described as "diarrhea" due to expedited intestinal transit, elevated temperature, and weight loss due to increased overall metabolic rate, ❸ ophthalmologic/ocular: in chronic cases particularly of the autoimmune variety, exophthalmos develops secondary to retro-orbital connective tissue proliferation and autoimmunity directed toward the extraocular muscles; the histologic abnormalities are chiefly characterized by increased accumulation of collagen (behind the eye and within the extraocular muscles, leading to muscle weakness), accumulation of glycosaminoglycans (GAGs), and the attendant edema.

- Clinical presentation of *hypo*thyroidism: In his classic book *Biochemical Individuality*, Williams[177] noted that "a wide variation in thyroid activity exists among 'normal' human beings." Clearly, some patients do not make enough thyroid hormone to function optimally[178]; or, perhaps more precisely, they make enough thyroid hormone (T4) but do not efficiently convert it to the active form (T3) in the periphery. Further complicating the picture is that some patients make appropriate amounts of TSH, T4, and T3 but they make excess of inactive reverse T3 (rT3) which puts them into a physiologic state of hypothyroidism despite adequate glandular function. Patients may have one or more of the following: fatigue, depression, **cold hands and feet** (excluding Raynaud's syndrome, peripheral vascular disease), dry skin, menstrual irregularities, infertility, premenstrual syndrome (PMS), uterine fibroids, excess menstrual bleeding, **low basal body temperature,** weak fingernails, sleep apnea and increased need for sleep (hypersomnia), slow heart rate (relative or absolute **bradycardia**), easy weight gain and difficult weight loss (thus, predisposition to overweight and obesity), hypercholesterolemia, slow healing, decreased memory and concentration, frog-like husky voice, low libido, recurrent infections, hypertension especially diastolic hypertension, poor digestion (due to insufficient gastric production of hydrochloric acid), **delayed Achilles return** (due to delayed muscle relaxation), carotenodermia, vitamin A deficiency, and gastroesophageal acid reflux, constipation, and predisposition to small intestine bacterial overgrowth (SIBO) due to slow intestinal transit. Of these manifestations, cold hands and feet, low basal body temperature, bradycardia, and delayed Achilles return are the most specific; some very competent physicians will—following proper patient evaluation—treat with thyroid hormone based on the clinical presentation of the patient and *with proper consideration of* and *without dependency upon* laboratory findings.
- Overview of thyroid tests:
  - Thyrotropin-releasing hormone (TRH): The hypothalamus releases TRH to stimulate pituitary production of TSH. TRH is not routinely tested in clinical practice, although abnormalities of TRH secretion are noted in patients with mental "depression."
  - Thyroid-stimulating hormone (TSH: 0.4 - 5.0 mIU/L [milli-international units per liter]): TSH is the most commonly performed test for evaluating thyroid status; its frequent (over)use owes more to habit and inexpensiveness than to aspirations for clinical excellence. TSH values greater than 2 mIU/L represent a disturbance of the thyroid-pituitary axis and an increased risk for future thyroid problems[179], and the American Association of Clinical Endocrinologists states, "The target TSH level should be between 0.3 and 3.0 μIU/mL."[180] Clinical rationale is available to support implementation of a therapeutic trial of thyroid hormone treatment in patients who are clinically hypothyroid even if they are biochemically euthyroid (per TSH) provided

[177] Williams RJ. *Biochemical Individuality: The Basis for the Genetotrophic Concept*. Austin and London: University of Texas Press, 1956 page 82
[178] Broda Barnes MD, Lawrence Galton, *Hypothyroidism: The Unsuspected Illness*. Ty Crowell Co; 1976
[179] Weetman AP. Fortnightly review: Hypothyroidism: screening and subclinical disease. *BMJ: British Medical Journal* 1997;314: 1175
[180] American Association of Clinical Endocrinologists. "The target TSH level should be between 0.3 and 3.0 μIU/mL." AACE Medical Guidelines for Clinical Practice for Evaluation and Treatment of Hyperthyroidism and Hypothyroidism. 2002, 2006 Amended Version. https://www.aace.com/sites/default/files/hypo_hyper.pdf Accessed Aug 2011

Thyroid status—laboratory assessments	

that treatment is implemented cautiously, in appropriately selected patients, and patients are appropriately informed.[181,182] If the clinical world were as perfect as it is portrayed in basic physiology textbooks, then a clinician might fancifully rely on TSH to perform the diagnosis *prima facie*, with reduced TSH values correlating with glandular overperformance and negative feedback suppressing TSH secretion, whilst an underperforming gland would require greater stimulation with elevated TSH levels; however, TSH has never been thus vested with infallible reliability, which explains in part why doctors need brains of their own and why better clinicians have developed the capacity for independent thought.

- Free thyroxine (free T4: 4.5 - 11.2 mcg/dL): Unbound T4 is tested to provide evidence of glandular production of thyroid hormone(s). Because T4 is the major thyroid hormone produced by the thyroid gland it serves as an excellent marker for glandular productivity but it reveals nothing about peripheral conversion of T4 to the active thyroid hormone triiodothyronine (T3); in the practice of medicine, conversion of T4 to the active T3 is assumed to reliably occur unabated despite evidence to the contrary, especially among symptomatic patients.

- Triiodothyronine (T3: 100 - 200 ng/dL[183]): In textbook-perfect physiology, T4 is converted by deiodinase enzymes type-1 and type-2 to the active thyroid hormone T3; in reality, this is only part of the story. Because T3 is the active form of the hormone responsible for the physiologic functions of thyroid physiology, a clinician desiring to assess a patient's thyroid status might reasonably ask the proper question by performing the proper test. T3 is tested as "total T3" or "free T3" in large part based on the clinician's preference; the current author prefers total T3 because it can be compared to the total level of reverse T3 (rT3) in a ratio, the optimal range of which is generally considered to be 10-14 as originally presented by McDaniel[184] and reviewed in the following pages. Patients with psychiatric depression have lower levels of T3 than do healthy controls and have been described as having "low T3 syndrome"[185]; very obviously—whether cause or effect—the low T3 levels in these patients would serve to promote and perpetuate their state of mental depression. Although the focus of this review within the subject of laboratory evaluation is not to describe the implementation of thyroid hormone treatment, clinicians should be aware that T3 administration increases hepatic production of sex hormone binding globulin (SHBG) and that therefore T3 administration can reduce cellular bioavailability of protein-bound hormones. Many authoritative and clinically-experienced sources recommend using a time-released (e.g., sustained-release) form of T3 due to its shorter half-life compared with T4. However, obtaining time-released T3 via a compounding pharmacy can be cumbersome and expensive for the patient; clearly some patients respond to once daily dosing of *non*-time-released preparations with good effects and without adverse effects. Some patients can divide the immediate-release dose into two servings per day for enhanced effect and lessened physiologic fluctuations, if necessary. Per Drugs.com[186] in August 2011, "Since liothyronine sodium (T3) is not firmly bound to serum protein, it is readily available to body tissues. The onset of activity of liothyronine sodium is rapid, occurring within a few hours. Maximum pharmacologic

[181] Skinner GR, Thomas R, Taylor M, Sellarajah M, Bolt S, Krett S, Wright A. Thyroxine should be tried in clinically hypothyroid but biochemically euthyroid patients. *BMJ: British Medical Journal* 1997 Jun 14; 314(7096): 1764

[182] McLaren EH, Kelly CJ, Pollack MA. Trial of thyroxine treatment for biochemically euthyroid patients has been approved. *BMJ* 1997; 315: 1463

[183] U.S. National Library of Medicine (NLM) and National Institutes of Health (NIH) http://www.nlm.nih.gov/medlineplus/ency/article/003687.htm Accessed August 2011

[184] McDaniel AB. Thyroid Assessment: Controversies and Conundrums. Institute for Functional Medicine 14th International Symposium. Tucson, Arizona. May 23-26, 2007

[185] "Out of 250 subjects with major psychiatric depression, 6.4% exhibited low T3 syndrome (mean serum T3 concentration 0.94 nmol/l vs normal mean serum concentration of 1.77 nmol/l)." Premachandra BN, Kabir MA, Williams IK. Low T3 syndrome in psychiatric depression. *J Endocrinol Invest*. 2006 Jun;29(6):568-72

[186] http://www.drugs.com/pro/cytomel.html Accessed August 2011.

response occurs within 2 or 3 days, providing early clinical response. The biological half-life is about 2.5 days." Very clearly, a significant portion of hypothyroid patients respond to T3 alone (either time-released, divided-dosing, or once-daily dosing) or a combination of T4 and T3 when other treatments have failed.[187,188]

- o Reverse triiodothyronine (rT3: 90 - 320 pg/mL[189]): T4 is converted by deiodinase enzymes type-1 and type-3 to the inactive thyroid hormone rT3; per a standard endocrinology textbook, "Approximately 70–80% of released T4 is converted by deiodinases to the biologically active T3, the remainder to reverse-T3 (rT3) which has no significant biological activity."[190] Clinicians must know that, "The prohormone T4 must be converted to T3 in the body before it can exert biological effects. **During periods of illness or stress, this conversion is often inhibited and can be diverted to the inactive reverse T3 (rT3) moiety.**"[191] Furthermore and very importantly, clinicians should appreciate that rT3 is not simply inactive but that it may actually impair production/utilization of normal T3; "T4-T3 and T4-rT3 conversion are provoked by different enzymes. The <u>elevation of rT3</u> might be a cause of the observed decrease in peripheral T3 generation in old [elderly] subjects, acting by an <u>inhibition of the T4-T3 conversion</u>."[192] During times of psychologic/physiologic stress and specific types of pharmacologic stress (e.g., propanolol[193] and corticosteroids), T4 metabolism is preferentially shunted away from T3 toward rT3; an anthropocentric explanation holds that by making less of the active T3 and more of the inactive rT3, the body is better able to conserve energy during times of stress by reducing overall metabolic rate, particularly resting energy expenditure and protein utilization. For example, caloric restriction and fasting result in a decrease in resting metabolic rate (RMR), and the reduced RMR persists for months after the fasting has ended and a normal diet is resumed.[194] This author (AV) terms this stress-induced impairment of thyroid hormone conversion "**metabolic hypothyroidism**" or "**functional hypothyroidism**" because the defect is in the metabolism (not the production) of thyroid hormone into its most active form; "**peripheral hypothyroidism**" might also be used to distinguish the fact that the defect is in the peripheral metabolism rather than located more centrally, within the thyroid gland itself. Because psychologic stress and certain pharmacologic exposures—as well as the thyro-metabolic stress of fasting and caloric restriction in which the counterregulatory hormone glucagon appears to trigger enhanced rT3 production—reduce T3 while simultaneously increasing rT3 levels, clinicians can appreciate that calculation of the T3/rT3 ratio will be more significantly altered (and thus a more sensitive indicator of metabolic disruption) than will be the isolated measurements of T3 or rT3 alone. Functional medicine clinicians[195] note the importance of the ratio of total T3 to reverse T3 (tT3:rT3 ratio) and consider the optimal range to be 10-14 with lower ratios indicating impaired formation or T3 and/or excess production of rT3.[196] Contrary to the previous view which held that rT3 was simply inactive, we now

[187] Bunevicius R, Kazanavicius G, Zalinkevicius R, Prange AJ Jr. Effects of thyroxine as compared with thyroxine plus triiodothyronine in patients with hypothyroidism. *N Engl J Med*. 1999 Feb 11;340(6):424-9
[188] Kelly T, Lieberman DZ. The use of triiodothyronine as an augmentation agent in treatment-resistant bipolar II and bipolar disorder NOS. *J Affect Disord*. 2009;116(3):222-6
[189] The reference range provided here for rT3 is a compilation from the laboratory reference ranges from the sample reports on the following pages, each of which is performed by either Quest Diagnostics or LabCorp, the two largest medical laboratories in the United States.
[190] Nussey S, Whitehead S. *Endocrinology: An Integrated Approach*. Oxford: BIOS Scientific Publishers; 2001. See also Box 3.29 Metabolism of thyroid hormones. http://www.ncbi.nlm.nih.gov/books/NBK28/box/A270/?report=objectonly Accessed July 2011
[191] *1998 Mosby's GenRX. Sixth Edition*. St. Louis Missouri; Mosby-Year Book, Inc., 1998
[192] Szabolcs I, Weber M, Kovács Z, Irsy G, Góth M, Halász T, Szilágyi G. The possible reason for serum 3,3'5'-(reverse) triiodothyronine increase in old people. *Acta Med Acad Sci Hung*. 1982;39(1-2):11-7
[193] "Propranolol administration (40 mg t.i.d. for a week) caused a similar rT3 elevation in old persons (n = 18) as in 12 young ones." Szabolcs I, Weber M, Kovács Z, Irsy G, Góth M, Halász T, Szilágyi G. The possible reason for serum 3,3'5'-(reverse) triiodothyronine increase in old people. *Acta Med Acad Sci Hung*. 1982;39(1-2):11-7
[194] Elliot DL, Goldberg L, Kuehl KS, Bennett WM. Sustained depression of the resting metabolic rate after massive weight loss. *Am J Clin Nutr* 1989 Jan;49(1):93-96
[195] The conclusion of this paragraph is derived from **Vasquez A**. *Musculoskeletal Pain: Expanded Clinical Strategies*. Published 2008 by The Institute for Functional Medicine. http://www.functionalmedicine.org/ifm_ecommerce/ProductDetails.aspx?ProductID=127
[196] McDaniel AB. Thyroid Assessment: Controversies and Conundrums. Institute for Functional Medicine 14th International Symposium. Tucson, Arizona. May 23-26, 2007

Thyroid status—laboratory assessments	
	appreciate that rT3 actually impairs normal thyroid hormone metabolism thus functioning as an thyrometabolic monkeywrench or "brake" on normal metabolism. Elevated rT3 levels predict mortality among critically ill patients.[197] Aberrancies in thyroid hormone levels may reflect organic disease, psychoemotional stress, or nutritional deficiency[198], and therefore such serologic abnormalities warrant consideration of underlying problems and direct treatment when possible. If no underlying cause is apparent, then a trial of thyroid hormone/hormones is reasonable in appropriately selected patients. Beyond stress reduction, allergen/gluten avoidance, and nutritional supplementation with iodine, selenium, and zinc (as indicated per patient), correction of overt, subclinical, and functional hypothyroidism generally centers on the administration of natural or synthetic thyroid hormones in the form of T4 and T3. Correction of functional hypothyroidism (relatively reduced total T3 and increased rT3) is accomplished with either time-released or twice-daily dosing of T3 *without T4* to suppress endogenous T4 conversion to T3, thereby allowing rT3 levels to fall precipitously. T3 administration allows temporary downregulation of transforming enzymes so that rT3 production is reduced following withdrawal of T3 replacement; thus, short-term and/or periodic T3 administration helps normalize or "reset" peripheral thyroid metabolism so that, following withdrawal of T3 administration, T4 can be converted to T3 without excess production of rT3. The safety and effectiveness of this approach—using T3 administration (often twice daily or in a sustained-release compounded tablet or capsule) to recalibrate peripheral thyroid hormone metabolism—has documented safety and effectiveness.[199] Alleviation of symptoms, restoration of morning body temperature to 98.6° F (oral or axillary) and other clinical objective improvements achieved by the judicious and safe administration of T3 are the criteria of success; physiologic improvement following T3 administration retrospectively confirms the diagnosis. o Antithyroid antibodies—antithyroglobulin (anti-TG) and anti-thyroid peroxidase (anti-TPO): Autoimmune thyroiditis (also called Hashimoto's disease or chronic lymphocytic thyroiditis) or is the most common cause of overt primary hypothyroidism. The diagnosis of autoimmune thyroiditis can be made clinically (i.e., without biopsy) upon detection of elevated blood levels of antibodies against thyroglobulin (anti-thyroglobulin antibodies) and anti-thyroid peroxidase (anti-TPO) antibodies. Autoimmune thyroiditis may present asymptomatically and with normal thyroid hormone levels; classically, patients may have a slightly hyperthyroid presentation as the inflamed gland releases extra thyroid hormone before becoming atrophic and hypofunctional.
Advantages:	▪ Thyroid disorders are quite common in general practice and are often undiagnosed, undertreated, or inappropriately treated. ▪ Consistent with the principle of beneficence, patients and doctors benefit when thyroid disorders are diagnosed and treated appropriately.
Limitations:	▪ A properly interpreted TSH may overlook problems of T4 production or conversion to active T3. Additionally, in some patients, all of these tests are normal but they may have thyroid

[197] Peeters RP, Wouters PJ, van Toor H, Kaptein E, Visser TJ, Van den Berghe G. Serum 3,3',5'-triiodothyronine (rT3) and 3,5,3'-triiodothyronine/rT3 are prognostic markers in critically ill patients and are associated with postmortem tissue deiodinase activities. *J Clin Endocrinol Metab.* 2005 Aug;90(8):4559-65
[198] Kelly GS. Peripheral metabolism of thyroid hormones: a review. Altern Med Rev. 2000 Aug;5(4):306-33
[199] Friedman M, Miranda-Massari JR, Gonzalez MJ. Supraphysiological cyclic dosing of sustained release T3 in order to reset low basal body temperature. *P R Health Sci J.* 2006 Mar;25(1):23-9

Thyroid status—laboratory assessments	
	autoimmunity (i.e., thyroid peroxidase antibodies, anti-TPO) and should receive treatment with thyroid hormone[200] or some other corrective treatment (e.g., selenium supplementation[201,202] and a gluten-free diet[203]) to normalize thyroid status.
Comments:	▪ Comprehensive thyroid laboratory testing including ❶ TSH, ❷ free T4, ❸ total T3, ❹ rT3, ❺ antithyroid antibodies, should be evaluated alongside the ❻ heart rate, ❼ cold extremities, ❽ basal body temperature, ❾ Achilles' return rate, and ❿ overall symptoms and clinical picture. ▪ The combination of T3 and T4 (as in the prescription Liotrix/Thyrolar or Armour thyroid) appears to have similar safety to T4 alone (Levothyroxine, Synthroid) and may result in greater improvements in mood and neuropsychological function.[204] ▪ Glandular thyroid supplements and Armour thyroid generally should *not* be used in patients with thyroid autoimmunity (Hashimoto's thyroiditis) because the bovine/porcine antigens will exacerbate the anti-thyroid immune response as evidenced by increased anti-TPO antibodies.

Optimal thyroid status

Concept by Dr Vasquez: Optimal thyroid status is not defined by basic laboratory testing with TSH and free T4. It is defined *per patient* based on the levels and ratios of all major thyroid-related hormones and antibodies—in association with other hormonal, psychologic, dysbiotic, nutritional and environmental factors— that work best for that particular unique biochemically-individual patient.

Laboratory interpretation by Dr McDaniel: "Optimal hormone balance is debatable. My observations: A few "well" people and patients treated successfully with T4 and T3 seem best with:

- TSH around 0.7–0.9µIU/mL
- fT4 around 0.7–0.8ng/dL
- fT3 optimally 3.4–3.8pg/mL
- **Total T3-RT3 ratio 12 +/-2**"

McDaniel AB. Thyroid Assessment: Controversies and Conundrums. Institute for Functional Medicine Fourteenth International Symposium. Tucson, Arizona. May 23-26, 2007

---

[200] Beers MH, Berkow R (eds). The Merck Manual. 17th Edition. Whitehouse Station; Merck Research Laboratories 1999 page 96

[201] Duntas LH, Mantzou E, Koutras DA. Effects of a six month treatment with selenomethionine in patients with autoimmune thyroiditis. *Eur J Endocrinol.* 2003 Apr;148(4):389-93 http://eje-online.org/cgi/reprint/148/4/389

[202] Gartner R, Gasnier BC. Selenium in the treatment of autoimmune thyroiditis. *Biofactors.* 2003;19(3-4):165-70

[203] Sategna-Guidetti C, Volta U, Ciacci C, Usai P, Carlino A, De Franceschi L, Camera A, Pelli A, Brossa C. Prevalence of thyroid disorders in untreated adult celiac disease patients and effect of gluten withdrawal: an Italian multicenter study. *Am J Gastroenterol.* 2001 Mar;96(3):751-7

[204] "CONCLUSIONS: In patients with hypothyroidism, partial substitution of triiodothyronine for thyroxine may improve mood and neuropsychological function; this finding suggests a specific effect of the triiodothyronine normally secreted by the thyroid gland." Bunevicius R, Kazanavicius G, Zalinkevicius R, Prange AJ Jr. Effects of thyroxine as compared with thyroxine plus triiodothyronine in patients with hypothyroidism. *N Engl J Med.* 1999 Feb 11;340(6):424-9

Presentation: 38yo male under extreme psychological stress with a complaint of constantly cold extremities—testing performed in February 2010 by LabCorp: Review the following labs and outline your treatment plan before reading the discussion below.

Date and Time Collected	Date Entered	Date and Time Reported	Physician Name	NPI	Pl
02/04/10 11:41	02/04/10	02/09/10 04:0(	EBAN		19(

Tests Ordered

Triiodothyronine (T3);Reverse T3;Triiodothyronine,Free,Serum

General Comments

PID: 8282293

TESTS	RESULT	FLAG	UNITS	REFERENCE INTERV
Triiodothyronine (T3)				
Triiodothyronine (T3)	57	**Low**	ng/dL	71-180
Reverse T3				
Reverse T3	312		pg/mL	90-350
Triiodothyronine,Free,Serum				
Triiodothyronine,Free,Serum	2.5		pg/mL	2.0-4.4

Discussion: In this case, because the T3 level is low, *prima facie* justification for administration of T3 is provided, assuming that the clinical picture is compatible and that no contraindications to treatment are present. To calculate the total T3/rT3 ratio, equilibrate the units (multiply total T3 in ng/dL x 10 to convert to pg/mL; 1 pg = 0.001 ng (1 ng = 1,000 pg); 1 dl = 100 ml). The total T3/rT3 ratio should be >10-14 (per McDaniel[205]), but in this patient's case 570/312 = 1.8. Remember, more T3 than rT3 is better; hence, the higher ratio is better. On-line calculators for this conversion have been developed[206] and surely more will be available in the future. This athletic and otherwise healthy 220-lb (100 kg) patient responded very well to T3 (liothyronine/Cytomel) with a starting dose of 150 mcg which was eventually tapered to 25 mcg and then to 12.5 mcg; in this patient's case, the initial high dose of T3 was well-tolerated because of the initially low level of T3, the elevated rT3 which appears to block T3 function, and the patient's overall excellent cardiovascular fitness. A reasonable dosage range for liothyronine/Cytomel supplementation is 12.5-50 mcg for most patients tapered to the constellation of patient tolerance, patient preference, heart rate, basal body temperature optimization to 98.6° F, suppression of TSH and T4, resolution of symptoms and objective markers, and clinician's impression and experience.

Step-by-step conversion from ng/dL to pg/mL—end result is multiply by 10 (i.e., 10x)

Original units	Convert ng to pg[207]	Convert dL to mL	Simplify the fraction
1 ng / 1 dL	1,000 pg/ 1 dL	1,000 pg/ 100 mL	10 pg/ 1 ml
57 ng/ 1 dL	57,000 pg / 1 dL	57,000 pg / 100 mL	570 pg / 1 mL

Contraindications to T3, liothyronine, Cytomel

Absolute contraindications:
- Anaphylaxis or severe hypersensitivity,
- Acute (current) myocardial infarction,
- Hyperthyroidism,
- Untreated adrenal insufficiency.

Relative contraindications and cautions:
- CAD, angina pectoris, or cardiac arrhythmia,
- Elderly patients—start with low dose and titrate as tolerated.

Reference: Epocrates.com August 2011

---

[205] McDaniel AB. Thyroid Assessment: Controversies and Conundrums. Institute for Functional Medicine Fourteenth International Symposium. Tucson, AZ. May 23-26, 2007
[206] http://www.stopthethyroidmadness.com/rt3-ratio/ Accessed—but not necessarily endorsed—August 2011
[207] Double-checked with http://www.unitconversion.org/weight/nanograms-to-picograms-conversion.html July 2011

Presentation: 42yo male with fatigue—testing performed by Quest Diagnostics in January 2010: Review the following labs and outline your treatment plan before reading the discussion below. Note that the "optimal ratio" provided by the laboratory in this example was performed using free T3 rather than total T3 and without converting to equal units.

```
FREE T3/REVERSE T3 RATIO
   FREE T3/REVERSE T3 RATIO                      0.93 L            1.05-1.91**
   FREE T3                          325                            230-420 pg/dL
   REVERSE T3                                    350 H            100-340*** pg/mL
              **Ratio= Free T3 in pg/dL : reverse T3 in pg/mL. Ratio for reference
              range is calculated by dividing the lower and upper end of free T3
              with the mean of reverse T3 (220 pg/mL).

              ***Observed reference range is reported for reverse T3 per client
              request.

              This test was performed using a kit that has not been approved or
              cleared by the FDA. The analytical performance characteristics of this
              test have been determined by Quest Diagnostics Nichols Institute, San
              Juan Capistrano. This test should not be used for diagnosis without
              confirmation by other medically established means.
```

Discussion: Note that if the T3 had been tested without rT3 the results would have been reported as "normal" and that a "depressed" patient so assessed would have likely been given an "antidepressant" medication and a diagnosis of depression rather than the proper treatment with T3 and a diagnosis of functional hypothyroidism. Luckily for this patient, his clinician tested rT3 and upon finding it impressively elevated treated with patient with T3 to suppress rT3 production by temporarily suppressing T4 production. The ratio calculation is provided and interpreted by the laboratory; notice that the "ideal ratio" for **total** T3/rT3 (>10) differs from that of **free** T3/rT3 (>1.05) *and that per the ratio provided by the labotatory does not equilibriate the measurement units.* This method is acceptable but is not the preferred method for determining functional thyroid status. The preferred method is the one presented by McDaniel[208] at the Institute for Functional Medicine's 14th International Symposium in 2007 wherein he advocated using total T3 (not free T3) in comparison with rT3 interpreted by an optimal ratio of 10-14.

Step-by-step conversion from pg/dL to pg/mL—end result is divide by 100 (i.e., 0.01x): Provided for the sake of completeness even though the conversion is not necessary per the laboratory interpretation provided above.

Original units	Convert dL to mL	Simplify the fraction
1 pg / 1 dL	1 pg/ 100 mL	0.01 pg/ 1 mL
325 pg/ 1 dL	325 pg / 100 mL	3.25 pg / 1 mL

---

[208] McDaniel AB. Thyroid Assessment: Controversies and Conundrums. Institute for Functional Medicine 14th International Symposium. Tucson, Arizona. May 23-26, 2007

Presentation: 31yo female with fatigue, a recent history of extreme emotional stress (death of first-degree family member), maternal history of Hashimotos thyroiditis, and a personal history of presumed gluten intolerance—testing performed in May 2010 by Quest Diagnostics: Outline your treatment plan before reading discussion.

Test Name	In Range	Out of Range	Reference Range
THYROGLOBULIN ANTIBODIES	<20		<20 IU/mL
THYROID PEROXIDASE ANTIBODIES		38 H	<35 IU/mL
T3, TOTAL	89		76-181 ng/dL
T3 UPTAKE		37 H	22-35 %
T4, FREE	1.6		0.8-1.8 ng/dL
T4 (THYROXINE), TOTAL			
T4 (THYROXINE), TOTAL	10.9		4.5-12.5 mcg/dL
FREE T4 INDEX (T7)		**4.0 H**	1.4-3.8
TSH, 3RD GENERATION	0.82		mIU/L

Reference Range

> or = 20 Years   0.40-4.50

Pregnancy Ranges
First trimester   0.20-4.70
Second trimester   0.30-4.10
Third trimester   0.40-2.70

T3, FREE	318		230-420 pg/dL
T3, REVERSE		**43 H**	11-32 ng/dL

This test was performed using a kit that has not been approved or cleared by the FDA. The analytical performance characteristics of this test have been determined by Quest Diagnostics Nichols Institute, San Juan Capistrano. This test should not be used for diagnosis without confirmation by other medically established means.

Discussion: Note that the TSH is completely normal and thus would give the impression of normalcy and "health" if the clinician had not ordered the additional tests. Thyroid peroxidase antibodies are minimally elevated; this is consistent with thyroid autoimmunity but titers this low are of limited clinical importance. Note that the rT3 level is abnormally elevated. Note that because the units provided for total T3 (89 ng/dL) and rT3 (43 ng/dL) are identical, no unit conversion is required, thereby making the calculation of the ideal ratio (range: 10-14) very simple. In this patient's case, the ratio comes to 2.06 which is obviously significantly lower than the proposed optimal of 10-14; the patient responded well to liothyronine/Cytomel supplementation with 15 mcg/d. Patients with thyroid autoimmunity often benefit from a gluten-free diet[209] and supplementation with selenium 200 mcg/d.[210] Finally, note that the reference range for total T3 provided by this laboratory is 76-181 ng/dL which contrasts significantly from the range recommended by the US National Institutes of Health (NIH) 100 to 200 ng/dL[211]; using the NIH's reference range, this patient's T3 production is inadequate.

---

[209] "Hypothyroidism, diagnosed in 31 patients (12.9%) and nine controls (4.2%), was subclinical in 29 patients and of nonautoimmune origin in 21. ... In most patients who strictly followed a 1-yr gluten withdrawal (as confirmed by intestinal mucosa recovery), there was a normalization of subclinical hypothyroidism. The greater frequency of thyroid disease among celiac disease patients justifies a thyroid functional assessment. In distinct cases, gluten withdrawal may single-handedly reverse the abnormality." Sategna-Guidetti C, Volta U, Ciacci C, et al. Prevalence of thyroid disorders in untreated adult celiac disease patients and effect of gluten withdrawal: an Italian multicenter study. *Am J Gastroenterol.* 2001 Mar;96(3):751-7

[210] "Patients with HT assigned to Se supplementation for 3 months demonstrated significantly lower thyroid peroxidase autoantibodies (TPOab) titers (four studies, random effects weighted mean difference: −271.09, 95% confidence interval: −421.98 to −120.19, p< 10⁻⁴) and a significantly higher chance of reporting an improvement in well-being and/or mood (three studies, random effects risk ratio: 2.79, 95% confidence interval: 1.21-6.47, p= 0.016) when compared with controls. .. On the basis of the best available evidence, Se supplementation is associated with a significant decrease in TPOab titers at 3 months and with improvement in mood and/or general well-being."Toulis KA, Anastasilakis AD, Tzellos TG, Goulis DG, Kouvelas D. Selenium supplementation in the treatment of Hashimoto's thyroiditis: a systematic review and a meta-analysis. *Thyroid.* 2010 Oct;20(10):1163-73

[211] U.S. National Library of Medicine and NIH www.nlm.nih.gov/medlineplus/ency/article/003687.htm Accessed Aug 2011

Toxic metal testing—emphasis on lead and mercury	

Overview and application:	• <u>Introduction</u>: Per the US Department of Labor's Occupational Safety and Health Administration (OSHA)[212], toxic metals, including "heavy metals", are individual metals and metal compounds that negatively affect people's health. While lists of toxic metals can vary per source, OSHA names the following: arsenic, beryllium, cadmium, hexavalent chromium, lead, and mercury; of these, lead and mercury are the most commonly observed problematic toxic metals in outpatient practice. The three most important clinical concepts with regard to testing for "heavy metals" or "toxic metals" are as follows:
	
	  1. <u>Heavy metal toxicity/accumulation is not uncommon in clinical practice</u>: Toxic/heavy metal accumulation is clinically important due both to its frequency and its pathophysiologic consequences. An article published in *Journal of the American Medical Association (JAMA)*[213] showed that approximately 8% of [1,709 American] women had [blood mercury] concentrations higher than the US Environmental Protection Agency's recommended reference dose (5.8 µg/L), below which exposures are considered to be without adverse effects; **stated more plainly, 8% of American women have (potentially) toxic levels of mercury** *even when evaluated by the least sensitive of laboratory methods—blood mercury,* **which represents only 5% of total body mercury.** Another study, also published in *JAMA*[214], showed a positive relationship between blood lead levels and hypertension, even at blood lead levels considered within the normal range; the authors wrote, "At levels well below the current US occupational exposure limit guidelines (40 µg/dL), **blood lead level is positively associated with both systolic and diastolic blood pressure and risks of both systolic and diastolic hypertension among women aged 40 to 59 years.**"
	
	  2. <u>The clinical presentation of heavy metal toxicity/accumulation is generally diverse and nonspecific</u>: Clinical presentations due to or associated with toxic metal accumulation can include dyscognition, fatigue, anemia, chronic pain from myalgia or neuropathy, hypertension, autism, and immune disorders including autoimmunity and allergy. In particular, autism[215,216,217] and hypertension[218,219] are noteworthy for their consistent associations with mercury and with mercury and lead, respectively.
	
	  3. <u>(Therefore), clinicians should test for and treat toxic metal accumulation</u>: When problems are clinically significant and not extremely unlikely, clinicians have an obligation to test for and treat such problems for the benefit of the patient. Therefore, because toxic metal accumulation is common, clinically significant, and because it is a reversible cause of numerous symptoms, syndromes, and a contributing factor to many other diagnosable conditions (e.g., hypertension, immune disorders, mood disorders), clinicians have an obligation to consider and test for toxic metals among their patients.
	
	• <u>Additional details—mercury</u>: Mercury is an established neurotoxin, immunotoxin, and nephrotoxin. Because pathophysiologic effects are noted even with very small doses of

---

[212] http://www.osha.gov/SLTC/metalsheavy/index.html Accessed July 2011.

[213] Schober SE, Sinks TH, Jones RL, Bolger PM, McDowell M, Osterloh J, Garrett ES, Canady RA, Dillon CF, Sun Y, Joseph CB, Mahaffey KR. Blood mercury levels in US children and women of childbearing age, 1999-2000. *JAMA* 2003;289:1667-74 http://jama.ama-assn.org/content/289/13/1667.long

[214] Nash D, Magder L, Lustberg M, Sherwin RW, Rubin RJ, Kaufmann RB, Silbergeld EK. Blood lead, blood pressure, and hypertension in perimenopausal and postmenopausal women. *JAMA*. 2003 Mar 26;289(12):1523-32. See also Muntner P, He J, Vupputuri S, Coresh J, Batuman V. Blood lead and chronic kidney disease in the general United States population: results from NHANES III. *Kidney Int*. 2003 Mar;63(3):1044-50 http://www.nature.com/ki/journal/v63/n3/pdf/4493526a.pdf

[215] Stamova B, Green PG, Tian Y, Hertz-Picciotto I, Pessah IN, Hansen R, Yang X, Teng J, Gregg JP, Ashwood P, Van de Water J, Sharp FR. Correlations between gene expression and mercury levels in blood of boys with and without autism. *Neurotox Res*. 2011;19:31-48. Epub 2009 Nov 24.

[216] "The results of the study indicated that the participants' overall ATEC scores and their scores on each of the ATEC subscales (Speech/Language, Sociability, Sensory/Cognitive Awareness, and Health/Physical/Behavior) were linearly related to urinary porphyrins associated with mercury toxicity. The results show an association between the apparent level of mercury toxicity as measured by recognized urinary porphyrin biomarkers of mercury toxicity and the magnitude of the specific hallmark features of autism as assessed by ATEC." Kern JK, Geier DA, Adams JB, Geier MR. A biomarker of mercury body-burden correlated with diagnostic domain specific clinical symptoms of autism spectrum disorder. *Biometals*. 2010 Dec;23(6):1043-51

[217] Kempuraj D, Asadi S, Zhang B, Manola A, Hogan J, Peterson E, Theoharides TC. Mercury induces inflammatory mediator release from human mast cells. *J Neuroinflammation*. 2010 Mar 11;7:20 http://www.jneuroinflammation.com/content/7/1/20

[218] Schober SE, Sinks TH, Jones RL, Bolger PM, McDowell M, Osterloh J, Garrett ES, Canady RA, Dillon CF, Sun Y, Joseph CB, Mahaffey KR. Blood mercury levels in US children and women of childbearing age, 1999-2000. *JAMA* 2003;289:1667-74 http://jama.ama-assn.org/content/289/13/1667.long

[219] Nash D, Magder L, Lustberg M, Sherwin RW, Rubin RJ, Kaufmann RB, Silbergeld EK. Blood lead, blood pressure, and hypertension in perimenopausal and postmenopausal women. *JAMA*. 2003 Mar 26;289(12):1523-32

Toxic metal testing—emphasis on lead and mercury

exposure, one could reasonably argue that no safe amount exists and therefore that any detected mercury is an indication for therapeutic intervention to remove this toxicant. According to an article by Schober et al[220] published in *JAMA—Journal of the American Medical Association* in 2003, "Approximately 8% of [1,709 American] women had [blood mercury] concentrations higher than the US Environmental Protection Agency's recommended reference dose (5.8 µg/L), below which exposures are considered to be without adverse effects." Sources of exposure include dental amalgams, vaccinations, airborne pollution, deep-water fish such as tuna, some cosmetics[221], and selected herbicides, fungicides, and germicides; recently, high-fructose corn syrup was shown to contain mercury in clinically meaningful amounts.[222] Mercury impairs catecholamine degradation and can thereby cause a clinical syndrome that can include hypertension, tremor, tachycardia, diaphoresis, and neurocognitive changes.[223] Per Shih and Gartner[224], "Mercury combines with the sulfhydryl group of S-adenosylmethionine, which is a cofactor for catecholamine-O-methyltransferase (COMT), and this inhibition of COMT allows accumulation of norepinephrine, epinephrine, and dopamine." The clinical presentation of mercury toxicity can include any of the following: diffuse erythematosus rash, dermatitis (acrodynia), anorexia, malaise, **fatigue**, **muscle pain**, proximal and/or distal muscle weakness, tremor, weight loss, **insomnia**, night sweats, burning peripheral neuropathy (axonal neuropathy), renal insufficiency/failure, **inattention**, neurocognitive compromise, personality changes, **depression**, diaphoresis, tachycardia, and **hypertension**. Mercury poisoning/accumulation can occur in humans as a result of consumption of contaminated foods—especially seafood such as shark, swordfish, king mackerel, tilefish, and albacore ("white") tuna.[225] The immunologic effects of organic and/or inorganic mercury include immunosuppression, immunostimulation, formation of antinucleolar antibodies targeting fibrillarin, and formation and deposition of immune-complexes, resulting in a syndrome called "mercury-induced autoimmunity" which can be induced by exposure of susceptible animals to mercury.[226] Mercury/"silver" amalgam dental fillings rank highly among the most significant source of mercury exposure in humans, and implantation of mercury-silver dental amalgams in susceptible animals causes chronic stimulation of the immune system with induction of systemic autoimmunity.[227] Besides being a neurotoxin with no safe exposure limit[228], mercury is known to modify/antigenize/haptenize endogenous proteins to promote autoimmunity[229], and mercury may also promote autoimmunity by contributing to a pro-inflammatory environment that awakens quiescent autoreactive immunocytes via bystander activation.[230] For example, administration of mercury

---

[220] Schober SE, Sinks TH, Jones RL, et al. Blood mercury levels in US children and women of childbearing age, 1999-2000. *JAMA*. 2003 Apr 2;289(13):1667-74 http://jama.ama-assn.org/content/289/13/1667.long

[221] "Most makeup manufacturers have phased out the use of mercury, but it's still added legally to some eye products as a preservative and germ-killer, said John Bailey, chief scientist with the Personal Care Products Council in Washington." Associated Press. Minnesota Bans Adding Mercury To Cosmetics. February 11, 2009. http://www.cbsnews.com/stories/2007/12/14/health/main3618048.shtml Accessed August 2011

[222] "Average daily consumption of high fructose corn syrup is about 50 grams per person in the United States. With respect to total mercury exposure, it may be necessary to account for this source of mercury in the diet of children and sensitive populations." Dufault R, LeBlanc B, Schnoll R, Cornett C, Schweitzer L, Wallinga D, Hightower J, Patrick L, Lukiw WJ. Mercury from chlor-alkali plants: measured concentrations in food product sugar. *Environ Health*. 2009 Jan 26;8:2. See also: "High fructose corn syrup has been shown to contain trace amounts of mercury as a result of some manufacturing processes, and its consumption can also lead to zinc loss." Dufault R, Schnoll R, Lukiw WJ, Leblanc B, Cornett C, Patrick L, Wallinga D, Gilbert SG, Crider R. Mercury exposure, nutritional deficiencies and metabolic disruptions may affect learning in children. *Behav Brain Funct*. 2009 Oct 27;5:44.

[223] Wössmann W, Kohl M, Grüning G, Bucsky P. Mercury intoxication presenting with hypertension and tachycardia. *Arch Dis Child*. 1999 Jun;80(6):556-7 http://www.ncbi.nlm.nih.gov/pmc/articles/PMC1717944/pdf/v080p00556.pdf

[224] Shih H, Gartner JC Jr. Weight loss, hypertension, weakness, and limb pain in an 11-year-old boy. *J Pediatr*. 2001 Apr;138(4):566-9

[225] See http://www.fda.gov/Food/FoodSafety/Product-SpecificInformation/Seafood/FoodbornePathogensContaminants/Methylmercury/ucm115662.htm for the white-washed version; see http://www.ewg.org/news/bamboozled-fish for a more accurate and complete perspective.

[226] Havarinasab S, Hultman P. Organic mercury compounds and autoimmunity. *Autoimmun Rev*. 2005;4(5):270-5 www.generationrescue.org/pdf/havarinasab.pdf Dec 2005

[227] "We hypothesize that under appropriate conditions of genetic susceptibility and adequate body burden, heavy metal exposure from dental amalgam may contribute to immunological aberrations, which could lead to overt autoimmunity." Hultman P, Johansson U, Turley SJ, Lindh U, Enestrom S, Pollard KM. Adverse immunological effects and autoimmunity induced by dental amalgam and alloy in mice. *FASEB J*. 1994 Nov;8(14):1183-90

[228] University of Calgary Faculty of Medicine. How Mercury Causes Brain Neuron Degeneration.http://commons.ucalgary.ca/mercury/ Current Aug 2011

[229] Havarinasab S, Hultman P. Organic mercury compounds and autoimmunity. *Autoimmun Rev*. 2005 Jun;4(5):270-5. www.generationrescue.org/pdf/havarinasab.pdf Dec 2005

[230] "It is therefore theoretically possible that compounds present in vaccines such as thiomersal or aluminium hydroxyde can trigger autoimmune reactions through bystander effects." Fournie GJ, Mas M, Cautain B, et al. Induction of autoimmunity through bystander effects. Lessons from immunological disorders induced by heavy metals. *J Autoimmun*. 2001 May;16(3):319-26

to "susceptible" mice induces autoimmunity via modification of the nucleolar protein *fibrillarin*[231]; noteworthy in this regard is the fact that antifibrillarin antibodies are characteristic of the human autoimmune disease scleroderma.[232] The mercury-based preservative thimerosol is a type-IV (delayed hypersensitivity) sensitizing agent[233], and recent research implicates mercury as a contributor to autism[234,235] and eczema.[236] A review and clinical report published by Bains et al[237], stated, "Eczematous eruptions may be produced through topical contact with mercury and by systemic absorption in mercury sensitive individuals. Mercury...may cause hypersensitivity leading to contact dermatitis or Coomb's Type IV hypersensitivity reactions. The typical manifestation is an urticarial or erythematous rash, and pruritus on the face and flexural aspects of limbs, followed by progression to dermatitis." Thus, this survey of the literature supports the notions that mercury toxicity—i.e., a level of mercury in human patients sufficient to cause adverse health effects—is ❶ common (e.g., 8% of American women), ❷ problematic via causation of or contribution to various health problems commonly encountered in clinical practice, ❸ diagnosable via laboratory testing followed by monitoring response to treatment, and ❹ treatable, most notably with DMSA but also to a lesser extent with potassium citrate, selenium, and phytochelatins.

- Additional details—lead: The International Agency for Research on Cancer (IARC, part of the World Health Organization [WHO]) classified lead as a "possible human carcinogen" in 1987. A 2003 review published in *British Medical Bulletin* by Järup[238] noted that lead exposure (which comes equally from air and food, particularly food served via lead-contaminated ceramics) should be avoided as much as possible because physiologic toxicity occurs with low-level exposure; "Blood levels in children should be reduced below the levels so far considered acceptable, recent data indicating that there may be neurotoxic effects of lead at lower levels of exposure than previously anticipated." Occupational exposure to lead occurs in mines, smelting plants, glass-manufacturing facilities, battery plants, and among workers who weld metals already painted with lead-containing paints; air emissions near such facilities and activities may also contaminate nonworkers. Air contamination frequently leads to water contamination, threatening wildlife and humans who are exposed to contaminated water. Children are particularly vulnerable to lead exposure due to very efficient (compared with adults) gastrointestinal absorption and a more permeable ("leaky") blood-brain barrier. Organic lead compounds such as tetramethyl lead and tetraethyl lead easily penetrate skin and blood-brain barrier of children as well as adults. Classic, large-dose, acute and subacute lead poisoning manifests as anemia, renal tubular damage, and dark blue line of lead sulphide at the gingival margin; clinicians awaiting this classic presentation prior to considering lead toxicity should fortify their knowledge of and reconsider their perspective on this topic. Other symptoms of acute lead poisoning are headache, irritability, abdominal pain and various neurologic-psychiatric symptoms generally referred to as "lead encephalopathy" characterized by sleeplessness, restlessness, confusion/dyscognition, behavioral disturbances,

---

[231] Nielsen JB, Hultman P. Mercury-induced autoimmunity in mice. *Environ Health Perspect.* 2002 Oct;110 Suppl 5:877-81 http://ehp.niehs.nih.gov/docs/2002/suppl-5/877-881nielsen/abstract.html

[232] "Since anti-fibrillarin antibodies are specific markers of scleroderma, the present animal model may be valuable for studies of the immunological aberrations which are likely to induce this autoimmune response." Hultman P, Enestrom S, Pollard KM, Tan EM. Anti-fibrillarin autoantibodies in mercury-treated mice. *Clin Exp Immunol.* 1989;78(3):470-7

[233] "Thimerosal is an important preservative in vaccines and ophthalmologic preparations. The substance is known to be a type IV sensitizing agent. High sensitization rates were observed in contact-allergic patients and in health care workers who had been exposed to thimerosal-preserved vaccines." Westphal GA, Schnuch A, Schulz TG, Reich K, Aberer W, Brasch J, Koch P, Wessbecher R, Szliska C, Bauer A, Hallier E. Homozygous gene deletions of the glutathione S-transferases M1 and T1 are associated with thimerosal sensitization. *Int Arch Occup Environ Health.* 2000 Aug;73(6):384-8

[234] Vojdani A, Pangborn JB, Vojdani E, Cooper EL. Infections, toxic chemicals and dietary peptides binding to lymphocyte receptors and tissue enzymes are major instigators of autoimmunity in autism. *Int J Immunopathol Pharmacol.* 2003 Sep-Dec;16(3):189-99

[235] Geier DA, Geier MR. A comparative evaluation of the effects of MMR immunization and mercury doses from thimerosal-containing childhood vaccines on the population prevalence of autism. *Med Sci Monit.* 2004 Mar;10(3):PI33-9. http://www.medscimonit.com/pub/vol_10/no_3/3986.pdf

[236] Weidinger S, Kramer U, Dunemann L, Mohrenschlager M, Ring J, Behrendt H. Body burden of mercury is associated with acute atopic eczema and total IgE in children from southern Germany. *J Allergy Clin Immunol.* 2004 Aug;114(2):457-9

[237] Bains VK, Loomba K, Loomba A, Bains R. Mercury sensitisation: review, relevance and a clinical report. *Br Dent J.* 2008 Oct 11;205(7):373-8 http://www.intolsante.com/documents/publications/-mercury-sensitisation-review-relevance-and-clinical-report-22.pdf Accessed August 2011

[238] Järup L. Hazards of heavy metal contamination. *Br Med Bull.* 2003;68:167-82

Toxic metal testing—emphasis on lead and mercury	
	particularly learning and concentration difficulties in children; more extreme manifestations can include acute psychosis and stupor. Per the previously cited review by Järup, "Individuals [chronically exposed to lead] with average blood lead levels under 3 µmol/l may show signs of peripheral nerve symptoms with reduced nerve conduction velocity and reduced dermal sensibility."
Overview and application:	▪ No universally accepted consensus exists for the most accurate testing methodology. However, from the science-based perspectives that **toxic metals have been proven to cause harm at levels previously believed to be "acceptable" and that—very importantly—toxic metals are exponentially more toxic when in combination than when present alone**, reasonable clinicians can therefore conclude that the best test for clinical use is the one that is most sensitive, along with being reasonably convenient for the patient as well as affordable. For these reasons, the current author and many other clinicians chose DMSA-provoked urine toxic metal testing. Hair and nails can also be tested for chronic exposure, as can blood which is generally only useful for recent and relatively high-level exposure. Our clinical concern in general outpatient practice is not with recent and relatively high-level exposure, and therefore blood is not necessarily optimal. Our clinical concern in general outpatient practice is with chronic low-level exposure which leads to adverse cellular effects despite the failure to "spike" the serum level into the detectable toxic range. Arguments in favor of allowing symptomatic patients to persist untreated in a state of toxic metal accumulation would be difficult to justify scientifically and ethically.
Advantages:	▪ Toxic metal accumulation is ❶ sufficiently common to warrant testing in selected patients, ❷ problematic via causation of or contribution to various health problems commonly encountered in clinical practice, ❸ diagnosable via laboratory testing followed by monitoring response to treatment, and ❹ treatable. Therefore, clinicians should establish pathways for the assessment and treatment of metal toxicity.
Limitations:	▪ Patients with toxic metal accumulation frequently have accumulation of chemical xenobiotics as well; thus testing for and treating toxicity due to metals only relieves one type of toxicity.
Comments:	▪ Clinicians should establish pathways for the assessment and treatment of toxic metal accumulation.

Presentation: Widespread musculoskeletal pain resembling fibromyalgia secondary to lead and mercury accumulation: This 54yo athletic female with healthy diet, lifestyle, and supportive relationship presented with chronic diffuse musculoskeletal pain. Health history was sigificant for decades of environmental illness/intolerance (EI) also known as multiple chemical sensitivity (MCS). Family history was positive for maternal temporal (giant cell) arteritis. Physical examination revealed numerous tender points consistent with fibromyalgia; yet the history and stool analysis with comprehensive bacteriology and parasitology were unsupportive of gastrointestinal dysbiosis, particularly of the subtype small intestine bacterial overgrowth, which is causal for fibromyalgia.[239] Laboratory investigations revealed normal results for hsCRP (high-sensitity c-reactive protein), CK (creatine kinase, a marker of muscle damage and myositis), ANA (anti-nuclear antibodies), vitamin D, calcium, phosphorus, and comprehensive thyroid evaluation. The patient was then (defensively) referred to an osteopathic internist who diagnosed fibromyalgia.

Date Completed: 10/22/2005

| Lead | 30 | < | 5 |
| Mercury | 21 | < | 3 |

Discussion: The patient, unsatisfied with the diagnosis of fibromyalgia, returned to the current author, who then performed urine heavy metal testing provoked with 10 mg per kilogram of dimercaptosuccinic acid (DMSA). Results revealed the highest levels of lead and mercury encountered in the author's practice at that time. As shown above, lead levels were 6x above the reference range and mercury levels were 7x above the reference range. The patient was commenced on DMSA 10 mg/kg/d on alternating weeks to avoid toxicity in general and bone marrow toxicity (neutropenia) in particular, selenium 800 mcg/d to promote excretion of toxic metals and to support renal and antoxidant protection, vegetable juices to provide potassium and citrate for urinary alkalinization and enhanced excretion of xenobiotics[240], and a proprietary phytochelatin (metal-binding peptides from plants[241]) concetrate to bind toxic metals in the gut and thereby promote their fecal excretion by blocking enterohepatic recycling/recirculation. The use of DMSA for children and adults is supported by peer-reviewed literature[242,243,244,245,246] and has been reviewed in more detail by this author in *Integrative Rheumatology*[247] and to a lesser extent in *Musculoskeletal Pain: Expanded Clinical Strategies*.[248] DMSA chelation is approved by the US Food and Drug Administration (FDA) for the treatment of lead toxicity in children.[249] After approximately 8 months of treatment, the patient was completely free of pain, and the clinical improvement was associated with a reduction in both lead and mercury of approximately 50% as demonstrated by follow-up laboratory testing. Testing was performed by Doctors Data. This case was published in peer-reviewed literature for continuing education credits.[250]

Date Completed: 6/30/2006

| Lead | 15 | < | 5 |
| Mercury | 8.2 | < | 4 |

[239] **Vasquez A.** Musculoskeletal Pain: Expanded Clinical Strategies. Institute for Functional Medicine. 2008

[240] Crinnion WJ. Environmental medicine, part three: long-term effects of chronic low-dose mercury exposure. *Altern Med Rev*. 2000 Jun;5(3):209-23 http://www.thorne.com/altmedrev/.fulltext/5/3/209.pdf

[241] Cobbett CS. Phytochelatins and their roles in heavy metal detoxification. *Plant Physiol*. 2000;123:825-32 plantphysiol.org/content/123/3/825

[242] Bradstreet J, Geier DA, Kartzinel JJ, Adams JB, Geier MR. A case-control study of mercury burden in children with autistic spectrum disorders. *Journal of American Physicians and Surgeons* 2003; 8: 76-79 http://www.jpands.org/vol8no3/geier.pdf

[243] Crinnion WJ. Environmental medicine, part three: long-term effects of chronic low-dose mercury exposure. *Altern Med Rev*. 2000 Jun;5(3):209-23

[244] Forman J, Moline J, Cernichiari E, Sayegh S, Torres JC, Landrigan MM, Hudson J, Adel HN, Landrigan PJ. A cluster of pediatric metallic mercury exposure cases treated with meso-2,3-dimercaptosuccinic acid (DMSA). *Environ Health Perspect*. 2000 Jun;108(6):575-7 http://ehp.niehs.nih.gov/docs/2000/108p575-577forman/abstract.html

[245] Miller AL. Dimercaptosuccinic acid (DMSA), a non-toxic, water-soluble treatment for heavy metal toxicity. *Altern Med Rev*. 1998 Jun;3(3):199-207 http://www.thorne.com/altmedrev/.fulltext/3/3/199.pdf

[246] DMSA. *Altern Med Rev*. 2000 Jun;5(3):264-7 http://thorne.com/altmedrev/.fulltext/5/3/264.pdf

[247] **Vasquez A.** Integrative Rheumatology. IBMRC 2006, 2007 and all future editions. http://optimalhealthresearch.com/rheumatology.html

[248] **Vasquez A.** Musculoskeletal Pain: Expanded Clinical Strategies. Institute for Functional Medicine. 2008

[249] "The Food and Drug Administration has recently licensed the drug DMSA (succimer) for reduction of blood lead levels >/= 45 micrograms/dl. This decision was based on the demonstrated ability of DMSA to reduce blood lead levels. An advantage of this drug is that it can be given orally." Goyer RA, Cherian MG, Jones MM, Reigart JR. Role of chelating agents for prevention, intervention, and treatment of exposures to toxic metals. *Environ Health Perspect*. 1995 Nov;103(11):1048-52 Http://ehp.niehs.nih.gov/docs/1995/103-11/meetingreport.html

[250] **Vasquez A.** Musculoskeletal Pain: Expanded Clinical Strategies. Institute for Functional Medicine. 2008

Presentation: Chronic "idiopathic" hypertension associated with lead and mercury accumulation (per DMSA-provoked urine testing): This 43yo male presents with recalcitrant stage-1 hypertension. His cardiologist prescribed drugs to "treat" (some would say "mask") his elevated blood pressure. Since hypertension always has an underlying cause, the ethical and appropriate course of action is to determine the cause of the problem rather than silencing the alarm that is alerting to an underlying dysfunction. While this case is currently in progress at the time of this writing (the patient's medical records arrived in July 2011), it does offer a model case for clinical decision-making. Clinicians should be aware that, per animal studies, the toxicity of lead and mercury are greatly enhanced when both toxins are present at the same time.

				Date Collected:	6/3/2010
Lead	8.5	<	2		
Mercury	17	<	3		

Mercury and hypertension: Mercury is an established neurotoxin, immunotoxin, and nephrotoxin. Because pathophysiologic effects are noted even with very small doses of exposure, one could reasonably argue that no safe amount exists and therefore that any detected mercury is an indication for therapeutic intervention to remove this toxicant. Sources of exposure include dental amalgams, vaccinations, airborne pollution, and fish; recently, high-fructose corn syrup was shown to contain mercury.[251] Mercury impairs catecholamine degradation and can thereby cause a clinical syndrome that can include hypertension, tremor, tachycardia, diaphoresis, and neurocognitive changes.[252] Per Shih and Gartner[253], "Mercury combines with the sulfhydryl group of S-adenosylmethionine, which is a cofactor for catecholamine-O-methyltransferase (COMT), and this inhibition of COMT allows accumulation of norepinephrine, epinephrine, and dopamine."

Lead and hypertension: In the United States, a consistent correlation has been found between body burden of lead and HTN, even when blood lead levels are well below the current US occupational exposure limit guidelines (40 microg/dl).[254] Harlan et al[255] analyzed data from the second National Health and Nutrition Examination Survey (1976-1980) and thereby found a direct relationship between blood lead levels and systolic and diastolic pressures for men and women and for white and black persons aged 12 to 74 years; they concluded, "Blood lead levels were significantly higher in younger men and women (aged 21 to 55 years) with high blood pressure, but not in older men or women (aged 56 to 74 years)." Schwartz and Stewart[256] found that blood lead was the assessment that most strongly correlated with HTN; they concluded, "Systolic blood pressure was elevated by blood lead levels as low as 5 microg/dl." Thus, clinicians might first measure blood lead levels, which do not measure total body burden but rather the lead that is mobile or *in transit* within the body and which appears to have the best correlation with HTN; the finding of normal blood lead results could then be followed with the more sensitive DMSA-provoked heavy metal testing before concluding that heavy metals are noncontributory to that particular patient's HTN. For heavy metal testing in various clinical scenarios, this author's preference is to use DMSA-provoked measurement of urine toxic metals. After a minimal test dose of DMSA (e.g., in the range of 50-100 mg) to screen for hypersensitivity, patients take oral DMSA 10 mg/kg as a single oral dose in the morning on an empty stomach after emptying the bladder and send a sample from the next urination for laboratory analysis; follow laboratory protocol if different from these instructions. Use of DMSA for lead and mercury chelation/detoxification and for diagnostic purposes is generally safe and effective[257,258,259]; detoxification procedures are reviewed in much greater detail in *Integrative Rheumatology*.[260]

---

[251] "Average daily consumption of high fructose corn syrup is about 50 grams per person in the United States. With respect to total mercury exposure, it may be necessary to account for this source of mercury in the diet of children and sensitive populations." Dufault R, LeBlanc B, Schnoll R, Cornett C, Schweitzer L, Wallinga D, Hightower J, Patrick L, Lukiw WJ. Mercury from chlor-alkali plants: measured concentrations in food product sugar. *Environ Health*. 2009 Jan 26;8:2. See also: "High fructose corn syrup has been shown to contain trace amounts of mercury as a result of some manufacturing processes, and its consumption can also lead to zinc loss." Dufault R, Schnoll R, Lukiw WJ, Leblanc B, Cornett C, Patrick L, Wallinga D, Gilbert SG, Crider R. Mercury exposure, nutritional deficiencies and metabolic disruptions may affect learning in children. *Behav Brain Funct*. 2009 Oct 27;5:44.

[252] Wössmann W, Kohl M, Grüning G, Bucsky P. Mercury intoxication presenting with hypertension and tachycardia. *Arch Dis Child*. 1999 Jun;80(6):556-7 http://www.ncbi.nlm.nih.gov/pmc/articles/PMC1717944/pdf/v080p00556.pdf

[253] Shih H, Gartner JC Jr. Weight loss, hypertension, weakness, and limb pain in an 11-year-old boy. *J Pediatr*. 2001 Apr;138(4):566-9

[254] Nash D, Magder L, Lustberg M, Sherwin RW, Rubin RJ, Kaufmann RB, Silbergeld EK. Blood lead, blood pressure, and hypertension in perimenopausal and postmenopausal women. *JAMA*. 2003 Mar 26;289(12):1523-32 http://jama.ama-assn.org/cgi/content/full/289/12/1523

[255] Harlan WR, Landis JR, Schmouder RL, Goldstein NG, Harlan LC. Blood lead and blood pressure. Relationship in the adolescent and adult US population. *JAMA*. 1985 Jan 25;253(4):530-4

[256] "Systolic blood pressure was elevated by blood lead levels as low as 5 microg/dl." Schwartz BS, Stewart WF. Different associations of blood lead, meso 2,3-dimercaptosuccinic acid (DMSA)-chelatable lead, and tibial lead levels with blood pressure in 543 former organolead manufacturing workers. *Arch Environ Health*. 2000 Mar-Apr;55(2):85-92

[257] Bradstreet J, Geier DA, Kartzinel JJ, Adams JB, Geier MR. A case-control study of mercury burden in children with autistic spectrum disorders. *Journal of American Physicians and Surgeons* 2003; 8: 76-79 http://www.jpands.org/vol8no3/geier.pdf

[258] Miller AL. Dimercaptosuccinic acid (DMSA), a non-toxic, water-soluble treatment for heavy metal toxicity. *Altern Med Rev*. 1998 Jun;3(3):199-207

[259] DMSA. *Altern Med Rev*. 2000 Jun;5(3):264-7 http://thorne.com/altmedrev/.fulltext/5/3/264.pdf

[260] **Vasquez A**. Integrative Rheumatology. IBMRC 2006, 2007 and all future editions. http://optimalhealthresearch.com/rheumatology.html

Antinuclear antibody: ANA

Overview and interpretation:	<ul><li>**Good screening test for autoimmune conditions**: SLE, Sjogren's syndrome, and various other connective tissue diseases.</li><li>Good and "highly sensitive" for initial assessment of SLE; positive in 95-98% of SLE patients; negative result strongly suggests against diagnosis of SLE.[261] Only 2% of patients with SLE have a negative ANA test—these patients may be identified by testing with anti-RO antibodies and CH50 (complement levels).</li><li>This test measures for the presence of antibodies that react to nucleoproteins. Some labs report titers of 1:20 or 1:40 as "positive"; however, low levels of ANA are common (5-15%) in the general population. Thus, ANA is not specific for any one disease; may be positive in SLE, RA, scleroderma, Sjogren's, also seen with elderly, infected patients, cancer, and certain medications. Titers less than 1:160 should be interpreted cautiously as they may not indicate the presence of *clinical* autoimmunity.[262] **Titers greater than 1:320 are considered indicative of clinically significant autoimmunity.**</li><li>Methodologies (indirect immunofluorescence is most popular), subtypes, and patterns reported for ANA results may be irrelevant or clinically meaningful; the most common descriptors are provided in the table below.</li></ul>

ANA patterns and descriptions[263,264]	*Clinical correlation*
Homogeneous, diffuse nuclear staining	Nonspecific
Speckled	Least specific
Rim or **peripheral staining**	Suggests SLE and warrants assessment for anti-dsDNA, which is specific for lupus
Anti-centromere: selective staining of the centromeres of nuclei in metaphase	Highly specific for the limited scleroderma subtype associated with CREST syndrome
Nucleolar	Correlated with diffuse scleroderma (systemic sclerosis)
FANA: fluorescent ANA	The standard ANA test in the US
Anti-Sm: anti-Smith[265]	<u>Virtually diagnostic of SLE</u>: Highly specific for SLE; insensitive: positive in 20-30% of SLE patients
Anti-dsDNA: anti-double stranded DNA	<u>Virtually diagnostic of SLE</u>: Highly specific for SLE and indicative of an increased likelihood of poor prognosis with major organ involvement[266] especially active renal disease
Anti-Ro (anti-SS-A)	Correlates with SLE, Sjögren's syndrome, and neonatal SLE
Anti-La (anti-SS-B)	Sjögren's syndrome or low risk of SLE nephritis
Anti-RNP	SLE and/or mixed connective tissue disease (MCTD)
Anti-Jo-1	Specific but not sensitive for polymyositis/dermatomyositis
Antihistone	SLE and especially drug-induced SLE
Antitopoisomerase (Scl-70)	Correlates with diffuse scleroderma, especially with interstitial lung disease

[261] Shojania K. Rheumatology: 2. What laboratory tests are needed? *CMAJ*. 2000 Apr 18;162(8):1157-63 http://www.cmaj.ca/cgi/content/full/162/8/1157
[262] Hardin JG, Waterman J, Labson LH. Rheumatic disease: Which diagnostic tests are useful? *Patient Care* 1999; March 15: 83-102
[263] Shojania K. Rheumatology: 2. What laboratory tests are needed? *CMAJ*. 2000 Apr 18;162(8):1157-63 http://www.cmaj.ca/cgi/content/full/162/8/1157
[264] Ward MM. Laboratory testing for systemic rheumatic diseases. *Postgrad Med.* 1998 Feb;103(2):93-100.
[265] Lane SK, Gravel JW Jr. Clinical utility of common serum rheumatologic tests. *Am Fam Physician.* 2002;65:1073-80 http://www.aafp.org/afp/20020315/1073.html
[266] Shojania K. Rheumatology: 2. What laboratory tests are needed? *CMAJ*. 2000 Apr 18;162(8):1157-63 http://www.cmaj.ca/cgi/content/full/162/8/1157

Antinuclear antibody: ANA—*continued*	
Advantages:	■ ANA has 98% sensitivity and 90% specificity for SLE in an unselected population. ■ The negative predictive value in an unselected population is greater than 99%. ANA is therefore an excellent test for *excluding* the diagnosis of SLE.
Limitations:	■ The positive predictive value in an unselected population is about 30%; **only 30% of unselected people with a positive result will have SLE**—this fact underscores the importance of patient selection and judicious interpretation of this test. ■ Positive ANA is seen in patients with conditions other than SLE, including rheumatoid arthritis, Sjogren's syndrome, scleroderma, polymyositis, vasculitis, juvenile rheumatoid arthritis (JRA), and infectious diseases.
Comments:	■ ANA is most often used to support the diagnosis of SLE in a patient with multisystemic illness and a clinical picture compatible with SLE. Nearly all patients with SLE will have positive ANA. **A positive ANA does not mean that the patient necessarily has SLE; be weary of paraneoplastic syndromes and viral hepatitis as underlying causative processes in patients with an unclear clinical picture.** ■ I view any "positive ANA" as an indicator of poor health in general and immune dysfunction in particular. The goal, then, is to restore health. I have seen ANA show a trend toward normalization or completely normalize with effective health restoration as detailed in *Integrative Rheumatology* (chapter 4). I realize that my experience in this regard contrasts sharply with the allopathic view that serial measurements of ANA are worthless because the result never normalizes once a patient is ANA-positive[267]; I consider this evidence of the effectiveness of my integrative-functional approach and the comparable failure of the allopathic approach.

Antineutrophilic cytoplasmic antibodies: ANCA	

Overview:	■ ANCA are autoantibodies to the cytoplasmic constituents of granulocytes and are characteristically found in vasculitic syndromes and also in (Chinese) patients with inflammatory bowel disease[268] and nearly all patients with hepatic amebiasis due to *Entamoeba histolytica.*[269]
	
	Two types:
	  ■ Cytoplasmic ANCA (C-ANCA): classically seen in **Wegener's granulomatosis**; also seen in some types of glomerulonephritis and vasculitis; this test is highly sensitive and specific for these conditions. In fact, a positive C-ANCA result can replace biopsy in a patient with a clinical picture of **Wegener's granulomatosis.**[270]
	  ■ Perinuclear ANCA (P-ANCA): considered a nonspecific finding[271] that correlates with SLE, drug induced lupus, and some types of glomerulonephritis and vasculitis. Shojania[272] stated that this test must be confirmed with antimyeloperoxidase antibodies to evaluate for Churg–Strauss syndrome, crescentic glomerulonephritis, and microscopic polyarteritis.

Advantages, limitations, and comments	■ Not to be used as a screening test, except in patients with idiopathic vasculitis or glomerulonephritis. ■ The fact that hepatic amebiasis due to *Entamoeba histolytica* induces production of C-ANCA antibodies in nearly 100% of infected patients may support the hypothesis that autoimmunity can be induced or exacerbated by parasitic infections.

[267] Shojania K. Rheumatology: 2. What laboratory tests are needed? *CMAJ.* 2000 Apr 18;162(8):1157-63 http://www.cmaj.ca/cgi/content/full/162/8/1157

[268] "Fourteen patients (73.5%) were positive, of which six (31.5%) showed a perinuclear staining pattern and eight (42%) demonstrated a cytoplasmic pattern." Sung JY, Chan KL, Hsu R, Liew CT, Lawton JW. Ulcerative colitis and antineutrophil cytoplasmic antibodies in Hong Kong Chinese. *Am J Gastroenterol.* 1993 Jun;88(6):864-9

[269] "ANCA was detected in 97.4% of amoebic sera; the pattern of staining was cytoplasmic, homogeneous, without central accentuation (C-ANCA)." Pudifin DJ, Duursma J, Gathiram V, Jackson TF. Invasive amoebiasis is associated with the development of anti-neutrophil cytoplasmic antibody. *Clin Exp Immunol.* 1994 Jul;97(1):48-5

[270] Shojania K. Rheumatology: 2. What laboratory tests are needed? *CMAJ.* 2000 Apr 18;162(8):1157-63 http://www.cmaj.ca/cgi/content/full/162/8/1157

[271] Shojania K. Rheumatology: 2. What laboratory tests are needed? *CMAJ.* 2000 Apr 18;162(8):1157-63 http://www.cmaj.ca/cgi/content/full/162/8/1157

[272] Shojania K. Rheumatology: 2. What laboratory tests are needed? *CMAJ.* 2000 Apr 18;162(8):1157-63 http://www.cmaj.ca/cgi/content/full/162/8/1157

RF: Rheumatoid Factor	
Overview and application:	• Rheumatoid factor—"anti-IgG antibodies"—are antibodies directed to the Fc portion of the patient's own IgG. Rheumatoid factors are anti-immunoglobulin antibodies, classically anti-IgG IgM. RF are found in low levels in most patients, and despite the "rheumatoid" name, RF is not specific for rheumatoid arthritis.[273] Current tests (latex fixation or nephelometry) detect IgM anti-immunoglobulin antibodies; however IgA-RF appears to have clinical superiority over other forms of RF because it correlates more strongly with clinical status.[274] • This test is most commonly used to support the diagnosis of rheumatoid arthritis in a patient with a compelling clinical picture: peripheral polyarthritis lasting >6 weeks.[275] A negative result with a compelling clinical presentation of RA is termed "seronegative rheumatoid arthritis" by allopathic textbooks whereas a more appropriate term might be oligoarthritis, a condition described as "idiopathic" by allopathic text books despite the clear evidence that the majority of patients have one or more subsets of dysbiosis.[276] • **Titers (latex fixation) of 1:160 are considered clinically significant, favoring the diagnosis of RA.**[277] However the positive predictive value is low—only 20-34% of people in an unselected population with a positive test result actually have RA.[278,279]
Advantages:	• Supports the diagnosis of rheumatoid arthritis: about 60-85% positive/sensitive in patients with rheumatoid arthritis (RA).[280,281] Quantitative titers of RF correlate with prognosis: a very high RF value portends a poor prognosis.
Limitations:	• **Positive findings are common in the following conditions: rheumatoid arthritis, viral hepatitis, Sjögren's syndrome, endocarditis, scleroderma, mycobacteria diseases, polymyositis and dermatomyositis, syphilis, systemic lupus erythematosus, old age, mixed connective tissue disease, sarcoidosis**; positive results may also been noted in: **cryoglobulinemia, parasitic infection, interstitial lung disease, asymptomatic relatives of people with autoimmune diseases.** • Febrile patients with arthralgia are more likely to have endocarditis than RA.[282] • Patients with iron overload present with a similar clinical picture (i.e., polyarthropathy with systemic complaints) and may have a positive RF. Thus, patients with positive RF and polyarthropathy should be tested for iron overload; use serum ferritin.[283,284]
Comments:	• This test should only be used to confirm the diagnosis of rheumatoid arthritis in patients with a compelling clinical picture of the disease: inflammatory peripheral polyarthropathy with systemic complaints for > 6 weeks. A negative result does not mean that the patient *does not* have rheumatoid arthritis; a positive result does not mean that the patient *does* have rheumatoid arthritis.[285] • CCP (cyclic citrullinated protein) antibodies appear to be more specific and sensitive for RA and is becoming the test of choice for RA as described on the following page.

[273] Shojania K. Rheumatology: 2. What laboratory tests are needed? *CMAJ*. 2000 Apr 18;162(8):1157-63 http://www.cmaj.ca/cgi/content/full/162/8/1157
[274] Jonsson T, Valdimarsson H. What about IgA rheumatoid factor in rheumatoid arthritis? *Ann Rheum Dis*. 1998 Jan;57(1):63-4
[275] Shojania K. Rheumatology: 2. What laboratory tests are needed? *CMAJ*. 2000 Apr 18;162(8):1157-63 http://www.cmaj.ca/cgi/content/full/162/8/1157
[276] See chapter 4 of *Integrative Rheumatology* and Vasquez A. Reducing Pain and Inflammation Naturally. Part 6: Nutritional and Botanical Treatments Against "Silent Infections" and Gastrointestinal Dysbiosis, Commonly Overlooked Causes of Neuromusculoskeletal Inflammation and Chronic Health Problems. *Nutr Perspect* 2006; Jan http://optimalhealthresearch.com/part6.html
[277] Beers MH, Berkow R (eds). The Merck Manual. Seventeenth Edition. Whitehouse Station; Merck Research Laboratories 1999 Page 417
[278] Ward MM. Laboratory testing for systemic rheumatic diseases. *Postgrad Med*. 1998 Feb;103(2):93-100.
[279] Shojania K. Rheumatology: 2. What laboratory tests are needed? *CMAJ*. 2000 Apr 18;162(8):1157-63 http://www.cmaj.ca/cgi/content/full/162/8/1157
[280] Tierney ML. McPhee SJ, Papadakis MA (eds). Current Medical Diagnosis and Treatment 2002, 41st Edition. New York: Lange Medical, 2002 p854
[281] Shojania K. Rheumatology: 2. What laboratory tests are needed? *CMAJ*. 2000 Apr 18;162(8):1157-63 http://www.cmaj.ca/cgi/content/full/162/8/1157
[282] Klippel JH (ed). Primer on the Rheumatic Diseases. 11th Edition. Atlanta: Arthritis Foundation. 1997 page 96
[283] Bensen WG, Laskin CA, Little HA, Fam AG. Hemochromatoic arthropathy mimicking rheumatoid arthritis. A case with subcutaneous nodules, tenosynovitis, and bursitis. *Arthritis Rheum* 1978; 21: 844-8
[284] **Vasquez A**. Musculoskeletal disorders and iron overload disease: comment on the American College of Rheumatology guidelines for the initial evaluation of the adult patient with acute musculoskeletal symptoms. *Arthritis Rheum* 1996;39: 1767-8
[285] Shojania K. Rheumatology: 2. What laboratory tests are needed? *CMAJ*. 2000 Apr 18;162(8):1157-63 http://www.cmaj.ca/cgi/content/full/162/8/1157

	CCP: Cyclic citrullinated protein antibody; Citrullinated protein antibodies (CPA); anti-CCP antibodies: anticyclic citrullinated peptide antibody	
Overview and use:	<ul><li>CCP—cyclic citrullinated protein antibodies; anticitrullinated protein antibodies: this is a relatively new auto-antibody marker that shows great promise and specificity for the early diagnosis of rheumatoid arthritis (RA). The test often becomes positive/present in asymptomatic patients years before the onset of clinical manifestations of RA.</li><li>As of the first inclusion of this information in my books in December 2006, the information on anti-CCP antibodies is so new that it is not even included in most 2006-edition medical and rheumatology reference textbooks; nonetheless, doctors nationwide are already starting to use this test for the early diagnosis of RA. This may be particularly important because some research has shown that *early* and *aggressive* treatment of RA has an important impact on long-term prognosis[286]; however, the importance of early intervention is debatable.[287]</li><li>Anti-CCP antibodies are directed toward several native proteins (e.g., filaggrin, fibrinogen, and vimentin) that have become posttranslationally modified by a uncharged citrulline in contrast to the normal positively charged arginine. This "citrullination" is catalyzed by a calcium-dependent enzyme, **peptidylarginine deiminase (PAD)**. These changes in protein charge and sequence make the native protein a target of auto-antibody attack by IgG antibodies in RA.[288] However, this does not necessarily imply that citrullination of native proteins is "the cause" of RA because citrullination of native proteins can also occur *de novo* in inflamed joints, which are then further targeted for inflammatory destruction. Until more information is available, we should withhold final judgment as to the ultimate role and origin of anti-CCP antibodies and in the meanwhile view them as a very strong and sensitive association with RA that facilitates the early diagnosis of this disease.</li></ul>
Advantages:	<ul><li>Anti-CCP antibodies have 98% specificity for RA[289] and is likely to become the future laboratory standard in the diagnosis and prognosis of RA.[290] Anti-CCP antibodies with a positive rheumatoid factor (RF) is termed "composite seropositivity" and appears to be more specific than isolated anti-CCP antibodies or RF.[291]</li></ul>
Limitations:	<ul><li>**The best current data indicates that anti-CCP antibodies are sensitive and specific for RA[292], and clinicians should use this test to diagnose and confirm RA.**</li></ul>
Comments:	<ul><li>Healthy people do not generally have anti-CCP antibodies. Asymptomatic patients with anti-CCP antibodies are at increased risk for clinical RA and are probably *en route* to the manifestation of clinical autoimmunity—RA, Sjogren's disease, or SLE. *Holistically intervene.*</li><li>I hypothesize that PAD may become upregulated in synovial joints exposed to allergens, xenobiotics, bacterial debris/toxins/lipopolysaccharides and that the subsequent citrullination of joint proteins may lead to an autoimmune arthropathy that persists, perhaps despite removal of the inciting immunogen. More obviously, given that PAD is calcium-dependent, it may be upregulated secondary to intracellular hypercalcinosis secondary to vitamin D deficiency, magnesium deficiency, or fatty acid imbalance.[293]</li></ul>

[286] "CONCLUSION: An initial 6-month cycle of intensive combination treatment that includes high-dose corticosteroids results in sustained suppression of the rate of radiologic progression in patients with early RA, independent of subsequent antirheumatic therapy." Landewe RB, et al. COBRA combination therapy in patients with early rheumatoid arthritis: long-term structural benefits of a brief intervention. *Arthritis Rheum.* 2002 Feb;46:347-56

[287] "By 5 years patients receiving early DMARDs had similar disease activity and comparable health assessment questionnaire scores to patients who received DMARDs later in their disease course." Scott DL. Evidence for early disease-modifying drugs in rheumatoid arthritis. *Arthritis Res Ther.* 2004;6(1):15-18 http://arthritis-research.com/content/6/1/15

[288] Hill J, Cairns E, Bell DA. The joy of citrulline. *J Rheumatol.* 2004 Aug;31(8):1471-3 http://www.jrheum.com/subscribers/04/08/1471.html

[289] Hill J, Cairns E, Bell DA. The joy of citrulline. *J Rheumatol.* 2004 Aug;31(8):1471-3

[290] "We conclude that, at present, the antibody response directed to citrullinated antigens has the most valuable diagnostic and prognostic potential for RA." van Boekel MA, Vossenaar ER, van den Hoogen FH, van Venrooij WJ. Autoantibody systems in rheumatoid arthritis: specificity, sensitivity and diagnostic value. *Arthritis Res.* 2002;4(2):87-93 http://arthritis-research.com/content/4/2/87

[291] "...our findings suggest that a positive anti-CCP antibody result does not necessarily exclude SLE in African American patients presenting with inflammatory arthritis. In such patients, the additional assessment of IgA-RF or IgM-RF isotypes may be of added value since composite seropositivity appears to be nearly exclusive to patients with RA." Mikuls TR, Holers VM, Parrish L, et al. Anti-cyclic citrullinated peptide antibody and rheumatoid factor isotypes in African Americans with early rheumatoid arthritis. *Arthritis Rheum.* 2006 Sep;54(9):3057-9

[292] "Serum antibodies reactive with citrullinated proteins/peptides are a very sensitive and specific marker for rheumatoid arthritis." Migliorini P, Pratesi F, Tommasi C, Anzilotti C. The immune response to citrullinated antigens in autoimmune diseases. *Autoimmun Rev.* 2005 Nov;4(8):561-4

[293] See optimalhealthresearch.com/archives/intracellular-hypercalcinosis and naturopathydigest.com/archives/2006/sep/vasquez.php for discussion

HLA-B27: Human leukocyte antigen B-27	

Overview and interpretation:	▪ A common (5-10% of general population) genetic marker strongly associated with seronegative* spondyloarthropathy (all of which occur more commonly in men[294]):
	   1. Ankylosing spondylitis (90-95% of 'whites' and 50% of 'blacks')[295]
	   2. Reactive arthritis [formerly called Reiter's syndrome] (85%)
	   3. Enteropathic spondyloarthropathy
	   4. Psoriatic spondylitis (<60%)
	
	* Recall that "seronegative" in this context implies that the *rheumatoid factor is negative*, even though *the HLA-B27 may be positive*.

Advantages: Limitations: Comments:	▪ *From a diagnostic perspective*: The clinical application and significance of this test is of limited value. All of the above-listed conditions are better assessed with the combination of clinical assessment and radiographs. In a patient with early and mild disease, this test may add evidence either supporting or refuting the diagnosis; but the test itself is not diagnostic of anything other than a genetic/histologic marker associated with various types of infection-induced arthropathy and autoimmunity (dysbiotic arthropathy[296]). ▪ *From an integrative/functional medicine perspective*: This test can be of some value if the result is positive and the patient has evidence of a systemic inflammatory/autoimmune disorder since it therefore more strongly suggests that a dysbiotic locus is the cause of disease.[297] A consistent theme in the rheumatology literature is that of "molecular mimicry"—the phenomenon by which structural similarities between human and microbial structures lead to targeting of human tissues by immune responses aimed at microbial antigens. This topic is explored in considerable detail in the section on multifocal dysbiosis in *Integrative Rheumatology*. The important link between microbe-induced autoimmunity and HLA-B27 is that many dysbiotic bacteria produce an HLA-B27-like molecule that appears to trigger an immune response which then erroneously affects human tissues, leading to the clinical picture of autoimmune inflammation. Many of these HLA-B27-producing bacteria colonize the gastrointestinal and genitourinary tracts, promoting musculoskeletal inflammation via molecular mimicry and other mechanisms.[298,299] A strong and growing body of research shows that HLA-B27 is a risk factor for microbe-induced autoimmunity. "Autoimmune" patients positive for HLA-B27 are presumed to have an occult infection—especially gastrointestinal, genitourinary, or sinorespiratory—until proven otherwise. ▪ **Keep in mind that HLA-B27 itself is not a disease** and therefore a "positive" result merely means that the patient has this particular human leukocyte antigen; this test is not and will never be diagnostic of a specific disease—it simply correlates with increased propensity toward dysbiotic arthropathy and suggests the need for dysbiosis testing and the (re)establishment of eubiosis.[300]

---

[294] "The major diseases associated with HLA-B27 (Reiter's disease, ankylosing spondylitis, acute anterior uveitis, and psoriatic arthritis) all occur much more commonly in men." James WH. Sex ratios and hormones in HLA related rheumatic diseases. *Ann Rheum Dis.* 1991 Jun;50(6):401-4

[295] Shojania K. Rheumatology: 2. What laboratory tests are needed? *CMAJ.* 2000 Apr 18;162(8):1157-63 http://www.cmaj.ca/cgi/content/full/162/8/1157

[296] See chapter 4 of *Integrative Rheumatology* and **Vasquez A**. Reducing Pain and Inflammation Naturally. Part 6: Nutritional and Botanical Treatments Against "Silent Infections" and Gastrointestinal Dysbiosis, Commonly Overlooked Causes of Neuromusculoskeletal Inflammation and Chronic Health Problems. *Nutr Perspect* 2006; Jan http://optimalhealthresearch.com/part6.html

[297] "The association between HLA-B27 and reactive arthritis (ReA) has also been well established… In a similar way, microbiological and immunological studies have revealed an association between Klebsiella pneumoniae in AS and Proteus mirabilis in RA." Ebringer A, Wilson C. HLA molecules, bacteria and autoimmunity. *J Med Microbiol.* 2000 Apr;49(4):305-11

[298] **Inman RD. Antigens, the gastrointestinal tract, and arthritis.** *Rheum Dis Clin North Am.* **1991 May;17(2):309-21**

[299] **Hunter JO. Food allergy--or enterometabolic disorder?** *Lancet.* **1991 Aug 24;338(8765):495-6**

[300] Dysbiotic arthropathy—joint inflammation and destruction as a result of a neuroimmune inflammatory response to microorganisms. Phrase coined by Alex Vasquez on December 15, 2005. No matching term on Medline or Google search. See chapter 4 of *Integrative Rheumatology* and **Vasquez A**. Reducing Pain and Inflammation Naturally. Part 6: Nutritional and Botanical Treatments Against "Silent Infections" and Gastrointestinal Dysbiosis, Commonly Overlooked Causes of Neuromusculoskeletal Inflammation and Chronic Health Problems. *Nutr Perspect* 2006; Jan http://optimalhealthresearch.com/part6.html

Complement C3 and C4	
Overview and interpretation:	▪ Complement proteins are consumed in the complement cascades (typically activated by immune complexes) and thus low levels of complement proteins provide indirect evidence of extensive consumption due to immune complex-mediated inflammation. **Low levels of complement are seen with immune complex disorders (such as SLE, vasculitis, mixed cryoglobulinemia, rheumatoid vasculitis, glomerulonephritis) and inherited complement deficiencies.** ▪ 10%–15% of Caucasian patients with SLE have an inherited complement deficiency.[301]
Advantages:	▪ Low complement levels provide indirect evidence of immune complex-mediated inflammation. ▪ Elevated levels of complement are seen in conditions of infection or inflammation.
Limitations:	▪ Some patients have a hereditary absence of complement proteins and thus their levels are always abnormally low; obviously the test cannot be used in these patients for monitoring inflammatory disease.

CIC: Circulating immune complexes	
Overview and interpretation:	▪ Antibodies/immunoglobulins are produced in several different "classes": IgG, IgA, IgM, IgE, IgD. IgA antibodies are produced mostly in response to mucosal infections, such as from gastrointestinal dysbiosis or overt infections. When antibodies (in the shape of the letter "Y" with 2 antigen-binding sites on one end and the immuno-reactive site on the other) combine with the target antigen (depicted here in the shape of an oval, such as a bacteria or globular protein), "immune complexes" are formed which are chain-like links of antigens and antibodies. ▪ Although formed in small amounts in healthy persons, in certain disease states, immune complexes may accumulate and initiate complement-dependent injury in various organs and tissues. This activation of complement may begin a series of potentially destructive events in the host, including anaphylatoxin production, cell lysis, leukocyte stimulation, and activation of macrophages and other cells. When immune complexes become fixed to vessel walls, destruction of normal tissue can occur, as in some types of glomerulonephritis and vasculitis. Predisposed to deposition in joints, vessels, and kidneys, immune complexes contribute directly to tissue injury in several autoimmune-inflammatory diseases.[302] **Immune Complexes, (Raji Cell), Quantitative** ▪ <u>Reference Range:</u> (Enzyme immunoassay [EIA]; cost $130) ▪ <u>Normal:</u> ≤15.0 μg Eq/mL ▪ <u>Equivocal:</u> 15.1-19.9 μg Eq/mL ▪ <u>Positive:</u> ≥20.0 μg Eq/mL
Advantages:	▪ This test allows for direct quantification of immune-complex production.
Limitations:	▪ This test has only recently become available to practicing clinicians; however, it is very well supported by many publications in peer-reviewed research.[303]

[301] Shojania K. Rheumatology: 2. What laboratory tests are needed? *CMAJ.* 2000 Apr 18;162(8):1157-63 http://www.cmaj.ca/cgi/content/full/162/8/1157
[302] Jancar S, Sánchez Crespo M. Immune complex-mediated tissue injury: a multistep paradigm. *Trends Immunol.* 2005 Jan;26(1):48-55
[303] Davies KA,etal. Immune complex processing in patients with systemic lupus erythematosus. *J Clin Invest* 1992;90:2075-83 jci.org/articles/view/116090

Lactulose-mannitol assay: assessment for intestinal hyperpermeability and malabsorption	
Overview and interpretation:	▪ The lactulose-mannitol assay is a highly validated assessment for the accurate determination of small intestine permeability. This test is used to diagnose "leaky gut", which is a common problem and contributor to systemic inflammation in patients with inflammation and immune dysfunction—see chapter 4 of *Integrative Rheumatology*. Intestinal hyperpermeability reflects inflammation of and damage to the small intestine mucosa and is seen in patients with parasite infections, food allergies, celiac disease, malnutrition, bacterial infections, systemic ischemia or inflammation, ankylosing spondylitis, Crohn's disease, eczema, psoriasis, and those who consume enterotoxins such as NSAIDs and excess ethanol.[304] ▪ Elevations of **lactulose** indicate increased **paracellular** permeability caused by intestinal damage and are diagnostic of "leaky gut." *Clinical pearl:* remember that the "L" in *lactulose* rhymes with *leaky*. ▪ Decrements in **mannitol** suggest impaired **transcellular** absorption and suggest malabsorption in general and villous atrophy in particular. *Clinical pearl:* remember that the "M" in *mannitol* rhymes with *malabsorption*. ▪ Classically, in patients with damaged intestinal mucosa, we generally see a combined ***increase in paracellular*** permeability (measured with lactulose) and a ***reduction in transcellular*** transport (measured with mannitol); these divergent effects result in an increased lactulose-to-mannitol ratio.
Advantages:	▪ This test is safe and affordable for the assessment of small intestine mucosal integrity. Abnormal results—"leaky gut" and/or malabsorption—generally indicate one or more of following: 1. <u>Malnutrition</u>: may be due to poor intake, catabolism, or malabsorption. 2. <u>Enterotoxins</u>: generally NSAIDs or ethanol 3. <u>Food allergies</u>: including celiac disease 4. <u>"Parasites"</u>: including yeast, bacteria, protozoa, amebas, worms, etc.[305] 5. <u>Systemic inflammation</u>: tissue hypoxia, trauma, recent surgery, etc. 6. <u>Genetic predisposition toward enteropathy</u>: check family history for IBD.
Limitations:	▪ Abnormalities and the identification of "leaky gut" are nonspecific and do not point to a specific or single diagnosis or treatment.
Comments:	▪ The value of this test is two-fold: 1) as a screening test for the above-mentioned disorders, and 2) as a method for determining the efficacy of treatment once the cause of the problem has been putatively identified and treated. ▪ This test can be used to promote compliance and to encourage the use of additional testing in patients who are otherwise prone to noncompliance or who resist other tests, such as stool testing. In other words, the clinician can gain an advantage by showing the patient an objective abnormality which then validates the need for treatment and additional testing. ▪ I only use this test on rare occasions because I more commonly either assume that a patient has leaky gut if he/she has one of the aforementioned conditions or we move directly to stool testing and comprehensive parasitology—clearly one of the most valuable tests in the management and treatment of systemic inflammation and immune dysfunction—otherwise known as "autoimmunity" and "allergy."

---

[304] Miller AL. The Pathogenesis, Clinical Implications, and Treatment of Intestinal Hyperpermeability. *Alt Med Rev 1997*:2(5):330-345 http://www.thorne.com/pdf/journal/2-5/intestinalhyperpermiability.pdf
[305] See chapter 4 of *Integrative Rheumatology* and **Vasquez A**. Reducing Pain and Inflammation Naturally. Part 6: Nutritional and Botanical Treatments Against "Silent Infections" and Gastrointestinal Dysbiosis, Commonly Overlooked Causes of Neuromusculoskeletal Inflammation and Chronic Health Problems. *Nutr Perspect* 2006; Jan http://optimalhealthresearch.com/part6.html

Presentation: Highly abnormal lactulose-mannitol ratio in a patient with idiopathic peripheral neuropathy prior to comprehensive stool analysis and parasitology showing intestinal dysbiosis: This 40-yo man presented with a multiyear history of periodic febrile exacerbations of peripheral neuropathy that would cause severe paresthesias and motor deficits. Patient had been evaluated by several board-certified medical neurologists to no avail. Laboratory, imaging, electrodiagnostic studies, and cerebrospinal fluid (CSF) analysis revealed nonspecific abnormalities that did not lead to an established diagnosis. From an integrative naturopathic and functional medicine perspective, food allergy and intestinal dysbiosis are the most obvious probable etiologies; these clinical suspicions were confirmed with laboratory testing showing increased intestinal permeability and gastrointestinal dysbiosis.

Patient:

Age: 40
Sex: M
MRN:

Order Number: 40220637
Completed: April 24, 2003
Received: April 22, 2003
Collected: April 21, 2003

HOUSTON OPTIMAL HEALTH
ALEX VASQUEZ DC ND

Houston, TX 77098

Intestinal Permeability

Lactulose Percent Recovery — Ref Range % — (1.51) — <= 0.80 — 2.00
Mannitol Percent Recovery — Ref Range % — (8) — 5 — 30
Lactulose/Mannitol Ratio — Ref Range — (0.19) — <= 0.03 — 0.20

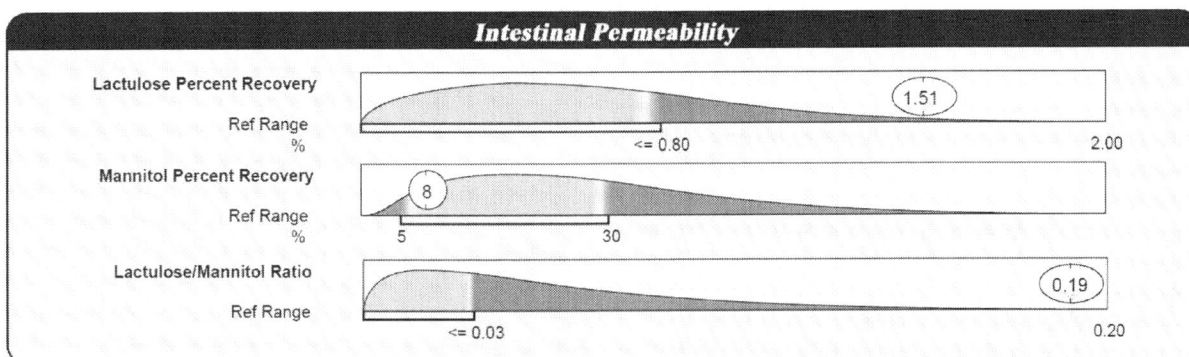

As expected, comprehensive parasitology showed intestinal dysbiosis, including insufficiency of *Lactobacillus* and presence of *Psuedomonas* and abnormal yeast species. Of particular note, *Psuedomonas aeruginosa* shows cross-reactivity with human neuronal tissues.[306,307] Eradication of the dysbiotic condition with a combination of dietary improvement, nutritional supplementation, hormonal optimization, and antimicrobial drugs and herbs lead to rapid and sustained remission of this "idiopathic peripheral neuropathy" which had defied standard medical diagnosis and treatment for many years.

Comprehensive Stool Analysis / Parasitology x3

MICROBIOLOGY

Bacteriology Culture

Beneficial flora		Imbalances		Dysbiotic flora	
Bifidobacter	4+	Haemolytic E. coli	4+	Pseudomonas sp.	4+
E. coli	4+	Gamma strep	2+		
Lactobacillus	2+				

Mycology (Yeast) Culture

Normal flora		Dysbiotic flora
Candida glabrata	1+	
Rhodotorula sp.	1+	

[306] Hughes LE, Bonell S, Natt RS, et al. Antibody responses to Acinetobacter spp. and Pseudomonas aeruginosa in multiple sclerosis: prospects for diagnosis using the myelin-acinetobacter-neurofilament antibody index. *Clin Diagn Lab* Immunol. 2001 Nov;8(6):1181-8 http://cvi.asm.org/content/8/6/1181.full.pdf
[307] Hughes LE, Smith PA, Bonell S, Natt RS, Wilson C, Rashid T, Amor S, Thompson EJ, Croker J, Ebringer A. Cross-reactivity between related sequences found in Acinetobacter sp., Pseudomonas aeruginosa, myelin basic protein and myelin oligodendrocyte glycoprotein in multiple sclerosis. *J Neuroimmunol*. 2003 Nov;144(1-2):105-15

Comprehensive stool analysis and comprehensive parasitology

Overview and interpretation:

- **This is clearly one of the most valuable tests in clinical practice when working with patients with chronic fatigue, systemic inflammation, and autoimmunity. Second only to routine laboratory assessments such as CBC, chemistry panel, and CRP, the importance of stool testing and comprehensive parasitology assessments must be appreciated by progressive clinicians of all disciplines.**

- Stool testing must be performed by a specialty laboratory because the quality of testing provided by most standard "medical labs" and hospitals is completely inadequate. Initial samples should be collected on three separate occasions by the patient and each sample should be analyzed separately by the laboratory.

- Important qualitative and quantitative markers include the following:

  1. **Beneficial bacteria ("probiotics")**: Microbiological testing should quantify and identify various beneficial bacteria, which should be present at "+4" levels on a 0-4 scale.

  2. **Harmful and potentially harmful bacteria, protozoans, amebas, etc.**: Questionable or harmful microbes should be eradicated even if they are not identified as true pathogens in the Paleo-classic Pasteurian/Kochian sense.[308]

  3. **Yeast and mycology**: At least two tests must be performed for a complete assessment: 1) yeast culture, and 2) microscopic examination for yeast elements. Both tests are necessary because some patients—perhaps those with the most severe symptomatology and the most favorable response to anti-yeast treatment—will have a negative yeast culture and positive findings on the microscopic examination. In other words, these patients have intestinal yeast that contributes to their disease/symptomatology but which does not grow on culture despite being clearly visible with microscopy; a similar pattern (using a swab of the rectal mucosa rather than microscopy) is referred to as "negative culture with positive smear."[309]

  4. **Microbial sensitivity testing**: An important component to parasitology testing is the determination of which anti-microbial agents (natural and synthetic) the microbe is sensitive to. This helps to guide and enhance the effectiveness of anti-microbial therapy.

  5. **Secretory IgA**: SIgA levels are elevated in patients who are having an immune response to either food or microbial antigens.[310] Thus, in a patient with minimal dysbiosis, say for example with *Candida albicans*, an elevated sIgA can indicate that the patient is having a hypersensitivity reaction to an otherwise benign microbe—in this case, eradication of the microbe is warranted and may result in a positive clinical response. Low sIgA suggests either primary or secondary immune defect such as selective sIgA deficiency[311] or malnutrition, stress, prednisone/corticosteroids, or possibly mycotoxicosis (immunosuppression due to fungal immunotoxins). In addition to addressing any systemic causative factors, a low sIgA may be addressed with the administration of bovine colostrum, glutamine, vitamin A, and *Saccharomyces boulardii*; the following doses may be considered for use in adults with proportionately smaller doses for children:

     - Bovine colostrum: 2.4 – 3.6 grams per day in divided doses for adults. No drug interactions are known. Side effects may include increased energy, insomnia, and

[308] **Vasquez A.** Reducing Pain and Inflammation Naturally. Part 6: Nutritional and Botanical Treatments Against "Silent Infections" and Gastrointestinal Dysbiosis, Commonly Overlooked Causes of Neuromusculoskeletal Inflammation and Chronic Health Problems. *Nutr Perspect* 2006; Jan http://optimalhealthresearch.com/part6.html

[309] "According to Galland, the best predictor of who will respond to anticandida medication is a negative stool culture combined with a positive smear of the rectal mucosa (for the identification of intracellular hyphal forms of the organism); however, even that test is not 100% reliable." Gaby AR. Before you order that lab test: part 2. *Townsend Letter for Doctors and Patients*. 2004; January findarticles.com/p/articles/mi_m0ISW/is_246/ai_112728028

[310] Quig DW, Higley M. Noninvasive assessment of intestinal inflammation: inflammatory bowel disease vs. irritable bowel syndrome. *Townsend Letter for Doctors and Patients* 2006;Jan:74-5

[311] "Selective IgA deficiency is the most common form of immunodeficiency. Certain select populations, including allergic individuals, patients with autoimmune and gastrointestinal tract disease and patients with recurrent upper respiratory tract illnesses, have an increased incidence of this disorder." Burks AW Jr, Steele RW. Selective IgA deficiency. *Ann Allergy*. 1986;57:3-13

Comprehensive stool analysis and comprehensive parasitology

stimulation. One study in particular used very large doses of 10 grams per day for four days in children and found no adverse effects[312]; another case report of a child involved the use of 50 grams per day for at least two weeks and showed no adverse effects.[313]

- Glutamine: 6 grams 3 times per day (18 grams per day) is a common dosage with significant literature support.
- Vitamin A: Correction of subclinical vitamin A deficiency improves mucosal integrity and increases sIgA production in humans.[314] Common doses used by integrative clinicians are in the range of 200,000 IU to 300,000 for a limited amount of time, generally 1-4 weeks; thereafter the dose is tapered. Patients are educated as to manifestations of toxicity (see the chapter on *Therapeutics* toward the end of this book) and the importance of limited duration of treatment.
- *Saccharomyces boulardii*: Common dose for adults is 250 mg thrice daily; ability of this treatment to increase sIgA levels and its anti-infective efficacy have been documented in human and animal studies.

6. **Short-chain fatty acids**: These are produced by intestinal bacteria. Quantitative excess indicates bacterial overgrowth of the intestines, while insufficiency indicates a lack of probiotics or an insufficiency of dietary substrate, i.e., soluble fiber. Abnormal patterns of individual short-chain fatty acids indicate qualitative/quantitative abnormalities in gastrointestinal microflora, particularly anaerobic bacteria that cannot be identified with routine bacterial cultures.

7. **Beta-glucuronidase**: This is an enzyme produced by several different intestinal bacteria. High levels of beta-glucuronidase in the intestinal lumen serve to nullify the benefits of detoxification (specifically glucuronidation) by cleaving the toxicant from its glucuronide conjugate. This can result in re-absorption of the toxicant through the intestinal mucosa which then re-exposes the patient to the toxin that was previously detoxified ("enterohepatic recirculation" or "enterohepatic recycling"[315]). This is an exemplary aspect of "auto-intoxication" that results in chronic fatigue and upregulation of Phase 1 detoxification systems (chapter 4 of *Integrative Rheumatology*).

8. **Lactoferrin**: The iron-binding glycoprotein lactoferrin is an inflammatory marker that helps distinguish functional disorders (i.e., IBS) from more serious diseases (i.e., IBD). Approximate values are as follows:
   - Healthy and IBS: 2 mcg/ml
   - Severe dysbiosis: up to 120 mcg/ml
   - Inactive IBD: 60-250 mcg/ml
   - Active IBD: > 400 mcg/ml.

9. **Lysozyme**: Elevated in proportion to intestinal inflammation in dysbiosis and IBD.

10. **Other markers**: Other markers of digestion, inflammation, and absorption are reported with the more comprehensive panels performed on stool samples. These tests are not always necessary, but such additional information is always helpful

---

[312] "In this double blind placebo-controlled trial, 80 children with rotavirus diarrhea were randomly assigned to receive orally either 10 g of IIBC (containing 3.6 g of antirotavirus antibodies) daily for 4 days or the same amount of a placebo preparation." Sarker SA, Casswall TH, Mahalanabis D, Alam NH, Albert MJ, Brussow H, Fuchs GJ, Hammerstrom L. Successful treatment of rotavirus diarrhea in children with immunoglobulin from immunized bovine colostrum. *Pediatr Infect Dis J*. 1998 Dec;17(12):1149-54

[313] Lactobin-R is a commercial hyperimmune bovine colostrum with some specificity for cryptosporidiosis; administration to a 4 year old child with AIDS and severe diarrhea resulted in significant clinical improvement in the diarrhea and "permanent elimination of the parasite from the gut as assessed through serial jejunal biopsy and stool specimens." Shield J, Melville C, Novelli V, Anderson G, Scheimberg I, Gibb D, Milla P. Bovine colostrum immunoglobulin concentrate for cryptosporidiosis in AIDS. *Arch Dis Child*. 1993 Oct;69(4):451-3

[314] "It can increase resistance to infection by increasing mucosal integrity, increasing surface immunoglobulin A (sIgA) and enhancing adequate neutrophil function. If infection occurs, vitamin A can act as an immune enhancer, increasing the adequacy of natural killer (NK) cells and increasing antibody production." Faisel H, Pittrof R. Vitamin A and causes of maternal mortality: association and biological plausibility. *Public Health Nutr*. 2000 Sep;3(3):321-7

[315] Parker RJ, Hirom PC, Millburn P.Enterohepatic recycling of phenolphthalein, morphine, lysergic acid diethylamide (LSD) and diphenylacetic acid in the rat. Hydrolysis of glucuronic acid conjugates in the gut lumen. *Xenobiotica*. 1980 Sep;10(9):689-70

Comprehensive stool analysis and comprehensive parasitology	
	when working with complex patients. These markers are relatively self-explanatory and/or are described on the results of the test by the laboratory.
Advantages:	▪ **Stool analysis in general and parasitology assessments in particular provide supremely valuable information in the comprehensive assessment and treatment of patients with complex illnesses such as chronic fatigue, irritable bowel syndrome, fibromyalgia, and all of the autoimmune/rheumatic diseases.**
Limitations:	▪ Tests vary in price from $250-$400. ▪ Anaerobic bacteria are difficult to culture. ▪ Specialty examinations, such as for *Helicobacter pylori* antigen and enterohemorrhagic *E. coli* cytotoxin, must be requested specifically at additional cost.
Comments:	▪ I have found stool testing to be the single most powerful diagnostic tool for helping chronically ill patients to attain improved health. Insights from stool/parasitology testing can be used to implement powerfully effective treatments. The value of this test in the treatment of patients with rheumatic disease must be appreciated and is extensively detailed in ***Integrative Rheumatology***.

Concept: Not all "Injury-related Problems" are "Injury-related Problems"

In the case of most acute injuries, the underlying problem is often the injury itself. However, the physician must conduct a thorough history and examination to assess for possible underling pathologies that cause or contribute to the problem that "appears" to be injury-related. Congenital anomalies, underlying pathology, previous injury, occult infections, and psychoemotional disorders may have been present *before* the "injury."

> **"Pediatric infections and neoplasms are notorious for masquerading as sport injuries."**
>
> "...Take the relevant history directly from the patient, and keep tumors and infections high on your list of differential diagnoses... For example, about 15% of children with leukemia present with musculoskeletal complaints..."
>
> Shaw BA, Gerardi JA, Hennrikus WL. How to avoid orthopedic pitfalls in children. *Patient Care* 1999 Feb

Just because the patient reports a problem such as pain following an injury does not mean that the injury is the *sole* cause of the pain. *Do not let a biased history lead you down the wrong path*. **In children and young adults, 5% of "sports-related" injuries are associated with preexisting infection, anomalies, or other conditions.** In adult women, "...between 9% and 20% of women with breast cancer attribute their symptoms to previous trauma to the breast. In these cases, the association of the breast mass with a traumatic event resulted in a delay in diagnosis ranging from four months to one year."[316]

A group of German physicians describe a man who presented with a soft-tissue pain following a soccer game; he was later diagnosed with a malignant tumor—synovial sarcoma.[317] Similarly, Wakeshima and Ellen[318] describe a young athletic woman who presented with chronic hip pain. The woman's history was significant for ulcerative colitis, but otherwise her radiographs were normal and her history and examination lead to a diagnosis of trochanteric bursitis. However, the patient's condition did not respond to routine treatment, and additional investigation over several months lead to a diagnosis of giant cell carcinoma. The authors concluded, "This case shows **the importance of repeat radiographic studies in patients whose joint pain does not respond or responds slowly to conservative therapy, despite initial normal findings."**

What you expect to find and hear when taking a trauma-related history is that **1) a healthy patient** with no previous health concerns was **2) exposed to a traumatic event**, the history and consequences of which perfectly coincide with the injury you are assessing in your office, and that **3) your physical examination findings are all consistent** and lead to a specific diagnosis, which then **4) responds to your treatment. If you find discrepancies between the history of the injury and your physical examination findings (e.g., fever after a "sports-related" injury), if the patient appears unhealthy in disproportion to the presenting complaint, or if the patient does not respond to your treatment, then you must consider the possibility of preexisting or concomitant disease.**

When treating children, be very careful to get an accurate history—this is difficult since your two sources of information are not very reliable: parents often think that they already have the problem figured out, and so their history will be biased toward convincing you of what they think is the problem and solution; children are often not good historians and can form illogical relationships between events that can be misleading.

Astute doctors search for and rule out preexisting and underlying pathology before ascribing the problem to the "obvious cause." Always assess for consistency between the history, examination findings, and response to treatment—inconsistencies suggest the need for additional investigation.

---

[316] Seifert S. Medical Illness Simulating Trauma (MIST) syndrome: case reports and discussion of syndrome. *Fam Med* 1993 Apr;25(4):273-6

[317] Engel C, Kelm J, Olinger A. Blunt trauma in soccer. The initial manifestation of synovial sarcoma. [Article in German] *Zentralbl Chir* 2001 Jan;126(1):68-71

[318] Wakeshima Y, Ellen MI. Atypical hip pain origin in a young athletic woman: a case report of giant cell carcinoma. *Arch Phys Med Rehabil* 2001 Oct;82(10):1472-5

```
                    ┌────────────────────────────────────────────────┐
                    │          Previous health history               │
                    │                    +                           │
                    │       History of the present complaint         │
                    │                    +                           │
                    │  Clinical observations and physicalexamination findings │
                    │                    +                           │
                    │           Response to treatment                │
                    │                                                │
                    │  If all 4 parts of the story do not add up perfectly, then you need to consider │
                    │   alternate diagnoses and take appropriate steps to ensure patient care.  │
                    └────────────────────────────────────────────────┘
```

Abuse: child abuse, adult abuse, elder abuse	Systemic illness: cancer, infection, rheumatic	Preexisting condition: metabolic disorder or congenital anomaly	Inadequate compliance with treatment

Assess and report to authorities as indicated

Discover and address cause of non-compliance

If you have a specific condition in mind, then test specifically for it. If you suspect preexisting/concomitant illness but are unsure of exact nature of the condition, gather additional information by:

1) taking a more detailed history,
2) ordering lab tests: CRP, CBC, chemistry panel, ferritin, ANA.
3) obtaining diagnostic imaging radiographs, bone scan, MRI, CT, US
4) reassessing patient within two weeks for progression of disease or crossing diagnostic threshold.
5) referral or co-management: if the patient does not respond to your treatment and/or you suspect an underlying serious pathology, refer the patient to another physician at least for co-management. Put your referral in writing and chart appropriately. "When in doubt, refer it out."

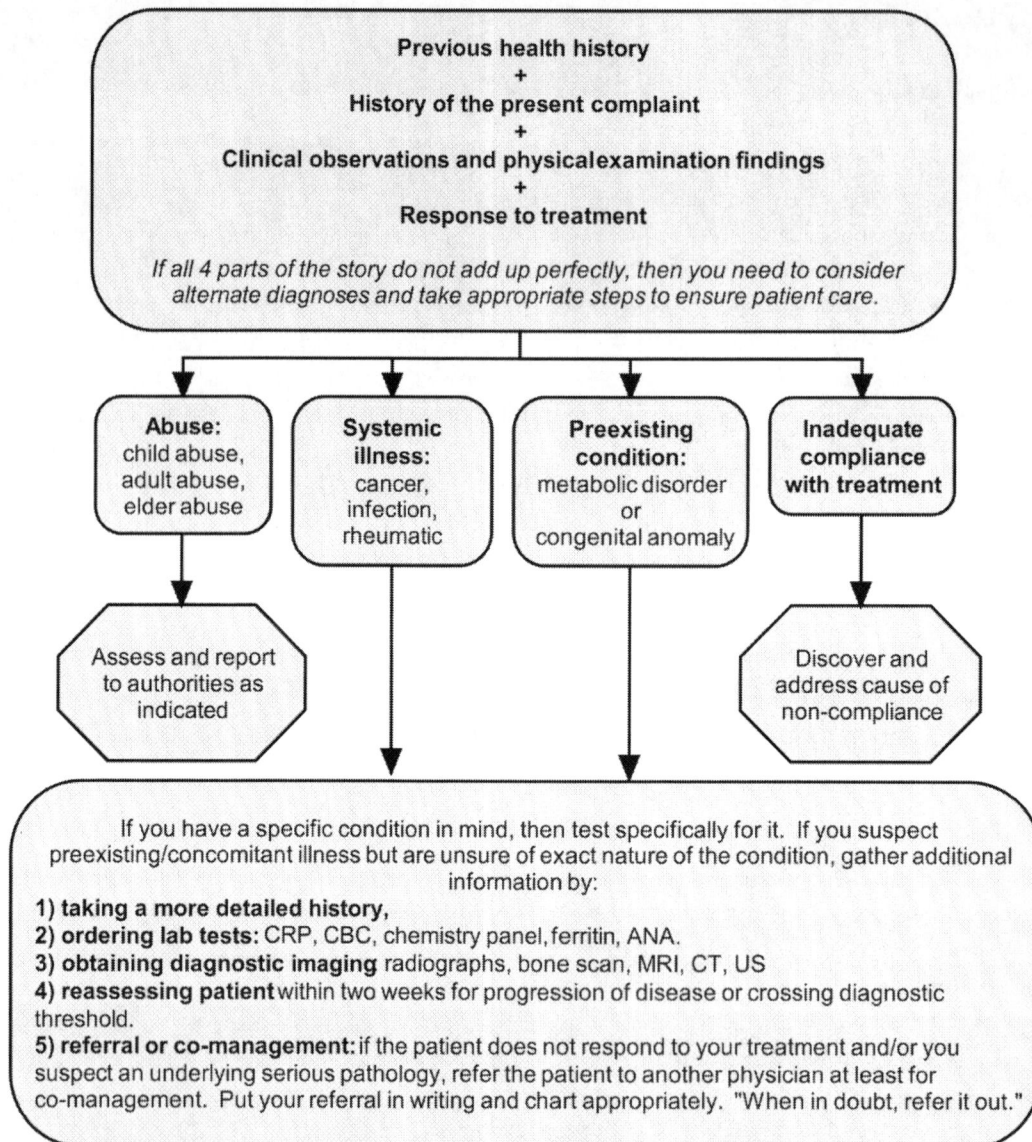

Clinical management: Inconsistencies between the history, exams, and response to treatment indicate the need for additional investigation and additional diagnostic considerations.

```
┌─────────────────────────┐
│  Patient presents with  │
│  musculoskeletal pain   │
└─────────────────────────┘
            │
            ▼
┌─────────────────────────────────┐
│ ● Presentation appears benign?  │
│                                 │
│ ● Doctor is confident with      │
│   diagnosis?                    │
│                                 │
│ ● Patient is young and appears  │
│   in excellent overall health?  │
│                                 │
│ ● No history of disease or drug │
│   or medication use?            │
│                                 │
│ ● Risk of complications is low? │
└─────────────────────────────────┘
```

answer NO to <u>any</u> question →

Perform additional investigation:
- <u>Perform additional/repeat physical examination</u>

- <u>Lab tests</u>: CBC, CRP, chemistry/metabolic panel, ferritin, TSH, and other tests as indicated such as joint aspiration or ANA

- <u>Imaging</u>: radiographs, ultrasound, CT, MRI

- <u>Treatment</u>: make significant modifications to treatment plan; ensure compliance

- <u>Referral</u> to specialist

answer YES to <u>all</u> questions

```
┌─────────────────────────┐
│ Begin with presumptive  │
│ diagnosis and initial   │
│ treatment plan          │
└─────────────────────────┘
            │
            ▼
┌─────────────────────────┐
│ Treatment is successful?│
└─────────────────────────┘
```

Treatment failure

Yes

```
┌─────────────────────────┐
│ Continue to treat until │
│ condition remits        │
└─────────────────────────┘
```

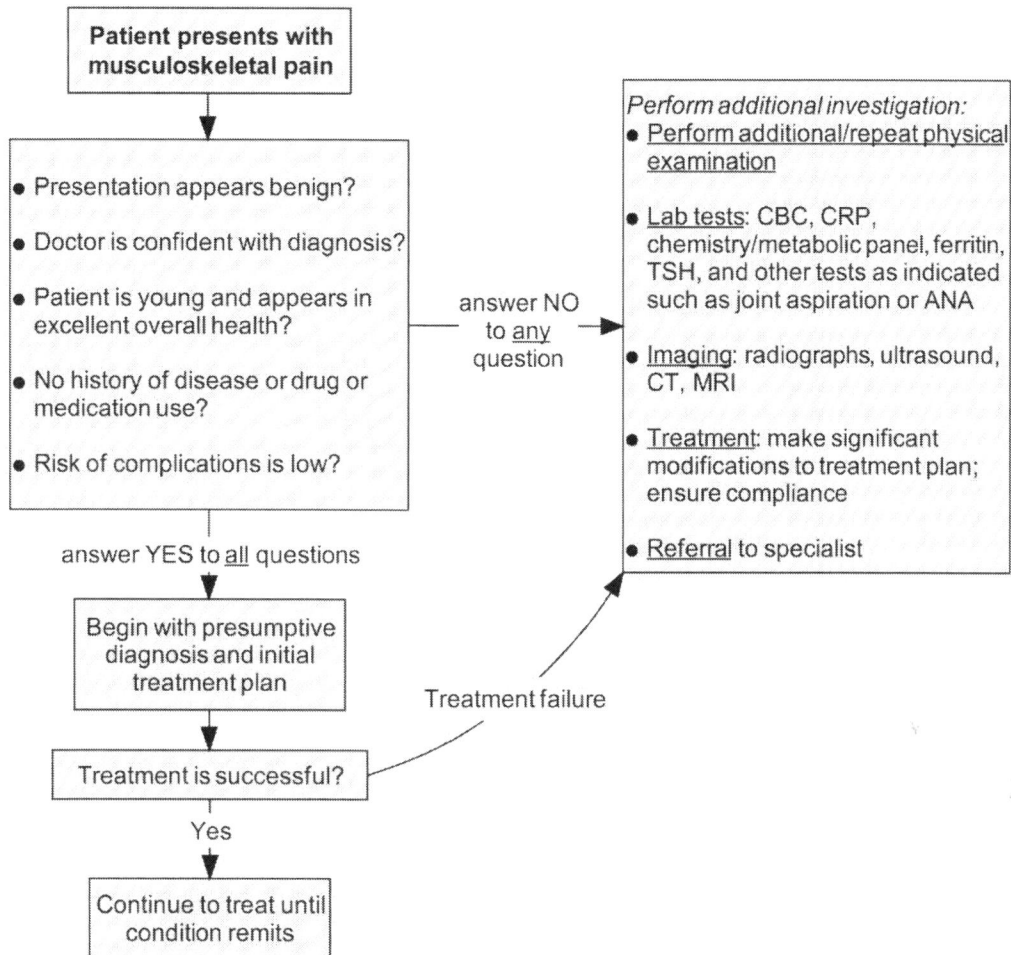

Clinical management: Inconsistencies between the history, exams, and response to treatment indicate the need for additional investigation and additional diagnostic considerations.

High-Risk Pain Patients:

When a patient has musculoskeletal pain and any of the following characteristics, radiographs should be considered as an appropriate component of comprehensive evaluation. These considerations are particularly—though not exclusively—relevant for spine and low-back pain.[319]

1.   **More than 50 years of age**
2.   **Physical trauma** (accident, fall, etc.)
3.   **Pain at night**
4.   **Back pain not relieved by lying supine**
5.   **Neurologic deficits** (motor or sensory)
6.   **Unexplained weight loss**
7.   **Documentation or suspicion of inflammatory arthropathy**[320]
     - **Ankylosing spondylitis**
     - **Lupus**
     - **Rheumatoid arthritis**
     - **Juvenile rheumatoid arthritis**
     - **Psoriatic arthritis**
8.   **Drug or alcohol abuse** (increased risk of infection, nutritional deficiencies, anesthesia)
9.   **History of cancer**
10. **Intravenous drug use**
11. **Immunosuppression, due to illness (e.g., HIV) or medications (e.g., steroids or cyclosporine)**
12. **History of corticosteroid use** (causes osteoporosis and increased risk for infection)
13. **Fever above 100° F or suspicion of septic arthritis or osteomyelitis**
14. **Diabetes** (increased risk of infection, nutritional deficiencies, anesthesia)
15. **Hypertension** (abdominal aneurysm: low back pain, nausea, pulsatile abdominal mass)
16. **Recent visit for same problem and not improved**
17. **Patient seeking compensation for pain/ injury** (increased need for documentation)
18. **Skin lesion** (psoriasis, melanoma, dermatomyositis, the butterfly rash of lupus, scars from previous surgery, accident, etc.…)
19. **Deformity or immobility**
20. **Lymphadenopathy** (suggests cancer or infection)
21. **Elevated ESR/CRP** (cancer, infection, inflammatory disorder)
22. **Elevated WBC count**
23. **Elevated alkaline phosphatase** (bone lesions, metabolic bone disease, hepatopathy, vitamin D deficiency)
24. **Elevated acid phosphatase** (occasionally used to monitor prostate cancer)
25. **Positive rheumatoid factor and/or CCP—cyclic citrullinated protein antibodies**
26. **Positive HLA-B27** (propensity for inflammatory arthropathies)
27. **Serum gammopathy** (multiple myeloma is the most common primary bone tumor)
28. **"High-risk for disease"** *examples:*
     - Long-term heavy smoking of cigarettes
     - Long-term exposure to radiation
     - Obesity
29. **Strong family history of inflammatory, musculoskeletal, or malignant disease**
30. **Others:**_____

_____

_____

_____

---

[319] Remember that metastasis often travel first from the primary site to bone, therefore bone pain may be an early manifestation of occult cancer. Most of the above are from "Table 1: The high-risk patient: clinical indications for radiography in low back pain patients." J Taylor, DC, DACBR, D Resnick, MD. Imaging decisions in the management of low back pain. Advances in Chiropractic. Mosby Year Book. 1994; 1-28

[320] Radiographs are often essential for diagnosis or to rule out complications of the disease. For example, in patients with inflammatory arthropathies such as these, spontaneous rupture of the transverse ligament (at the odontoid process) has been reported; although rare, this complication could be life-threatening if mismanaged or undiagnosed.

Concept: Safe Patient + Safe Treatment = Safe Outcome

The purpose of performing the history and physical examination on a new *or established* patient is to determine their current health status—including their mental and emotional health and their physical health, particularly as this relates to important and life-threatening possibilities such as cancer, infections, fractures, systemic diseases, and neurologic compromise. The questions that lead this investigation are: "**What is this patient's current status?**" "**Does this patient have a serious disease, neurologic injury, or are they at high risk for developing a serious complication in the near future that can be prevented with appropriate care** *now*?"

"Is this patient safe?"
- ♦ The question to ask yourself is, "Is this patient's health problem or current complaint/exacerbation a manifestation of an underlying condition that could result in a negative outcome?
- ♦ If a patient comes to you with a headache, and you neglect to find that their blood pressure is 230/130, then you missed the opportunity to help them avoid the stroke that they could have after leaving your office.
- ♦ If a patient comes to you with a complaint of low back pain, and you neglect to perform a neurologic examination to find that *the patient already has a neurologic deficit even before you treated them*, then you have lost the opportunity to defend yourself in court when the patient later claims that *your* treatment and *your* management of their case is the reason that they now have a permanent neurologic deficit.

Is your treatment safe?: Have you been perfectly clear with the patient about the risks and benefits of your treatment plan? **Have you obtained informed consent**? Have you charted **"PAR-B"** to indicate that you have discussed the Procedures, Alternatives, Risks, and Benefits of your treatment plan? Have you been clear about the duration of treatment and the need for appropriate follow-up? If you are prescribing nutrition or botanical medicines, have you informed the patient about the duration of treatment? **Have you looked for contraindications to your otherwise brilliant treatment plan**? What about the fact that this patient was on corticosteroids for the past 15 years and only discontinued prednisone 2 months before arriving at your office? *The patient may have steroid-induced osteoporosis even though he is no longer on prednisone.* When you recommend that your patient take 100,000 IU of vitamin A to treat her throat infection, what happens when she presents to your office 8 months later with signs of vitamin A toxicity because she continued her treatment plan indefinitely

> Double-check to ensure that your patient is safe (no forthcoming complications or predictable emergencies) and that your treatment is safe (appropriate, effective, clearly communicated, and time-limited with instructions to return for office visit).

rather than using it only for 7 days as you had intended? *Be sure to put a time limit on your treatment plans.* Every treatment plan should be 1) given to the patient in legible print and clear statements, 2) be copied for the chart, 3) include "what to do if things get worse" in the event of adverse treatment effect or exacerbation of problem, and 4) include patient's responsibility for returning to office/clinic for follow-up and reassessment.

Informed consent: From a legal standpoint, doctors can only treat a patient after the patient has given *consent to treatment*. Patients can only authoritatively consent to treatment after they have been educated about the treatment—thereafter, they can provide *informed consent*. Educating the patient requires discussion (and documentation) of each of the following:
- Procedures—what may take place, what is required; duration, costs, follow-up,
- Alternatives—what options are available,
- Risks—what risks are involved,
- Benefits—what benefits can be reasonably expected,
- Questions—allow for the patient to ask questions and receive answers.

This is commonly charted as "**PARB—no questions**" or "**PARB—questions answered**" once the patient gives consent to treatment; alternatively and more humorously, this may be charted as "**PAR-B-Q**".

Concept: Four Clues to Discovering Underlying Problems

When I taught Orthopedics at Bastyr University I encouraged students to search for specific **sets of clues** when evaluating patients. These clues—often insignificant in isolation but meaningful in combination—were often the "red flags" that could help make the difference between an accurate diagnosis and a missed diagnosis. These four categories can be recalled with the mnemonic "*S.C.I.N.*" or "*S.C.I.M.*" These four areas of assessment/safety emphasis differ from the "vindicates" mnemonic which is used for differential diagnosis.

Vindicates: a popular mnemonic for differential diagnosis	
V	Vascular
	Visceral referral
I	Infectious
	Inflammatory
	Immunologic
N	Neurologic
	Nutritional
	New growth: neoplasia or pregnancy
D	Deficiency
	Degenerative
I	Iatrogenic (drug related)
	Intoxication
	Idiosyncratic
C	Congenital
	Cardiac or circulatory
A	Allergy / Autoimmune
	Abuse: drugs, alcohol, physical
T	Trauma
	Toxicity
E	Endocrine
	Exposure
S	Subluxation
	Somatic dysfunction
	Structural
	Stress
	Secondary gain

- **Systemic symptoms and signs**: Ask about systemic signs and symptoms such as fever, weight loss, lymphadenopathy, or skin rash in patients who present with pain because these "whole body" manifestations might indicate an underlying or concomitant disease that deserves attention, either independently from the musculoskeletal pain, or as a cause of the musculoskeletal pain. For example, "headache" may appear benign, whereas "headache with fever and skin rash" suggests meningitis—a medical emergency. "Low-back pain" is a common occurrence; yet "low-back pain with weight loss and fever" might suggest occult malignancy, osteomyelitis, or other systemic disease.

- **Complications:** We ask about and look for already existing complications, such as "numbness, weakness, tingling in the arms or hands, legs or feet" to rapidly screen for neurologic deficits and we follow this up with screening assessments such as "squat and rise", toe walk, heel walk, and reflexes for spinal cord and lower extremity neuromuscular integrity. Additionally, when dealing with patients with spine-related complaints or injuries, we also ask about changes or loss of function in bowel and bladder control and numbness near the anus or genitals, which may be the *only* clinical clues to cauda equina syndrome—a medical emergency. Ask about effects of the condition on ADL (activities of daily living) to attain a more comprehensive view of the condition and to ensure that the patient's story is consistent.

- **Indicators from the history**: We look for specific "red flags" and "yellow flags" such as trauma, risk factors (such as smoking, prednisone, alcohol), or a positive history of chronic infections or cancer. Nonmechanical musculoskeletal pain in a patient with a history of or high risk for cancer is highly suspicious and mandates thorough investigation.

- **Non-Mechanical pain**: Non-mechanical pain suggests a pathologic etiology rather than simple joint dysfunction. Pain at night, pain that occurs without an inciting injury, pain that is not strongly affected by motion and is not powerfully provoked by your physical examination assessments suggests the possibility of underlying disorder such as cancer, neuropathy, or infection. However, the ability to elicit an exacerbation of pain with "mechanical" maneuvers does not indicate that the pain is "mechanical" and therefore "non-pathologic." Mechanical pain can still be pathologic pain, such as the exquisite pain felt by patients with spinal fractures—they may be neurologically intact, they do have pain worse with motion, but they are not safe to manipulate, and they require appropriate treatment and referral on an urgent basis.

> Keeping these four assessment categories in mind can serve as a useful "checkpoint" to ensure that your patient is safe, and that your treatment is appropriate and therefore safe, too.

Concept: Special Considerations in the Evaluation of Children

> "Pediatric infections and neoplasms are notorious for masquerading as sport injuries. … There is only one way to avoid this trap: Take the relevant history directly from the patient, and keep tumors and infections high on your list of differential diagnoses."[321]

- **Consider the possibility of child abuse when a child presents with an injury:** As a non-naïve physician, you always have to consider the possibility of child abuse when a child presents with an injury. Be detailed in your history taking, and be sure to search for discrepancies between 1) the child's version of the incident, 2) the adult's version of the incident, and 3) what is realistic (based on your practical life experience and clinical training). As a primary care physician, you are obligated to report your *suspicion* of child abuse to law enforcement agencies and/or child protective services.
- **Children heal quickly:** This rapid healing is good as long as tissues are approximated. But if a fractured bone is displaced and not correctly replaced, then problematic malunion deformities may result *within **days***.
- **Children are more susceptible to rapidly progressing infections than are adults:** Soft tissue, joint, and bone infections need to be diagnosed expeditiously and treated aggressively.
- **Children are radiographically different from adults:** Make sure that your radiographs are interpreted by a competent radiologist with experience in the interpretation of *pediatric radiographs*. Radiographic considerations specific to children include:
  - **Epiphyseal growth plates**
  - **Secondary ossification centers**
  - **Variants in trabecular patterns and bone densities**
  - **Specific conditions that happen only in children, such as slipped capital femoral epiphysis**
  - **Congenital anomalies**
  - **Difficulty following directions with positioning** (applies to some adults, too!)
  - **Bone scans can be difficult to interpret in children:** Bone scans derive their value from the demonstration of a focal increase in uptake of radioactive isotopes, which demonstrates and localizes an area of increased metabolic activity. In adults, this increased and localized activity generally indicates pathology, especially malignant disease in bone (primary or metastatic) and recent fracture. In children, however, since their bones are already highly metabolically active due to the normal growth process, bone scans are difficult to interpret and are not highly reliable for the demonstration of focal lesions.

> Always consider the possibility of abuse, cancer, infection, or congenital anomaly as a cause of musculoskeletal pain in children, even if the injury appears to be related to injury or trauma. Strongly consider lab tests, as well as radiographs (interpreted by a pediatric radiologist). When in doubt, refer for second opinion. If you suspect abuse, you have a legal and ethical obligation to report your *suspicion*.

---

[321] Shaw BA, Gerardi JA, Hennrikus WL. How to avoid orthopedic pitfalls in children. *Patient Care* 1999; Feb 28: 95-116

Concept: Differences between Primary Healthcare and Spectator Sports

In baseball, "errors" have been defined as "a defensive mistake that allows a batter to stay at the plate or reach first base, or that advances a base runner."[322] In baseball, a few errors can make the difference between winning and losing a particular game or season. However, a few errors in a game are to be expected, and ultimately the team can start over at the next game or season and try to do better.

Healthcare, however, is not a game, and even relatively minor errors such as the doctor's forgetting to ask a particular question or perform a specific test can result in a patient's catastrophic injury or death. In healthcare, when we are dealing with serious injuries and illnesses, even a single "error" is not allowed. "Failure to diagnose" is one of the biggest reasons for malpractice claims against doctors; such judgments often result in loss of licensure and awards of hundreds of thousands of dollars. "Failure to treat" results when the patient is injured because the doctor failed to

> While your compassion for human suffering and your love of nutrition and exercise may have directed you into healthcare, your professional success and survival will depend in large part on your ability to manage the technical and defensive aspects of clinical practice.
>
> Neuromusculoskeletal disorders and autoimmune diseases are "big league" clinical problems, and they need to be taken seriously.

effectively treat the patient or when the doctor failed to provide the appropriate referral to a specialist in a timely manner. Such failures are not only capable of destroying a physician's career and forcing the liquidation of his/her possessions, but such cases can also greatly damage the integrity of whole professions, especially the naturopathic and chiropractic professions which are generally guilty until proven innocent due to the double standards imposed by those adherent to the "always right" dogma of the medical paradigm.[323] Stated differently, **if the doctor does not ask the right questions and perform the right tests, then the doctor may miss an emergency diagnosis. Missing an emergency diagnosis can result in patient death. Patient death may result in litigation, loss of license for the doctor, and irreparable harm to the profession.** The upcoming section on **Musculoskeletal Emergencies** represents *core competencies* that every clinician must keep present in his/her mind during each interaction with a patient with musculoskeletal complaints, especially patients who are elderly, on medications such as prednisone, and those with known autoimmune or immunosuppressive disorders.

Concept: "Disease Treatment" is Different from "Patient Management"

> "The key to successful intervention for orthopedic problems in a primary care practice is to know what conditions to refer and when and to whom to refer the refractory patient."[324]

Treating a problem is one thing, managing a patient is something different. "Problems" such as "low back pain" are abstract concepts, and we automatically form mental lists of treatments for problems that are irrespective of the patient who has the condition. However this list may be of only very limited applicability to the individual patient with whom you are working. Management of patients includes ❶ assessing and reassessing the differential diagnoses, ❷ monitoring compliance with treatments, including the treatments of other healthcare providers, ❸ co-treating with other healthcare providers, ❹ assessing for contraindications, ❺ monitoring patient status and effectiveness of treatments, and also ❻ the office-related tasks of charting, documentation, billing, and correspondence. The management of emergency conditions often involves transport to the nearest hospital. In some situations, the patient will be able to drive himself/herself without difficulty. In other situations, the patient should be driven by friend, family, or taxi. In the most extreme, the patient should be transported by ambulance. When in doubt about the mode of transport, do not hesitate to call 911 for an ambulance. If the taxi driver gets lost on the way to the hospital, or your patient goes into shock while being driven by a friend, the liability will come back to haunt the *doctor*, not the *friend* or the *taxi driver*.

---

[322] http://www.nocryinginbaseball.com/glossary/glossary.html Accessed November 11, 2006
[323] Micozzi MS. Double standards and double jeopardy for CAM research. *J Altern Complement Med.* 2001 Feb;7(1):13-4
[324] Brier S. Primary Care Orthopedics. St. Louis: Mosby, 1999 page ix

Concept: Clinical Practice Involves Much More than "Diagnosis and Treatment"

Emergency room and hospital-based physicians are appropriately able to focus solely on diagnosis and treatment as their primary spheres of activity and interaction with patients. However, those of us in private practice learn that *healthcare* involves much more than simply being a "good doctor." From an integrative perspective we have to go beyond diagnosis and treatment *for each health disorder* with each patient. Beyond *diagnosis* and *treatment* are *understanding* and *integration*. Orchestrating all of this into a treatment plan that the patient can actually implement requires creativity, resourcefulness, and the ability to enroll patients in the process of *redesigning*—often *rebuilding*—their lives.

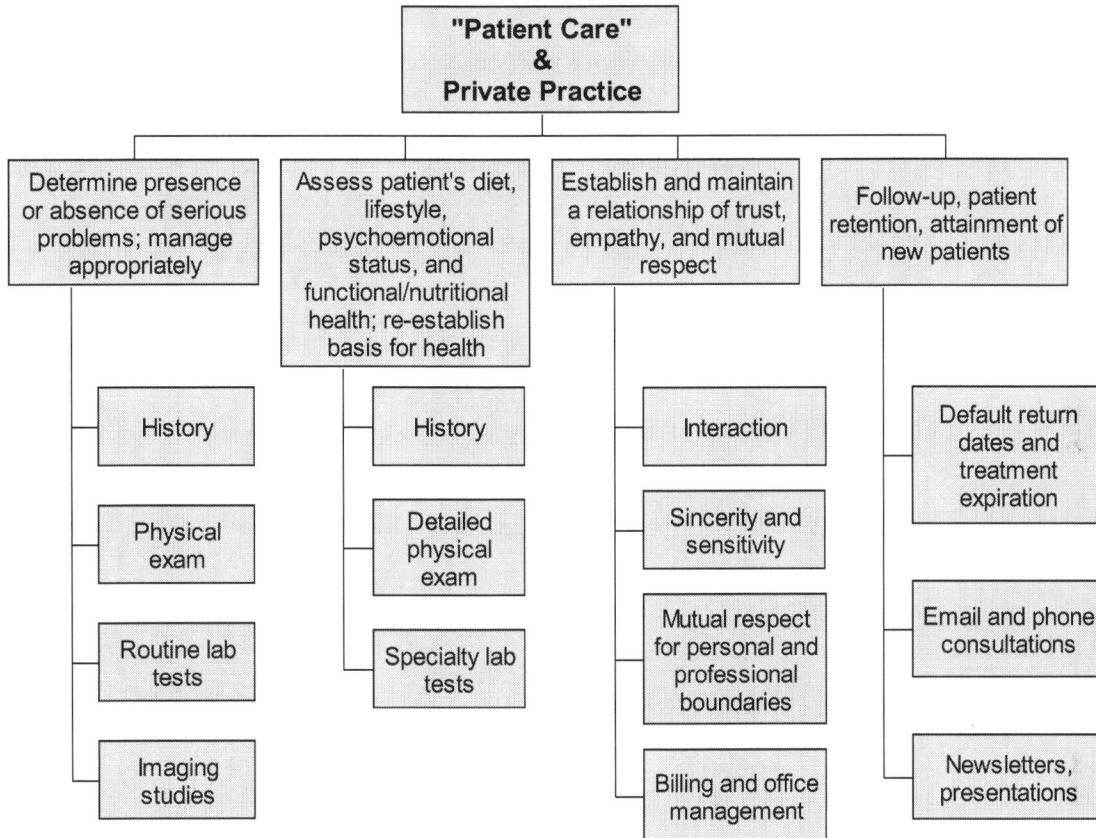

Recall that **28% of malpractice claims involve mistakes made by medical office staff**; this includes unreturned phone calls which can culminate in malpractice by way of "patient abandonment." Similarly, inability to get a timely consultation may result in sufficient "sense of harm" that a patient may decide to sue; this is a factor in 10% of malpractice cases.[325]

---

[325] James R. Hall, Ph.D., L.Psych., FABMP, FGICPP. Departments of Internal Medicine and Psychology, UNT Health Science Center at Fort Worth. "Communication and Medico-Legal Issues." October 19, 2006

Risk Management: A Note Especially to Students and Recent Licensees

Even if you are a board-certified rheumatologist and an assertive and astute clinician with years of experience, the consideration of these guidelines may help protect **you** from malpractice liability and **your patient** from harm. Practicing "good medicine" is inherently defensive and in the best interests of the patient and the doctor.

1. **Document the specifics of your treatment plan and the rationale behind it.**
2. **Do not tell your patient to discontinue their anti-rheumatic drugs unless these drugs are in your scope of practice *and* discontinuing such drugs is therapeutically appropriate.**
3. **Give your patient written instructions, and specifically delineate time parameters for the next visit to monitor for therapeutic effectiveness, adverse effects, and disease progression/regression.**
4. **Always have an internist or rheumatologist (or appropriate specialist) on-board as part of the clinical team in case the patient experiences an exacerbation and needs to be hospitalized or acutely immunosuppressed.**
5. **When working with patients that have potentially serious diseases such as most of the autoimmune diseases, you should have a back-up plan integrated into your treatment plan from day one.** You might consider having patients sign a consent form that includes language consistent with the following:
   - *"Due to the uniqueness of each disease and each individual, including his or her willingness and ability to implement the treatment plan, no guarantees of successful treatment can be offered."*
   - *"Dr.___ may not be available on a 24-hour basis at all times. If you have a serious health problem that requires immediate attention, you should call your other doctors(s), call 911, or have someone take you to the nearest hospital emergency room. If you notice an adverse effect from one of the components of your health plan, you should discontinue it then call Dr.__ and inform him/her of what occurred."*
   - *"Treatments with other physicians or healthcare providers are not necessarily to be discontinued. Please let Dr.__ know if you are being treated by other healthcare providers (physicians, counselors, therapists, etc.). Consult your prescribing doctor before discontinuing medications."*
6. **Test responsibly.**
7. **Treat responsibly.**
8. **Re-test to document effectiveness of your intervention.**
9. **When in doubt, refer the patient for co-management.** If you are working with a serious life-threatening disease, and *your plan* or *the patient's implementation of it* is unable to produce *documentable results*, then you should refer the patient for allopathic/osteopathic/specialist co-management for the sake of protecting the patient from harm and for protecting yourself from undue liability.
10. **Practice defensively.** You will thereby safeguard your patient and your livelihood.

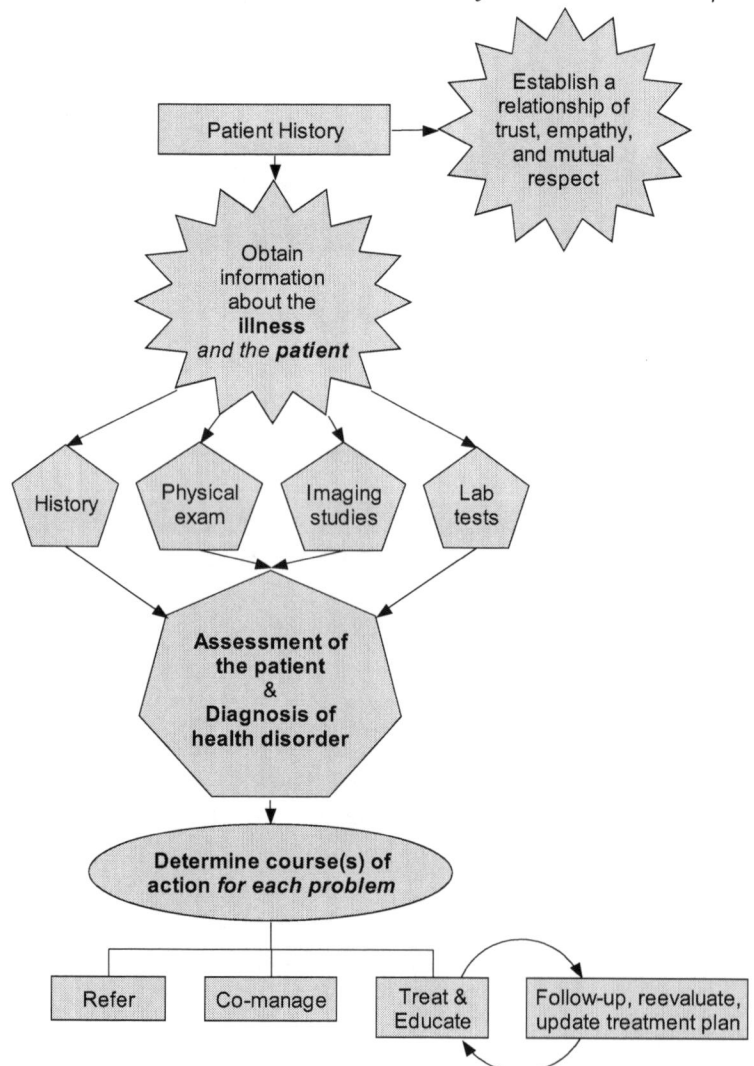

Musculoskeletal Emergencies

These are some of the "core competencies" that clinicians can never afford to miss, and these are pertinent to patients with musculoskeletal disorders, whether structural/orthopedic or metabolic/rheumatic. With these conditions, clinicians are wise to err on the side of caution— *"When in doubt, refer out"*—and implement the appropriate referral on an expedient basis. These are organized in a clinical/logical manner rather than listed alphabetically.

Neurovascular Disorders

Problem	Presentation	Assessment	Management
<u>Neuropsychiatric lupus</u>	▪ Psychosis ▪ Seizures ▪ Transient ischemic attacks ▪ Severe depression ▪ Delirium, confusion	▪ Neuropsychiatric manifestations with history of lupus	▪ Emergency or prompt referral as indicated
<u>Giant cell arteritis, Temporal arteritis</u>: Considered a medical emergency since it may rapidly progress to blindness due to associated involvement of the ophthalmic artery: *"Loss of vision is the most feared manifestation and occurs quite commonly."*[326]	Presentation typically includes the following: ▪ Headache, scalp tenderness ▪ Jaw claudication ▪ Changes in vision ▪ Systemic manifestations of rheumatic disease: fever, weight loss, muscle aches	▪ Palpation of the temporal artery may reveal a "cord-like" artery ▪ Elevated ESR ▪ CBC may show anemia ▪ Temporal artery biopsy is diagnostic	▪ Standard medical treatment is with immediate prednisone ▪ Implement treatment that is immediately effective or refer patient for medical treatment
<u>Acute red eye</u>: General term including acute iritis and scleritis; despite the name of this condition, redness may actually be rather minimal, and it is typically accompanied by cloudy changes in region of the iris and lens	▪ Eye pain and redness ▪ May have facial pain ▪ May be the presenting manifestation of rheumatic disease	▪ Red eye ▪ Photophobia ▪ Reduced vision ▪ May have fixed pupil ▪ Differential diagnosis includes acute glaucoma, bacterial/amebic/ viral conjunctivitis or keratitis, allergy, and irritation due to contact lens	▪ "The **acute** onset of a **painful**, **red** eye, even in the absence of visual upset, should be regarded primarily as an ophthalmological emergency."[327] ▪ **Granulomatous uveitis** occurs in 15% of patients with sarcoidosis and can result in bilateral blindness—this must be managed as a medically urgent condition

[326] Tierney ML. McPhee SJ, Papadakis MA (eds). <u>Current Medical Diagnosis and Treatment, 41st Edition</u>. New York: Lange Medical ; 2002. P999-1005
[327] McInnes I, Sturrock R. Rheumatological emergencies. *Practitioner*. 1994 Mar;238(1536):220-4

Neural canal compression

Problem	Presentation	Assessment	Management
Atlantoaxial instability: Excess mobility between the atlas and axis (commonly due to lesion of the dens or transverse ligament) makes the spinal cord vulnerable to compressive injury when the atlas translates anteriorly on the axis especially during cervical flexion; may progress to neurologic compromise including respiratory and somatic paralysis	▪ Post-traumatic neck injury ▪ Down's syndrome ▪ May present spontaneously (without trauma) in patients with inflammatory rheumatic disease, especially rheumatoid arthritis and ankylosing spondylitis ▪ May have gradual or sudden onset of myelopathy: upper motor neuron lesion (UMNL) signs (e.g., spastic weakness), changes in bowel-bladder function, numbness	▪ Clinical suspicion is followed by lateral cervical and APOM (anteroposterior open mouth) radiographs to assess ADI (atlantodental interval) and dens ▪ MRI should be performed in patients with suspected myelopathy ▪ Neurologic examination of the upper and lower extremities ▪ Do not force neck flexion; do not perform the Soto Hall test	▪ **Urgent neurosurgical consultation is recommended; stabilizing surgery is the best option for the prevention of neurologic catastrophes**[328] ▪ Onset of myelopathy mandates referral to ER and/or neurosurgeon; immobilize with spine board or hard cervical collar and transport appropriately ▪ Asymptomatic and mild increases in ADI (< 5mm) might be managed conservatively with activity restriction, exercises, and bracing/collars) ▪ PAR discussion and referral for surgical consultation is necessary for informed consent and safe management
Myelopathy, spinal cord compression or lesion: May occur due to infection, edema, tumor, spinal fracture, stenosis, or inflammatory disease	▪ **Spastic weakness** ▪ Bowel-bladder dysfunction ▪ Numbness ▪ Problems are distal to cord lesion	▪ Hyperreflexia ▪ Rigidity ▪ Muscle weakness ▪ MRI (with and without contrast) should be performed in patients with suspected myelopathy; CT may also be indicated	▪ Obtain MRI to confirm diagnosis ▪ Immobilize spine and transport if necessary ▪ Acute myelopathy is a medical emergency that can result in rapid-onset paralysis
Cauda equina syndrome: Compression of the sacral nerve roots due to lumbar disc herniation **Cauda equina syndrome is a surgical emergency.**	▪ History of sciatic low back pain ▪ Urinary retention, perineal numbness, and fecal incontinence are common ▪ May have lower extremity weakness	▪ Assess for bladder distention ▪ Assess anal sphincter strength with rectal exam ▪ Lower extremity neurologic examination	▪ Urgent referral for CT/MRI to confirm diagnosis ▪ If diagnosis is confirmed or strongly suspected clinically, urgent referral for surgical decompression is mandatory

---

[328] "When atlantoaxial stability is lost...it is thought that surgical stabilisation of the atlantoaxial joint is more reasonable and beneficial than conservative management. Minimal trauma of an unstable atlantoaxial joint can lead to serious neurological injury." Moon MS, Choi WT, Moon YW, Moon JL, Kim SS. Brooks' posterior stabilization surgery for atlantoaxial instability: review of 54 cases. *J Orthop Surg* (Hong Kong). 2002 Dec;10(2):160-4. http://www.josonline.org/PDF/v10i2p160.pdf

Acute peripheral nerve compression

Problem	Presentation	Assessment	Management
Acute compartment syndrome: acute onset of *potentially irreversible* muscle and/or nerve compression injury due to inflammation, swelling, or bleeding within a fascial compartment **Acute compartment syndrome is a surgical emergency.**	▪ Most commonly occurs in the anterior leg; may also occur in the posterior leg as well as forearm—these are the areas most notable anatomically for the investment of muscle in tight and resilient fascial sheaths ▪ Onset generally follows strenuous exercise that leads to reactive hyperemia and secondary edema ▪ May occur following trauma or fracture	Assess for: ▪ Pulselessness ▪ Palor ▪ Painful passive stretch ▪ Weakness ▪ **Numbness** ▪ Assessment and treatment should be performed on an emergency basis since irreversible nerve damage begins within 6 hours of intracompartmental hypertension	▪ Decompressive fasciotomy is the standard treatment for acute compartment syndrome that could result in permanent muscle necrosis and/or permanent nerve death ▪ Acute compartment syndrome can be fatal if rhabdomyolysis precipitates renal failure[329]

Musculoskeletal infections

Problem	Presentation	Assessment	Management
Septic arthritis: intraarticular bacterial infection; complications of septic arthritis are 1) articular destruction and 2) **death in 5-10% of patients**[330] **Septic arthritis is a medical emergency**	▪ **Febrile** patient has **acute/subacute mono/oligo-arthritis** ▪ Some patients may not have fever ▪ Other possible findings: Immuno-suppression due to medications, concomitant disease (RA, DM), elderly ▪ In some patients with concomitant disease or medications, the clinical picture can be blurred.	▪ **Warm, swollen, tender joint** ▪ Clinical assessment with **immediate referral for joint aspiration**, which reveals manifestations of infection such as WBC's and bacteria ▪ Differential diagnosis includes trauma, gout, CPPD, hemochromatosis	▪ **Immediate referral for joint aspiration** ▪ **An aggressive and prolonged course of IV and oral antimicrobials** ▪ "Immune support" such as vitamin A and glutamine and general measures to improve health and prevent recurrence
Osteomyelitis, infectious discitis: considered a medical emergency[331] **Osteomyelitis—especially vertebral osteomyelitis—is a medical emergency**	▪ Febrile patient with bone pain ▪ Assess for constitutional manifestations such as weight loss, night sweats, and malaise	▪ Exacerbation of bone pain when stress/percussion is applied to the bone ▪ Lab: CRP & WBC may be elevated ▪ MRI is more sensitive than CT, bone scan, or radiography[332]	▪ Emergency referral for vertebral osteomyelitis, since **up to 15% of patients will develop nerve lesions or cord compression**[333] ▪ Urgent referral for other types of osteomyelitis

[329] Paula R. Compartment Syndrome, Extremity. *eMedicine* June 22, 2006 http://www.emedicine.com/emerg/topic739.htm Accessed November 26, 2006
[330] Tierney ML. McPhee SJ, Papadakis MA. Current Medical Diagnosis and Treatment. 35th edition. Stamford: Appleton & Lange, 1996 page 759
[331] American College of Rheumatology Ad Hoc Committee on Clinical Guidelines. Guidelines for the initial evaluation of the adult patient with acute musculoskeletal symptoms. *Arthritis Rheum.* 1996;39(1):1-8
[332] Tierney ML. McPhee SJ, Papadakis MA (eds). Current Medical Diagnosis and Treatment 2002, 41st Edition. New York: Lange Medical; 2002. p 883
[333] King RW, Johnson D. Osteomyelitis. Updated July 13, 2006. *eMedicine* http://www.emedicine.com/emerg/topic349.htm Accessed Dec 24, 2006

Acute Nontraumatic Monoarthritis and Septic Arthritis

- "Acute monoarthritis is a potential medical emergency that must be investigated and treated promptly."[334]
- "Monoarthropathies should initially be investigated to exclude sepsis. ... Diagnostic joint aspiration ... should be carried out immediately."[335]
- "In acute monoarthritis, it is essential that infection of a joint be diagnosed or excluded, and this can only be done by joint aspiration and synovial fluid culture."[336]
- "Acute monoarthritis should be considered infectious until proven otherwise."[337]

Clinical presentations:

- Patient presents with acute joint pain in one joint (occasionally more than one joint may be involved).
- May or may not have fever and other systemic manifestations of infection.

> **Clinical Pearl**
>
> The primary goal of this section is to solidify your awareness of septic arthritis, its differential diagnoses, and the method and importance of assertive diagnosis and management.
>
> Septic arthritis is a medical emergency, and some authoritative textbooks report a mortality rate of 5-10%.
>
> Septic arthritis must be diagnosed urgently with joint aspiration, and it must be treated with antibiotics in order to preserve the joint and prevent spread of the infection.

Major Differential Diagnoses for Nontraumatic Monoarthritis

Problem	Presentation	Assessment & Management
Septic arthritis: intraarticular bacterial infection; complications of septic arthritis are 1) articular destruction and 2) **death in 5-10% of patients**[338]	▪ **Febrile** patient has **acute/subacute mono/oligo-arthritis** ▪ **Onset over hours or days** Other possible findings: ▪ Immuno-suppression due to medications, concomitant disease (RA, DM), elderly ▪ Some patients may not have fever ▪ In some patients with a previous or concomitant disease process, the clinical picture can be blurred	▪ **Warm, swollen, red, painful joint** ▪ Clinical assessment with **immediate referral for joint aspiration**, which reveals characteristic manifestations of infection such as WBCs and bacteria ▪ **Immediate joint aspiration** ▪ An aggressive and prolonged course of IV and oral antimicrobials ▪ "Immune support" and general measures to improve health and prevent recurrence **"Septic arthritis is still a life-threatening disease with a mortality of 2–5% and high morbidity."** Zacher J, Gursche A. Regional musculoskeletal conditions: 'hip' pain. *Best Practice & Research Clinical Rheumatology*. 2003 Feb;17:71-85

---

[334] Cibere J. Rheumatology: 4. Acute monoarthritis. CMAJ (*Canadian Medical Association Journal*). 2000;162(11):1577-83 www.cmaj.ca/cgi/content/full/162/11/1577 Jan 2004
[335] McInnes I, Sturrock R. Rheumatological emergencies. Practitioner. 1994 Mar;238(1536):220-4
[336] American College of Rheumatology Ad Hoc Committee on Clinical Guidelines. Guidelines for the initial evaluation of the adult patient with acute musculoskeletal symptoms. *Arthritis Rheum*. 1996 Jan;39(1):1-8
[337] Cibere J. Rheumatology: 4. Acute monoarthritis. CMAJ (*Canadian Medical Association Journal*). 2000;162(11):1577-83 www.cmaj.ca/cgi/content/full/162/11/1577 Jan 2004
[338] Tierney ML. McPhee SJ, Papadakis MA. Current Medical Diagnosis and Treatment. 35th edition. Stamford: Appleton and Lange, 1996 page 759

Major differential diagnoses for non-traumatic monoarthritis—*continued*

Problem	Presentation	Assessment & Management
Osteochondritis dissecans: A disorder of unclear etiology (trauma and/or avascular necrosis) which results in the death and subsequent fragmentation of subchondral bone[339]	▪ Primarily affects ages 10-30 years ▪ **Most common in the knees and elbows** ▪ Locking and crepitus due to intraarticular loose bodies ("joint mice") ▪ Some patients are almost asymptomatic, while others have acute pain ▪ Swelling of the affected joint	▪ Radiographs—consider to assess both knees as the condition is bilateral in 30% ▪ MRI is used to assess severity and need for surgical intervention ▪ Stable and nondisplaced lesions may be managed nonsurgically; larger and displaced fragments require surgical repair to reduce long-term complications[340]
Transient synovitis, irritable hip: Non-specific short-term inflammation and effusion of the hip joint	▪ Acute onset of painful hip and limp ▪ Decreased pain with hip in flexion and abduction ▪ Considered the most common cause of hip pain in children[341] ▪ More common in boys, age 3-6 years and generally younger than 10 years ▪ May have recent history of viral infection, and some children (1.5-10%) eventually manifest RA or AVN[342]	▪ May have slight elevation of ESR ▪ Normal WBC ▪ <u>No</u> fever; the child appears healthy ▪ "...radiography is indicated to exclude osseous pathological conditions..."[343] ▪ **Joint aspiration is indicated if septic arthritis is suspected**[344] ▪ Conservative treatment, restricted exertion and weight-bearing for several weeks
Legg-Calve-Perthe's disease: Idiopathic ischemic necrosis of the femoral head occurring in children **Avascular necrosis (AVN) of the femoral head, osteonecrosis**: Ischemic necrosis of the femoral head	Perthe's disease: ▪ 80% occur in children generally between ages of 4-9 years; more common in boys; may present with hip pain or knee pain AVN: ▪ Ages 20-40 years ▪ Unilateral hip pain ▪ May have knee pain ▪ History of trauma is common AVN associations: ▪ Steroid use, prednisone ▪ Hyperlipidemia ▪ Alcoholism ▪ Pancreatitis ▪ Hemoglobinopathies ▪ Smoking ▪ Fatty liver disease: "fat globules from the liver"[345]	▪ Limited ROM ▪ **Radiographs**; if normal and clinical suspicion is high order MRI or bone scan ▪ **Crutches** ▪ **Orthopedic referral is recommended** although not all patients will require surgery and some may be managed conservatively[346]

[339] Tatum R. Osteochondritis dissecans of the knee: a radiology case report. *J Manipulative Physiol Ther* 2000 Jun;23(5):347-51
[340] Browne RF, Murphy SM, Torreggiani WC, Munk PL, Marchinkow LO. Radiology for the surgeon: musculoskeletal case 30. Osteochondritis dissecans of the medial femoral condyle. *Can J Surg*. 2003;46(5):361-3 cma.ca/multimedia/staticContent/HTML/N0/l2/cjs/vol-46/issue-5/pdf/pg361.pdf
[341] Maroo S. Diagnosis of hip pain in children. *Hosp Med* 1999 Nov;60(11):788-93
[342] Souza TA. <u>Differential Diagnosis for the Chiropractor: Protocols and Algorithms</u>. Gaithersberg, Maryland: Aspen Publications. 1997 page 265
[343] Maroo S. Diagnosis of hip pain in children. *Hosp Med* 1999 Nov;60(11):788-93
[344] Maroo S. Diagnosis of hip pain in children. *Hosp Med* 1999 Nov;60(11):788-93

Problem	Presentation	Assessment & Management
<u>Gout</u>	<ul><li>**Febrile** patient has **acute/subacute mono/oligo-arthritis**</li><li>**Onset over hours or days**</li><li>"A history of discreet attacks, usually affecting one joint, that precede the onset of fixed symmetric arthritis is the major clue."[347]</li><li>May have fever, chills, tachycardia, leukocytosis—just like septic arthritis</li></ul>	<ul><li>Clinical presentation may be sufficient for DX; however septic arthritis should be excluded</li><li>Serum uric acid is generally meaningless for the diagnosis of gout since many gout patients will have normal serum uric acid</li><li>Medical treatment is rest, NSAID's, and allopurinol</li><li>Fluid loading: >3 liters per day; monitor for electrolyte imbalances and hyponatremia as needed</li><li>Integrative assessment and treatment for insulin resistance, hormonal imbalances, and nutritional deficiencies</li></ul>
<u>CPPD</u>: Calcium pyrophosphate dihydrate deposition disease	<ul><li>Idiopathic</li><li>May be caused by iron overload in some patients</li><li>Presentation may be acute or subacute</li></ul>	<ul><li>Medical diagnosis is by synovial biopsy</li><li>Radiographs reveal chondrocalcinosis</li><li>Allopathic treatment is NSAIDs; phytonutritional anti-inflammatory treatments may also be used (see chapter 3 of *Integrative Orthopedics/Rheumatology*)</li><li>Oral colchicine 0.5 to 1.5 mg per day prevents attacks[348]</li></ul>
<u>Hemarthrosis</u>: Generally associated with trauma, anticoagulation (i.e., coumadin), leukemia, hemophilia	<ul><li>Monoarthralgia with limited motion</li><li>May follow direct trauma</li><li>Nontraumatic hemarthrosis may be due to anticoagulation, leukemia, hemophilia</li></ul>	<ul><li>Synovial fluid analysis reveals blood</li><li>Treatment of underlying disorder; refer as indicated</li></ul>
<u>Slipped capital femoral epiphysis (SCFE)</u>: The most common cause of hip pain in adolescents[349]	<ul><li>Seen in adolescents generally 8-17 years of age</li><li>Classic presentation is a tall overweight boy with **hip pain**, knee pain, and/or a painful limp: "*Slipped femoral capital epiphysis is a developmental injury that must be considered in any adolescent who presents with hip pain.*"[350]</li></ul>	<ul><li>**Radiographs** of both hips (bilateral SCFE in 40%): "<u>**AP and frog lateral views are recommended in all children over age of 9 years with hip pain**</u>."[351]</li><li>Orthopedic referral—"*...the patient should be referred immediately to an orthopedist for surgical stabilization.*" [352]</li></ul>

[345] Skinner HB, Scherger JE. Identifying structural hip and knee problems. Patient age, history, and limited examination may be all that's needed. *Postgrad Med* 1999;106(7):51-2, 55-6, 61-4

[346] Souza TA. <u>Differential Diagnosis for the Chiropractor: Protocols and Algorithms</u>. Gaithersberg, Maryland: Aspen Publications. 1997 page 263

[347] Hardin JG, Waterman J, Labson LH. Rheumatic disease: Which diagnostic tests are useful? *Patient Care* 1999; March 15: 83-102

[348] Beers MH, Berkow R (eds). <u>The Merck Manual. Seventeenth Edition</u>. Whitehouse Station; Merck Research Laboratories 1999 Page

[349] Maroo S. Diagnosis of hip pain in children. *Hosp Med* 1999 Nov;60(11):788-93

[350] O'Kane JW. Anterior hip pain. *Am Fam Physician* 1999 Oct 15;60(6):1687-96

Clinical assessment:

- History and orthopedic assessment of the joint
- Laboratory tests must be performed if you have a suspicion of infection

History/subjective:

- Acute or subacute joint pain with or without systemic manifestations and fever.
- History or may not be significant; other than the obvious risk factor of immunosuppression, septic arthritis can occur with impressive spontaneity and randomness

Differential physical examination and objective findings:

- **Septic arthritis**: pain and limitation of motion, swelling, redness; patient may have systemic symptoms of fever and malaise
- **Gout**: pain and limitation of motion, swelling, redness; patient may have systemic symptoms of fever and malaise
- **Pseudogout and calcium pyrophosphate dihydrate deposition disease (CPDD/CPPD)**: pain and limitation of motion, swelling, redness; patient may have systemic symptoms of fever and malaise
- **Ischemic necrosis**: pain and limitation of motion; swelling, redness and systemic symptoms are less likely.
- **Hemarthrosis**: pain and limitation of motion; often associated with trauma, use of anticoagulant medications[353], or hemophilia and other hematologic abnormalities[354]
- **Tumor**: assess with history, imaging, and biopsy if possible
- **Injury**: Meniscal injury, fracture, ligament injury; physical examination procedures are described in the chapters that follow

Imaging and laboratory assessments:

- **Septic arthritis**: joint aspiration; STAT CBC (for WBC count) and CRP
- **Gout**: joint aspiration; CBC (for WBC count) and CRP
- **Pseudogout and PPDD**: rule out septic arthritis with joint aspiration, CBC, and CRP; radiographs often show chondrocalcinosis
- **Ischemic necrosis**: radiographs are diagnostic
- **Hemarthrosis**: joint aspiration and assessment for underlying disease or medication, especially if the condition was not trauma-induced
- **Tumor**: assess with radiographs
- **Injury**: rule out infection; consider imaging with radiography or MRI.

Establishing the diagnosis:

- The aforementioned examinations and lab assessments should establish the exact diagnosis. **The priorities are 1) first exclude life-threatening illness (i.e., septic arthritis), then 2) to exclude serious injury or illness,** and finally 3) to help manage the exact problem.

Complications:

- **Septic arthritis can result in death 5-10% of patients. "Five to 10 percent of patients with an infected joint die, chiefly from respiratory complications of sepsis. The mortality rate is 30% for patients with polyarticular sepsis. Bony ankylosis and articular destruction commonly also occur if the treatment is delayed or inadequate."[355]** Complications vary per location, infecting organism, severity, and patient.

---

[351] Maroo S. Diagnosis of hip pain in children. *Hosp Med* 1999 Nov;60(11):788-93
[352] O'Kane JW. Anterior hip pain. *Am Fam Physician* 1999 Oct 15;60(6):1687-96
[353] Riley SA, Spencer GE. Destructive monarticular arthritis secondary to anticoagulant therapy. *Clin Orthop*. 1987 Oct;(223):247-51
[354] Jean-Baptiste G, De Ceulaer K. Osteoarticular disorders of haematological origin. *Baillieres Best Pract Res Clin Rheumatol*. 2000 Jun;14(2):307-23
[355] Tierney ML. McPhee SJ, Papadakis MA. <u>Current Medical Diagnosis and Treatment. 35th edition</u>. Stamford: Appleton & Lange, 1996 page 759

Clinical management:

- **Suspected septic arthritis requires referral for joint aspiration and antimicrobial drugs.**
- Referral if clinical outcome is unsatisfactory or if serious complications are evident.
- Treatment of other conditions that cause acute monoarthritis (such as gout and calcium pyrophosphate dihydrate deposition disease) is based on the problem and individual patient.

Treatments:

- **Septic arthritis requires IV/oral antimicrobial drugs:** Intravenous antibiotics are generally started before culture results are available. After results and culture from synovial fluid analysis have been considered, the dose, combination, and administration of antibiotics can be fine-tuned. Frequently, antibiotics are administered intravenously for at least 3-4 weeks. Surgical/endoscopic drainage/debridement and immobilization during the acute phase may also be implemented.[356]

- **Immunonutrition considerations:** Immunonutritional considerations are listed below; doses listed are for adults. Although studies have not been performed specifically in patients with bone/joint infections, general benefits derived from the use of immunonutrition are reductions in severity/frequency/duration of major infections, abbreviated hospitalization (i.e., early discharge due to expedited healing and recovery), reductions in the need for medications, significant improvements in survival, and hospital savings.[357,358,359,360,361,362,363]

  o **Paleo-Mediterranean diet:** as detailed later in this text and elsewhere[364,365]

  o **Vitamin and mineral supplementation:** anti-infective benefits shown in elderly diabetics[366]

  o **High-dose vitamin A:** Vitamin A shows potent immunosupportive benefits, and vitamin A stores are depleted by the stress of infection and injury. Consider 200,000-300,000 IU per day of retinol palmitate for 1-4 weeks, then taper; reduce dose or discontinue with onset of toxicity symptoms such as skin problems (dry skin, flaking skin, chapped or split lips, red skin rash, hair loss), joint pain, bone pain, headaches, anorexia (loss of appetite), edema (water retention, weight gain, swollen ankles, difficulty breathing), fatigue, and/or liver damage.

  o **Arginine:** Dose for adults is in the range of 5-10 grams daily

---

[356] Brusch JL. Septic Arthritis (Last Updated: October 18, 2005). *eMedicine.* http://www.emedicine.com/med/topic3394.htm Accessed Nov 25, 2006

[357] "To evaluate the metabolic and immune effects of dietary arginine, glutamine and omega-3 fatty acids (fish oil) supplementation, we performed a prospective study... CONCLUSIONS: The feeding of Neomune in critically injured patients was well tolerated as Traumacal and significant improvement was observed in serum protein. Shorten ICU stay and wean-off respirator day may benefit from using the immunonutrient formula." Chuntrasakul C, Siltham S, Sarasombath S, Sittapairochana C, Leowattana W, Chockvivatanavanit S, Bunnak A. Comparison of a immunonutrition formula enriched arginine, glutamine and omega-3 fatty acid, with a currently high-enriched enteral nutrition for trauma patients. *J Med Assoc Thai.* 2003 Jun;86(6):552-6

[358] "CONCLUSIONS: In conclusion, arginine-enhanced formula improves fistula rates in postoperative head and neck cancer patients and decreases length of stay." de Luis DA, Izaola O, Cuellar L, Terroba MC, Aller R. Randomized clinical trial with an enteral arginine-enhanced formula in early postsurgical head and neck cancer patients. *Eur J Clin Nutr.* 2004;58(11):1505-8

[359] "In this prospective, randomised, double-blind, placebo-controlled study, we randomly assigned 50 patients who were scheduled to undergo coronary artery bypass to receive either an oral immune-enhancing nutritional supplement containing L-arginine, omega3 polyunsaturated fatty acids, and yeast RNA (n=25), or a control (n=25) for a minimum of 5 days... Intake of an oral immune-enhancing nutritional supplement for a minimum of 5 days before surgery can improve outlook in high-risk patients who are undergoing elective cardiac surgery." Tepaske R, Velthuis H, Oudemans-van Straaten HM, Heisterkamp SH, van Deventer SJ, Ince C, Eysman L, Kesecioglu J. Effect of preoperative oral immune-enhancing nutritional supplement on patients at high risk of infection after cardiac surgery: a randomised placebo-controlled trial. *Lancet.* 2001 Sep 1;358(9283):696-701

[360] "The feeding of IMMUNE FORMULA was well tolerated and significant improvement was observed in nutritional and immunologic parameters as in other immunoenhancing diets. Further clinical trials of prospective double-blind randomized design are necessary to address the so that the necessity of using immunonutrition in critically ill patients will be clarified." Chuntrasakul C, Siltharm S, Sarasombath S, Sittapairochana C, Leowattana W, Chockvivatanavanit S, Bunnak A. Metabolic and immune effects of dietary arginine, glutamine and omega-3 fatty acids supplementation in immunocompromised patients. *J Med Assoc Thai.* 1998 May;81(5):334-43

[361] "enteral diet supplemented with arginine, dietary nucleotides, and omega-3 fatty acids (IMPACT, Sandoz Nutrition, Bern, Switzerland)" Senkal M, Mumme A, Eickhoff U, Geier B, Spath G, Wulfert D, Joosten U, Frei A, Kemen M. Early postoperative enteral immunonutrition: clinical outcome and cost-comparison analysis in surgical patients. *Crit Care Med* 1997;25(9):1489-96

[362] "supplemented diet with glutamine, arginine and omega-3-fatty acids... It was clearly established in this trial that early postoperative enteral feeding is safe in patients who have undergone major operations for gastrointestinal cancer. Supplementation of enteral nutrition with glutamine, arginine, and omega-3-fatty acids positively modulated postsurgical immunosuppressive and inflammatory responses." Wu GH, Zhang YW, Wu ZH. Modulation of postoperative immune and inflammatory response by immune-enhancing enteral diet in gastrointestinal cancer patients. *World J Gastroenterol.* 2001 Jun;7(3):357-62 http://www.wjgnet.com/1007-9327/7/357.pdf

[363] "using a formula supplemented with arginine, mRNA, and omega-3 fatty acids from fish oil (Impact). CONCLUSIONS: Immune-enhancing enteral nutrition resulted in a significant reduction in the mortality rate and infection rate in septic patients admitted to the ICU. These reductions were greater for patients with less severe illness." Galban C, Montejo JC, Mesejo A, Marco P, Celaya S, Sanchez-Segura JM, Farre M, Bryg DJ. An immune-enhancing enteral diet reduces mortality rate and episodes of bacteremia in septic intensive care unit patients. *Crit Care Med.* 2000 Mar;28(3):643-8

[364] **Vasquez A.** A Five-Part Nutritional Protocol that Produces Consistently Positive Results. *Nutritional Wellness* 2005 September http://optimalhealthresearch.com/protocol

[365] **Vasquez A.** Implementing the Five-Part Nutritional Wellness Protocol for the Treatment of Various Health Problems. *Nutritional Wellness* 2005 November. http://optimalhealthresearch.com/protocol

[366] "CONCLUSIONS: A multivitamin and mineral supplement reduced the incidence of participant-reported infection and related absenteeism in a sample of participants with type 2 diabetes mellitus and a high prevalence of subclinical micronutrient deficiency." Barringer TA, Kirk JK, Santaniello AC, Foley KL, Michielutte R. Effect of a multivitamin and mineral supplement on infection and quality of life. A randomized, double-blind, placebo-controlled trial. *Ann Intern Med.* 2003 Mar 4;138(5):365-71 http://www.annals.org/cgi/reprint/138/5/365

- o **Fatty acid supplementation**: In contrast to the higher doses used to provide an anti-inflammatory effect in patients with autoimmune/inflammatory disorders, doses used for immunosupportive treatments should be kept rather modest to avoid the *relative* immunosuppression that has been controversially reported in patients treated with EPA and DHA. Reasonable doses are in the following ranges for adults: EPA+DHA: 500-1,500, and GLA: 300-500 mg.

- o **Glutamine**: Glutamine enhances bacterial killing by neutrophils[367], and administration of 18 grams per day in divided doses to patients in intensive care units was shown to improve survival, expedite hospital discharge, and reduce total healthcare costs.[368] Another study using glutamine 12-18 grams per day showed no benefit in overall mortality but significant benefits in terms of reduced healthcare costs (-30%) and significantly reduced need for medical interventions.[369] After administering glutamine 26 grams/d to severely burned patients, Garrel et al[370] concluded that glutamine reduced the risk of infection by 3-fold and that oral glutamine "may be a life-saving intervention" in patients with severe burns. A dose of 30 grams/d was used in a recent clinical trial showing hemodynamic benefit in patients with sickle cell anemia.[371] The highest glutamine dose that the current author is aware of is the study by Scheltinga et al[372] who used 0.57 gm/kg/day in cancer patients following chemotherapy administration; for a 220-lb-pt, this would be approximately 57 grams of glutamine per day.

- o **Melatonin**: 20-40 mg hs (*hora somni*—Latin: sleep time). Immunostimulatory anti-infective action of melatonin was demonstrated in a small clinical trial wherein septic newborns administered 20 mg melatonin showed significantly increased survival over nontreated controls.[373]

[367] Furukawa S, Saito H, Fukatsu K, Hashiguchi Y, Inaba T, Lin MT, Inoue T, Han I, Matsuda T, Muto T. Glutamine-enhanced bacterial killing by neutrophils from postoperative patients. *Nutrition* 1997;13(10):863-9. *In vitro* study.
[368] Griffiths RD, Jones C, Palmer TE. Six-month outcome of critically ill patients given glutamine-supplemented parenteral nutrition. *Nutrition* 1997;13(4):295-302
[369] "There was no mortality difference between those patients receiving glutamine-containing enteral feed and the controls. However, there was a significant reduction in the median postintervention ICU and hospital patient costs in the glutamine recipients $23 000 versus $30 900 in the control patients." Jones C, Palmer TE, Griffiths RD. Randomized clinical outcome study of critically ill patients given glutamine-supplemented enteral nutrition. *Nutrition.* 1999 Feb;15(2):108-15
[370] The glutamine dose in this study was "a total of 26 g/day" administered in four divided doses. CONCLUSION: "The results of this prospective randomized clinical trial show that enteral G reduces blood culture positivity, particularly with P. aeruginosa, in adults with severe burns and may be a life-saving intervention." Garrel D, Patenaude J, Nedelec B, et al. Decreased mortality and infectious morbidity in adult burn patients given enteral glutamine supplements: a prospective, controlled, randomized clinical trial. *Crit Care Med.* 2003 Oct;31(10):2444-9
[371] Niihara Y, Matsui NM, Shen YM, et al. L-glutamine therapy reduces endothelial adhesion of sickle red blood cells to human umbilical vein endothelial cells. *BMC Blood Disord.* 2005 Jul 25;5:4 http://www.biomedcentral.com.proxy.hsc.unt.edu/1471-2326/5/4
[372] "Subjects with hematologic malignancies in remission underwent a standard treatment of high-dose chemotherapy and total body irradiation before bone marrow transplantation. After completion of this regimen, they were randomized to receive either standard parenteral nutrition (STD, n = 10) or an isocaloric, isonitrogenous nutrient solution enriched with crystalline L-glutamine (0.57 g/kg/day, GLN, n = 10)." Scheltinga MR, Young LS, Benfell K, Bye RL, Ziegler TR, Santos AA, Antin JH, Schloerb PR, Wilmore DW. Glutamine-enriched intravenous feedings attenuate extracellular fluid expansion after a standard stress. *Ann Surg.* 1991 Oct;214(4):385-93; discussion 393-5 pubmedcentral.nih.gov/articlerender.fcgi?tool=pubmed&pubmedid=1953094 For additional review, see Ziegler TR. Glutamine supplementation in cancer patients receiving bone marrow transplantation and high dose chemotherapy. J Nutr. 2001 Sep;131(9 Suppl):2578S-84S http://jn.nutrition.org/cgi/content/full/131/9/2578S
[373] Gitto E, et al. Effects of melatonin treatment in septic newborns. *Pediatr Res.* 2001;50:756-60 pedresearch.org/cgi/content/full/50/6/756

Brief Overview of Integrative Healthcare Disciplines

Chiropractic

"Doctors of Chiropractic are physicians who consider man as an integrated being and give special attention to the physiological and biochemical aspects including structural, spinal, musculoskeletal, neurological, vascular, nutritional, emotional and environmental relationships." *American Chiropractic Association, 2004*[374]

"The human body represents the actions of three laws—spiritual, mechanical, and chemical—united as one triune. As long as there is perfect union of these three, there is health." *Daniel David Palmer, founder of the modern chiropractic profession*[375]

The basic philosophical model which is taught in many chiropractic colleges is to envision health, disease, and patient care from a conceptual model named the "triad of health" which gives its attention to the three fundamental foundations for well-being: namely, the physical/structural, mental/emotional, and biochemical/nutritional aspects of health. Revolutionary at the time of its inception in the early 1900's, this model now forms the foundation for the increasingly dominant and very popular paradigm of "holistic medicine." It remains a powerful contrast and an attractive alternative to the reductionistic allopathic approach, which generally approaches the human body as if it were simply a conglomerate of independent organ systems that have little or no functional relationship to each other.[376]

Using the state of the sciences before the year 1910, chiropractic was founded with a profound appreciation of the integrated nature of health, and the therapeutic focus was on spinal

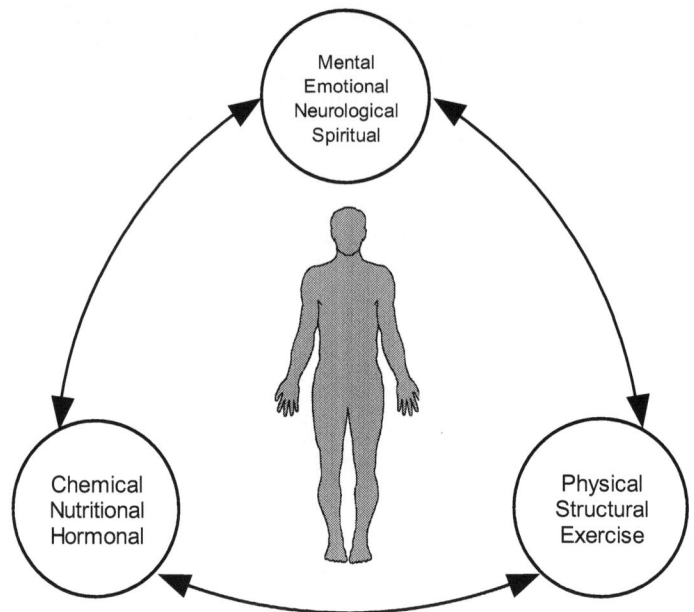

The chiropractic "triad of health"

manipulation. In describing the chiropractic model of health, DD Palmer[377] wrote, "The human body represents the actions of three laws—spiritual, mechanical, and chemical—united as one triune. As long as there is perfect union of these three, there is health." While the therapeutic focus of the profession has been spinal manipulation, from its inception the chiropractic profession has emphasized a holistic, integrative model of therapeutic intervention, health, and disease, and chiropractic was the first healthcare profession in America to specifically claim that the optimization of health requires attention to spiritual-emotional-psychological, mechanical-physical-structural, and biochemical-nutritional-hormonal-chemical considerations. Accordingly, these cornerstones are fundamental to the 2005 definition of the chiropractic profession articulated by the American Chiropractic Association[378]: "Doctors of Chiropractic are physicians who consider man as an integrated being and give special attention to the physiological and biochemical aspects including structural, spinal, musculoskeletal, neurological, vascular, nutritional, emotional, and environmental relationships."

---

[374] American Chiropractic Association. http://www.amerchiro.org/media/whatis/ Accessed March 13, 2004
[375] Palmer DD. The Science, Art, and Phiosophy, of Chiropractic. Portland, OR; Portland Printing House Company, 1910: 107
[376] Beckman JF, Fernandez CE, Coulter ID. A systems model of health care: a proposal. *J Manipulative Physiol Ther*. 1996 Mar-Apr; 19(3): 208-15
[377] Palmer DD. The Science, Art, and Phiosophy, of Chiropractic. Portland, OR; Portland Printing House Company, 1910: 107
[378] American Chiropractic Association. What is Chiropractic? http://amerchiro.org/media/whatis/ Accessed January 9, 2005

From its inception, chiropractic was a philosophy of healing that considered the entire health of the patient by addressing the interconnected aspects of our chemical-spiritual-physical being. Later, intraprofessional factions polarized between holistic and vitalistic paradigms; the latter has been presumed to be the philosophy of the entire profession by organizations such as the American Medical Association[379] that have sought to contain and eliminate chiropractic and other forms of natural healthcare[380] by falsifying research[381,382], intentionally misleading the public and manipulating politicians[383,384,385], arriving at illogical conclusions which support the medical paradigm and refute the value of manual therapies[386], and exploiting weaknesses within the profession for its own financial profitability and political advantage.[387] Intentional misrepresentation and defamation of chiropractic continues to occur today, as documented by the 2006 review by Wenban.[388]

Chiropractic Training and Clinical Benefits: In addition to the basic sciences and foundational skills of laboratory and clinical diagnosis, chiropractic physicians receive extensive training in manual physical manipulation, rehabilitation, therapeutic exercise, and clinical nutrition.

An irony exists in the observation that chiropractic education emphasizes anatomy, musculoskeletal therapeutics, and nutrition while these are the very topics that are neglected in allopathic and osteopathic education; the majority medical students and medical physicians who have graduated from allopathic and osteopathic medical schools lack competence in their knowledge of clinical anatomy and musculoskeletal medicine[389,390,391,392,393,394] as well as diet and nutrition.[395,396,397] In contrast to this replicable data showing that osteopathic and allopathic students and graduates generally fail to demonstrate competence in musculoskeletal medicine and nutrition, one study with 123 chiropractic students and 10 chiropractic doctors showed that chiropractic training in musculoskeletal medicine is significantly superior to allopathic and osteopathic musculoskeletal training.[398]

In accord with the comprehensive chiropractic training in musculoskeletal management, numerous sources of evidence demonstrate that chiropractic management of the most common spinal pain syndromes is safer and less expensive than allopathic medical treatment, particularly for the treatment of low-back pain. In

[379] American Medical Association. Report 12 of the Council on Scientific Affairs (A-97) Full Text. http://www.ama-assn.org/ama/pub/category/13638.html Accessed Sep 10, 2005
[380] Getzendanner S. Permanent injunction order against AMA. *JAMA*. 1988 Jan 1;259(1):81-2
[381] Terrett AG. Misuse of the literature by medical authors in discussing spinal manipulative therapy injury. *J Manipulative Physiol Ther*. 1995 May;18(4):203-10
[382] Morley J, Rosner AL, Redwood D. A case study of misrepresentation of the scientific literature: recent reviews of chiropractic. *J Altern Complement Med*. 2001 Feb;7(1):65-78
[383] Spivak JL. The Medical Trust Unmasked. Louis S. Siegfried Publishers; New York: 1961
[384] Trever W. In the Public Interest. Los Angeles; Scriptures Unlimited; 1972. This is probably the most authoritative documentation of the illegal actions of the AMA up to 1972; contains numerous photocopies of actual AMA documents and minutes of official meetings with overt intentionality of destroying Americans' healthcare options so that the AMA and related organizations would have a monopoly in healthcare.
[385] Wolinsky H, Brune T. The Serpent on the Staff: The Unhealthy Politics of the American Medical Association. GP Putnam and Sons, New York, 1994
[386] Mein EA, Greenman PE, McMillin DL, Richards DG, Nelson CD. Manual medicine diversity: research pitfalls and the emerging medical paradigm. *J Am Osteopath Assoc*. 2001 Aug;101(8):441-4
[387] Wilk CA. Medicine, Monopolies, and Malice: How the Medical Establishment Tried to Destroy Chiropractic. Garden City Park: Avery, 1996
[388] Wenban AB. Inappropriate use of the title 'chiropractor' and term 'chiropractic manipulation' in the peer-reviewed biomedical literature. *Chiropr Osteopat*. 2006;14:16 http://chiroandosteo.com/content/14/1/16
[389] "In summary, seventy (82 per cent) of eighty-five medical school graduates failed a valid musculoskeletal competency examination. We therefore believe that medical school preparation in musculoskeletal medicine is inadequate." Freedman KB, Bernstein J. The adequacy of medical school education in musculoskeletal medicine. *J Bone Joint Surg Am*. 1998;80(10):1421-7
[390] "CONCLUSIONS: According to the standard suggested by the program directors of internal medicine residency departments, a large majority of the examinees once again failed to demonstrate basic competency in musculoskeletal medicine on the examination. It is therefore reasonable to conclude that medical school preparation in musculoskeletal medicine is inadequate." Freedman KB, Bernstein J. Educational deficiencies in musculoskeletal medicine. *J Bone Joint Surg Am*. 2002;84-A(4):604-8
[391] Joy EA, Hala SV. Musculoskeletal Curricula in Medical Education: Filling In the Missing Pieces. *The Physician and Sportsmedicine* 2004; 32: 42-45
[392] "CONCLUSIONS: Seventy-nine percent of the participants failed the basic musculoskeletal cognitive examination. This suggests that training in musculoskeletal medicine is inadequate in both medical school and nonorthopaedic residency training programs." Matzkin E, Smith ME, Freccero CD, Richardson AB. Adequacy of education in musculoskeletal medicine. *J Bone Joint Surg Am*. 2005 Feb;87-A(2):310-4
[393] "Despite generally improved levels of competency with each year at medical school, less than 50% of fourth-year students showed competency. … These results suggested that the curricular approach toward teaching musculoskeletal medicine at this medical school was insufficient and that competency increased when learning was reinforced during the clinical years." Schmale GA. More evidence of educational inadequacies in musculoskeletal medicine. *Clin Orthop Relat Res*. 2005 Aug;(437):251-9
[394] "RESULTS: When the minimum passing level as determined by orthopedic program directors was applied to the results of these examinations, 70.4% of graduating COM students (n=54) and 82% of allopathic graduates (n=85) failed to demonstrate basic competency in musculoskeletal medicine." Stockard AR, Allen TW. Competence levels in musculoskeletal medicine: comparison of osteopathic and allopathic medical graduates. *J Am Osteopath Assoc*. 2006 Jun;106(6):350-5
[395] "CONCLUSIONS: Internal medicine interns' perceive nutrition counseling as a priority, but lack the confidence and knowledge to effectively provide adequate nutrition education." Vetter ML, Herring SJ, Sood M, Shah NR, Kalet AL. What do resident physicians know about nutrition? An evaluation of attitudes, self-perceived proficiency and knowledge. *J Am Coll Nutr*. 2008 Apr;27(2):287-98
[396] "CONCLUSIONS: The amount of nutrition education that medical students receive continues to be inadequate." Adams KM, Kohlmeier M, Zeisel SH. Nutrition education in U.S. medical schools: latest update of a national survey. *Acad Med*. 2010 Sep;85(9):1537-42
[397] CONCLUSIONS: This survey suggests that multiple barriers exist that prevent the primary care practitioner from providing dietary counseling. A multifaceted approach will be needed to change physician counseling behavior." Kushner RF. Barriers to providing nutrition counseling by physicians: a survey of primary care practitioners. *Prev Med*. 1995 Nov;24(6):546-52
[398] Humphreys BK, Sulkowski A, McIntyre K, Kasiban M, Patrick AN. An examination of musculoskeletal cognitive competency in chiropractic interns. *J Manipulative Physiol Ther*. 2007;30(1):44-9

their extensive review of the literature, Manga et al[399] published in 1993 that chiropractic management of low-back pain is superior to allopathic medical management in terms of greater safety, greater effectiveness, and reduced cost; they concluded, "There is an overwhelming body of evidence indicating that chiropractic management of low-back pain is more cost-effective than medical management" and "There would be highly significant cost savings if more management of LBP [low-back pain] was transferred from medical physicians to chiropractors." In a randomized trial involving 741 patients, Meade et al[400] showed, "Chiropractic treatment was more effective than hospital outpatient management, mainly for patients with chronic or severe back pain... The benefit of chiropractic treatment became more evident throughout the follow up period. Secondary outcome measures also showed that chiropractic was more beneficial." A 3-year follow-up study by these same authors[401] in 1995 showed, "At three years the results confirm the findings of an earlier report that when chiropractic or hospital therapists treat patients with low-back pain as they would in day to day practice, those treated by chiropractic derive more benefit and long term satisfaction than those treated by hospitals." More recently, in 2004 Legorreta et al[402] reported that the availability of chiropractic care was associated with significant cost savings among 700,000 patients with chiropractic coverage compared to 1 million patients whose insurance coverage was limited to allopathic medical treatments. Simple extrapolation of the average savings per patient in this study ($208 annual savings associated with chiropractic coverage) to the US population (295 million citizens in 2005[403]) suggests that, if fully implemented in a nation-wide basis, America could save $61,360,000,000 (more than $61 billion per year) in annual healthcare expenses by ensuring chiropractic for all citizens in contrast to failing to provide such coverage; obviously extrapolations such as this should consider other variables, such as the relatively higher prevalence of injury and death among patients treated with drugs and surgery.[404,405] Furthermore, whether the cost savings associated with chiropractic availability are due to 1) improved overall health and reduced need for pharmacosurgical intervention, 2) greater safety and lower cost of chiropractic treatment versus pharmacosurgical treatment, and/or 3) self-selection by wellness-oriented, perhaps healthier, and higher-income patients, remains to be determined.

A literature review by Dabbs and Lauretti[406] showed that spinal manipulation is safer than the use of NSAIDs in the treatment of neck pain. Contrasting the rates of manipulation-associated cerebrovascular accidents to the dangers of medical and surgical treatments for spinal disorders, Rosner[407] noted, "These rates are 400 times lower than the death rates observed from gastrointestinal bleeding due to the use of nonsteroidal anti-inflammatory drugs and 700 times lower than the overall mortality rate for spinal surgery." Similarly, in his review of the literature comparing the safety of chiropractic manipulation in patients with low-back pain associated with lumbar disc herniation, Oliphant[408] showed that, "The apparent safety of spinal manipulation, especially when compared with other [medically] accepted treatments for [lumbar disk herniation], should stimulate its use in the conservative treatment plan of [lumbar disk herniation]."

The clinical benefits and cost-effectiveness of chiropractic management of musculoskeletal conditions is extensively documented, and that spinal manipulation generally shows superior safety to drug and surgical treatment of back and neck pain is also well established.[409,410,411,412,413,414,415] Adjunctive therapies such as post-

[399] Manga P, Angus D, Papadopoulos C, et al. The Effectiveness and Cost-Effectiveness of Chiropractic Management of Low-Back Pain. Richmond Hill, Ontario: Kenilworth Publishing; 1993
[400] Meade TW, Dyer S, Browne W, Townsend J, Frank AO. Low-back pain of mechanical origin: randomised comparison of chiropractic and hospital outpatient treatment. BMJ. 1990;300(6737):1431-7
[401] Meade TW, Dyer S, Browne W, Frank AO. Randomised comparison of chiropractic and hospital outpatient management for low-back pain: results from extended follow up. BMJ. 1995;311(7001):349-5
[402] Legorreta AP, Metz RD, Nelson CF, Ray S, Chernicoff HO, Dinubile NA. Comparative analysis of individuals with and without chiropractic coverage: patient characteristics, utilization, and costs. Arch Intern Med. 2004;164:1985-92
[403] US Census Bureau http://factfinder.census.gov/home/saff/main.html?_lang=en Accessed January 12, 2005
[404] Rosner AL. Evidence-based clinical guidelines for the management of acute low-back pain: response to the guidelines prepared for the Australian Medical Health and Research Council. J Manipulative Physiol Ther. 2001;24(3):214-20
[405] Topol EJ. Failing the public health--rofecoxib, Merck, and the FDA. N Engl J Med. 2004 Oct 21;351(17):1707-9
[406] Dabbs V, Lauretti WJ. A risk assessment of cervical manipulation vs. NSAIDs for the treatment of neck pain. J Manipulative Physiol Ther. 1995;18:530-6
[407] Rosner AL. Evidence-based clinical guidelines for the management of acute low-back pain: response to the guidelines prepared for the Australian Medical Health and Research Council. J Manipulative Physiol Ther. 2001;24(3):214-20
[408] Oliphant D. Safety of spinal manipulation in the treatment of lumbar disk herniations: a systematic review and risk assessment. J Manipulative Physiol Ther. 2004;27:197-210
[409] Dabbs V, Lauretti WJ. A risk assessment of cervical manipulation vs. NSAIDs for the treatment of neck pain. J Manipulative Physiol Ther. 1995;18:530-6
[410] Rosner AL. Evidence-based clinical guidelines for the management of acute low-back pain: response to the guidelines prepared for the Australian Medical Health and Research Council. J Manipulative Physiol Ther. 2001 Mar-Apr;24(3):214-20
[411] Oliphant D. Safety of spinal manipulation in the treatment of lumbar disk herniations: a systematic review and risk assessment. J Manipulative Physiol Ther. 2004;27:197-210
[412] Meade TW, Dyer S, Browne W, Townsend J, Frank AO. Low-back pain of mechanical origin: randomised comparison of chiropractic and hospital outpatient treatment. BMJ. 1990;300(6737):1431-7
[413] Meade TW, Dyer S, Browne W, Frank AO. Randomised comparison of chiropractic and hospital outpatient management for low-back pain: results from extended follow up. BMJ. 1995;311(7001):349-5

isometric relaxation[416] and correction of myofascial dysfunction[417] can lead to tremendous and rapid reductions in musculoskeletal pain without the hazards and expense associated with pharmaceutical drugs. Nonmusculoskeletal benefits of musculoskeletal/spinal manipulation include improved pulmonary function and/or quality of life in patients with asthma[418,419,420,421] and—according to a series of cases published by an osteopathic ophthalmologist—improvement or restoration of vision in patients with post-traumatic and acute-onset visual loss.[422,423,424,425,426,427,428,429] More research is required to quantify the potential benefits of spinal manipulation in patients with wide-ranging conditions such as epilepsy[430,431], attention-deficit hyperactivity disorder[432,433], and Parkinson's disease.[434] Given that most pharmaceutical drugs work on single biochemical pathways, spinal manipulation is discordant with the medical/drug paradigm because its effects are numerous (rather than singular) and physical and physiological (rather than biochemical). Thus, when viewed through the allopathic/pharmaceutical lens, spinal manipulation (like acupuncture and other physical modalities) "does not make sense" and will be viewed as "unscientific" simply because it is based in physiology rather than pharmacology. In this case, the fault lies with the viewer and the lens, not with the object.

Research documenting the systemic and "nonmusculoskeletal" benefits of spinal manipulation mandates that our concept of "musculoskeletal" must be expanded to appreciate that **musculoskeletal interventions benefit nonmusculoskeletal body systems and physiologic processes**. This conceptual expansion applies also to soft tissue therapeutics such as massage, which can reduce adolescent aggression[435], improve outcome in preterm infants[436], alleviate premenstrual syndrome[437], and increase serotonin and dopamine levels in patients with low-back pain.[438]

[414] Manga P, Angus D, Papadopoulos C, et al. The Effectiveness and Cost-Effectiveness of Chiropractic Management of Low-Back Pain. Richmond Hill, Ontario: Kenilworth Publishing; 1993
[415] Legorreta AP, Metz RD, Nelson CF, Ray S, Chernicoff HO, Dinubile NA. Comparative analysis of individuals with and without chiropractic coverage: patient characteristics, utilization, and costs. *Arch Intern Med*. 2004;164:1985-92
[416] Lewit K, Simons DG. Myofascial pain: relief by post-isometric relaxation. *Arch Phys Med Rehabil*. 1984;65(8):452-6
[417] Ingber RS. Iliopsoas myofascial dysfunction: a treatable cause of "failed" low-back syndrome. *Arch Phys Med Rehabil*. 1989 May;70(5):382-6
[418] Nielson NH, Bronfort G, Bendix T, Madsen F, Wecke B. Chronic asthma and chiropractic spinal manipulation: a randomized clinical trial. *Clin Exp Allergy* 1995;25:80-8
[419] Mein EA, Greenman PE, McMillin DL, Richards DG, Nelson CD. Manual medicine diversity: research pitfalls and the emerging medical paradigm. *J Am Osteopath Assoc*. 2001 Aug;101(8):441-4
[420] "There were small increases (7 to 12 liters per minute) in peak expiratory flow in the morning and the evening in both treatment groups,... Symptoms of asthma and use of beta-agonists decreased and the quality of life increased in both groups, with no significant differences between the groups." Balon J, Aker PD, Crowther ER, Danielson C, Cox PG, O'Shaughnessy D, Walker C, Goldsmith CH, Duku E, Sears MR. A comparison of active and simulated chiropractic manipulation as adjunctive treatment for childhood asthma. *N Engl J Med*. 1998 Oct 8;339(15):1013-20
[421] Bronfort G, Evans RL, Kubic P, Filkin P. Chronic pediatric asthma and chiropractic spinal manipulation: a prospective clinical series and randomized clinical pilot study. *J Manipulative Physiol Ther*. 2001 Jul-Aug;24(6):369-77
[422] Stephens D, Pollard H, Bilton D, Thomson P, Gorman F. Bilateral simultaneous optic nerve dysfunction after periorbital trauma: recovery of vision in association with chiropractic spinal manipulation therapy. *J Manipulative Physiol Ther*. 1999 Nov-Dec;22(9):615-21
[423] Stephens D, Gorman F, Bilton D. The step phenomenon in the recovery of vision with spinal manipulation: a report on two 13-yr-olds treated together. *J Manipulative Physiol Ther*. 1997;20(9):628-33
[424] Stephens D, Gorman F. The association between visual incompetence and spinal derangement: an instructive case history. *J Manipulative Physiol Ther*. 1997 Jun;20(5):343-50.
[425] Stephens D, Gorman RF. Does 'normal' vision improve with spinal manipulation? *J Manipulative Physiol Ther*. 1996 Jul-Aug;19(6):415-8
[426] Gorman RF. Monocular scotomata and spinal manipulation: the step phenomenon. *J Manipulative Physiol Ther*. 1996 Jun;19(5):344-9
[427] Gorman RF. Monocular visual loss after closed head trauma: immediate resolution associated with spinal manipulation. *J Manipulative Physiol Ther*. 1995 Jun;18(5):308-14
[428] Gorman RF. The treatment of presumptive optic nerve ischemia by spinal manipulation. *J Manipulative Physiol Ther*. 1995;18(3):172-7
[429] Gorman RF. Automated static perimetry in chiropractic. *J Manipulative Physiol Ther*. 1993 Sep;16(7):481-7
[430] Elster EL. Treatment of bipolar, seizure, and sleep disorders and migraine headaches utilizing a chiropractic technique. *J Manipulative Physiol* Ther. 2004 Mar-Apr;27(3):E5
[431] Alcantara J, Heschong R, Plaugher G, Alcantara J. Chiropractic management of a patient with subluxations, low-back pain and epileptic seizures. *J Manipulative Physiol Ther*. 1998;21(6):410-8
[432] Giesen JM, Center DB, Leach RA. An evaluation of chiropractic manipulation as a treatment of hyperactivity in children. *J Manipulative Physiol Ther*. 1989 Oct;12(5):353-63
[433] Bastecki AV, Harrison DE, Haas JW. Cervical kyphosis is a possible link to attention-deficit/hyperactivity disorder. *J Manipulative Physiol Ther*. 2004 Oct;27(8):e14
[434] Elster EL. Upper cervical chiropractic management of a patient with Parkinson's disease: a case report. *J Manipulative Physiol Ther*. 2000 Oct;23(8):573-7
[435] Diego MA, Field T, Hernandez-Reif M, Shaw JA, Rothe EM, Castellanos D, Mesner L. Aggressive adolescents benefit from massage therapy. *Adolescence* 2002 Fall;37(147):597-607
[436] Mainous RO. Infant massage as a component of developmental care: past, present, and future. *Holist Nurs Pract* 2002 Oct;16(5):1-7
[437] Hernandez-Reif M, Martinez A, Field T, Quintero O, Hart S, Burman I. Premenstrual symptoms are relieved by massage therapy. *J Psychosom Obstet Gynaecol* 2000 Mar;21(1):9-15
[438] "RESULTS: By the end of the study, the massage therapy group, as compared to the relaxation group, reported experiencing less pain, depression, anxiety and improved sleep. They also showed improved trunk and pain flexion performance, and their serotonin and dopamine levels were higher." Hernandez-Reif M, Field T, Krasnegor J, Theakston H. Lower back pain is reduced and range of motion increased after massage therapy. *Int J Neurosci* 2001;106(3-4):131-45

<u>Spinal Manipulation: Mechanistic Considerations</u>: Applied to either the spine or peripheral joints, high-velocity low-amplitude (HVLA) joint manipulation appears to have numerous physical and physiological effects, including but not limited to the following:

1. Releasing entrapped intraarticular menisci and synovial folds,
2. Acutely reducing intradiscal pressure, thus promoting replacement of decentralized disc material,
3. Stretching of deep periarticular muscles to break the cycle of chronic autonomous muscle contraction by lengthening the muscles and thereby releasing excessive actin-myosin binding,
4. Promoting restoration of proper kinesthesia and proprioception,
5. Promoting relaxation of paraspinal muscles by stretching facet joint capsules,
6. Promoting relaxation of paraspinal muscles via "postactivation depression", which is the temporary depletion of contractile neurotransmitters,
7. Temporarily elevating plasma beta-endorphin,
8. Temporarily enhancing phagocytic ability of neutrophils and monocytes,
9. Activation of the diffuse descending pain inhibitory system located in the periaqueductal gray matter—this is an important aspect of nociceptive inhibition by intense sensory/mechanoreceptor stimulation, which will be discussed in a following section for its relevance to neurogenic inflammation, and
10. Improving neurotransmitter balance and reducing pain (soft-tissue manipulation).[439]

While the above list of mechanisms-of-action is certainly not complete, for purposes of this paper it is sufficient for the establishment that—indeed—joint manipulation in general and spinal manipulation in particular have objective mechanistic effects that correlate with their clinical benefits. Additional details are provided in numerous published reviews and primary research[440,441,442,443,444,445,446] and by Leach[447], whose extensive description of the mechanisms of action of spinal manipulative therapy is unsurpassed. Given such a wide base of experimental and clinical support published in peer-reviewed journals and widely-available textbooks, denigrations directed toward spinal manipulation on the grounds that it is "unscientific" or "unsupported by research" are unfounded and are indicative of selective ignorance.

---

[439] "RESULTS: By the end of the study, the massage therapy group, as compared to the relaxation group, reported experiencing less pain, depression, anxiety and improved sleep. They also showed improved trunk and pain flexion performance, and their serotonin and dopamine levels were higher." Hernandez-Reif M, Field T, Krasnegor J, Theakston H. Lower back pain is reduced and range of motion increased after massage therapy. *Int J Neurosci* 2001;106(3-4):131-45

[440] Maigne JY, Vautravers P. Mechanism of action of spinal manipulative therapy. *Joint Bone Spine*. 2003;70(5):336-41

[441] Brennan PC, Triano JJ, McGregor M, Kokjohn K, Hondras MA, Brennan DC. Enhanced neutrophil respiratory burst as a biological marker for manipulation forces: duration of the effect and association with substance P and tumor necrosis factor. *J Manipulative Physiol Ther*. 1992 Feb;15(2):83-9

[442] Brennan PC, Kokjohn K, Kaltinger CJ, Lohr GE, Glendening C, Hondras MA, McGregor M, Triano JJ. Enhanced phagocytic cell respiratory burst induced by spinal manipulation: potential role of substance P. *J Manipulative Physiol Ther*. 1991 Sep;14(7):399-408

[443] Heikkila H, Johansson M, Wenngren BI. Effects of acupuncture, cervical manipulation and NSAID therapy on dizziness and impaired head repositioning of suspected cervical origin: a pilot study. *Man Ther*. 2000 Aug;5(3):151-7

[444] Rogers RG. The effects of spinal manipulation on cervical kinesthesia in patients with chronic neck pain: a pilot study. *J Manipulative Physiol Ther*. 1997;20(2):80-5

[445] Bergman, Peterson, Lawrence. <u>Chiropractic Technique</u>. New York: Churchill Livingstone 1993. An updated edition is now availabe from Mosby.

[446] Herzog WH. Mechanical and physiological responses to spinal manipulative treatments. *JNMS: J Neuromusculoskeltal System* 1995; 3: 1-9

[447] Leach RA. (ed). <u>The Chiropractic Theories: A Textbook of Scientific Research, Fourth Edition</u>. Baltimore: Lippincott, Williams & Wilkins, 2004

Mechanoreceptor-Mediated Inhibition of Neurogenic Inflammation: A Possible Mechanism of Action of Spinal Manipulation: Neurogenic inflammation causes catabolism of articular structures and thus promotes joint destruction[448,449], a phenomena that the current author has termed "neurogenic chondrolysis."[450] The biologic and scientific basis for this concept rests on the following sequence of events which ultimately form a self-perpetuating and multisystem cycle:

1. Using joint pain as an example, we know that acute or chronic joint injury results in the release of inflammatory mediators in local tissues as **immunogenic inflammation**.

2. Nociceptive input is received centrally and results in release of inflammatory mediators *from sensory neurons* termed **neurogenic inflammation**[451] and results in a neurologically-mediated catabolic effect in articular cartilage[452,453] termed here as **neurogenic chondrolysis**.

3. As immunogenic and neurogenic inflammation synergize to promote joint destruction, pain from degenerating joints further increases nociceptive afferent transmission to further increase neurogenic and thus immunogenic inflammation. Thus, a *positive feedback* vicious cycle of immunogenic and neurogenic inflammation promotes and perpetuates joint destruction.

4. Further complicating this *regional* cycle of neurogenic-immunogenic inflammation and tissue destruction would be any pain or inflammation *in distant parts of the body*, since pain in one part of the body can exacerbate neurogenic inflammation in another part of the body via **neurogenic switching**[454,455] and immunologic reactivity such as allergy or autoimmunity in one part of the body may be transmitted *via the nervous system* to cause immunogenic inflammation in another part of the body via **immunogenic switching**.[456]

The clinical relevance of neurogenic inflammation and immunogenic switching is that when combined they provide a means *beyond biochemistry* by which to understand how and why inflammation ❶ is *transmitted and perpetuated by the nervous system* and ❷ must be treated with a body-wide *holistic* approach.

The current author is the first to propose the concept of **mechanoreceptor-mediated inhibition of neurogenic inflammation**.[457] Since neurogenic chondrolysis is inhibited by interference with C-fiber (type IV) mediated afferent transmission[458] and since chiropractic high-velocity low-amplitude (HVLA) manipulation appears to inhibit C-fiber mediated nociception[459,460], then chiropractic-type HVLA manipulation may reduce neurogenic inflammation and may promote articular integrity by inhibiting neurogenic chondrolysis. Further, mechanoreceptor-mediated inhibition of neurogenic inflammation would, for example, help explain the benefits of spinal manipulation in the treatment of asthma[461,462,463], since asthma is known to be mediated in large part by

---

[448] Gouze-Decaris E, Philippe L, Minn A, Haouzi P, Gillet P, Netter P, Terlain B. Neurophysiological basis for neurogenic-mediated articular cartilage anabolism alteration. *Am J Physiol Regul Integr Comp Physiol*. 2001;280(1):R115-22

[449] Decaris E, Guingamp C, Chat M, Philippe L, Grillasca JP, Abid A, Minn A, Gillet P, Netter P, Terlain B. Evidence for neurogenic transmission inducing degenerative cartilage damage distant from local inflammation. *Arthritis Rheum*. 1999;42(9):1951-60

[450] Vasquez A. *Integrative Orthopedics: Exploring the Structural Aspect of the Matrix*. Applying Functional Medicine in Clinical Practice. Tampa, Florida November 29-December 4, 2004. Hosted by the Institute for Functional Medicine: www.FunctionalMedicine.org

[451] Meggs WJ.Mechanisms of allergy and chemical sensitivity. *Toxicol Ind Health*. 1999 Apr-Jun;15(3-4):331-8

[452] Gouze-Decaris E, Philippe L, Minn A, Haouzi P, Gillet P, Netter P, Terlain B. Neurophysiological basis for neurogenic-mediated articular cartilage anabolism alteration. *Am J Physiol Regul Integr Comp Physiol*. 2001;280(1):R115-22

[453] Decaris E, Guingamp C, Chat M, Philippe L, Grillasca JP, Abid A, Minn A, Gillet P, Netter P, Terlain B. Evidence for neurogenic transmission inducing degenerative cartilage damage distant from local inflammation. *Arthritis Rheum*. 1999;42(9):1951-60

[454] Meggs WJ. Neurogenic Switching: A Hypothesis for a Mechanism for Shifting the Site of Inflammation in Allergy and Chemical Sensitivity. *Environ Health Perspect* 1995; 103:54-56

[455] Meggs WJ. Mechanisms of allergy and chemical sensitivity. *Toxicol Ind Health*. 1999 Apr-Jun;15(3-4):331-8

[456] "...—immunogenic switching—... In this scenario, the afferent stimulation from the cranial vasculature, which is inflamed during a migraine because of neurogenic processes, is rerouted by the CNS to produce immunogenic inflammation at the nose and sinuses." Cady RK, Schreiber CP. Sinus headache or migraine? Considerations in making a differential diagnosis. *Neurology*. 2002;58(9 Suppl 6):S10-4

[457] Vasquez A. *Integrative Orthopedics: Exploring the Structural Aspect of the Matrix*. Applying Functional Medicine in Clinical Practice. Tampa, Florida November 29-December 4, 2004. Hosted by the Institute for Functional Medicine: www.FunctionalMedicine.org

[458] Gouze-Decaris E, Philippe L, Minn A, Haouzi P, Gillet P, Netter P, Terlain B. Neurophysiological basis for neurogenic-mediated articular cartilage anabolism alteration. *Am J Physiol Regul Integr Comp Physiol*. 2001;280(1):R115-22

[459] Gillette R. A speculative argument for the coactivation of diverse somatic receptor populations by forceful chiropractic adjustments. *Man Med* 1987; 3:1-14

[460] Boal RW, Gillette RG. Central neuronal plasticity, low-back pain and spinal manipulative therapy. *J Manipulative Physiol Ther*. 2004;27(5):314-26

[461] Nielson NH, Bronfort G, Bendix T, Madsen F, Wecke B. Chronic asthma and chiropractic spinal manipulation: a randomized clinical trial. *Clin Exp Allergy* 1995;25:80-8

[462] "There were small increases (7 to 12 liters per minute) in peak expiratory flow in the morning and the evening in both treatment groups,... Symptoms of asthma and use of beta-agonists decreased and the quality of life increased in both groups, with no significant differences between the groups." Balon J, Aker PD, Crowther ER, Danielson C, Cox PG, O'Shaughnessy D, Walker C, Goldsmith CH, Duku E, Sears MR. A comparison of active and simulated chiropractic manipulation as adjunctive treatment for childhood asthma. *N Engl J Med*. 1998 Oct 8;339(15):1013-20

[463] Bronfort G, Evans RL, Kubic P, Filkin P. Chronic pediatric asthma and chiropractic spinal manipulation: a prospective clinical series and randomized clinical pilot study. *J Manipulative Physiol Ther*. 2001 Jul-Aug;24(6):369-77

neurogenic inflammation.[464,465] Thus, spinal manipulation appears to provide a means—*in addition to the use of other anti-inflammatory interventions such as diet, lifestyle and phytonutritional interventions*—by which pain and inflammation can be treated naturally, without drugs and surgery.

A science-based comprehensive protocol can be implemented against pain and inflammation by using ❶ an anti-inflammatory diet, ❷ frequent exercise, ❸ lifestyle and bodyweight optimization, ❹ nutritional supplementation, ❺ botanical supplementation[466,467], ❻ spinal manipulation (with its kinesthetic, analgesic, *directly* and *indirectly* anti-inflammatory, and *probably* piezoelectric benefits[468]), ❼ stress reduction[469,470], ❽ anti-dysbiosis protocols[471], ❾ hormonal correction ("orthoendocrinology"), and ❿ ancillary treatments such as acupuncture.[472,473] Additional details and citations for these interventions are provided in chapter 3 of *Integrative Orthopedics*[474] and chapter 4 of *Integrative Rheumatology*.[475] Pain and inflammation are self-perpetuating vicious cycles, well suited to intervention with comprehensive and multicomponent treatment plans as profiled above.

Wilk vs American Medical Association

The following two pages provide the transcript of the judgment in 1987 that supposedly ended the American Medical Association's antitrust violations and attempt to destroy the chiropractic profession.

A PDF copy of this document is available online: http://www.optimalhealthresearch.com/archives/wilk.html

---

[464] Renz H. Neurotrophins in bronchial asthma. *Respir Res*. 2001;2(5):265-8

[465] Groneberg DA, Quarcoo D, Frossard N, Fischer A. Neurogenic mechanisms in bronchial inflammatory diseases. *Allergy*. 2004 Nov; 59(11): 1139-52

[466] Jancso N, Jancso-Gabor A, Szolcsanyi J. Direct evidence for neurogenic inflammation and its prevention by denervation and by pretreatment with capsaicin. *Br J Pharmacol*. 1967 Sep;31(1):138-51

[467] Miller MJ, Vergnolle N, McKnight W, Musah RA, Davison CA, Trentacosti AM, Thompson JH, Sandoval M, Wallace JL. Inhibition of neurogenic inflammation by the Amazonian herbal medicine sangre de grado. *J Invest Dermatol*. 2001;117(3):725-30

[468] Lipinski B. Biological significance of piezoelectricity in relation to acupuncture, Hatha Yoga, osteopathic medicine and action of air ions. *Med Hypotheses*. 1977;3(1):9-12 See also: Athenstaedt H. Pyroelectric and piezoelectric properties of vertebrates. *Ann N Y Acad Sci*. 1974;238:68-94 See also: Athenstaedt H. "Functional polarity" of the spinal cord caused by its longitudinal electric dipole moment. *Am J Physiol*. 1984;247(3 Pt 2):R482-7

[469] Lutgendorf S, Logan H, Kirchner HL, Rothrock N, Svengalis S, Iverson K, Lubaroff D. Effects of relaxation and stress on the capsaicin-induced local inflammatory response. *Psychosom Med*. 2000;62:524-34

[470] "Couples who demonstrated consistently higher levels of hostile behaviors across both their interactions healed at 60% of the rate of low-hostile couples. High-hostile couples also produced relatively larger increases in plasma IL-6 and tumor necrosis factor alpha..." Kiecolt-Glaser JK, Loving TJ, Stowell JR, Malarkey WB, Lemeshow S, Dickinson SL, Glaser R. Hostile marital interactions, proinflammatory cytokine production, and wound healing. *Arch Gen Psychiatry*. 2005 Dec;62(12):1377-84

[471] Chapter 4 of Integrative Rheumatology and Vasquez A. Reducing Pain and Inflammation Naturally. Part 6: Nutritional and Botanical Treatments Against "Silent Infections" and Gastrointestinal Dysbiosis, Commonly Overlooked Causes of Neuromusculoskeletal Inflammation and Chronic Health Problems. *Nutr Perspect* 2006; Jan http://optimalhealthresearch.com/part6.html

[472] Joos S, Brinkhaus B, Maluche C, Maupai N, Kohnen R, Kraehmer N, Hahn EG, Schuppan D. Acupuncture and moxibustion in the treatment of active Crohn's disease: a randomized controlled study. *Digestion*. 2004;69(3):131-9

[473] "These results demonstrate an unorthodox new type of neurohumoral regulatory mechanism of sensory fibres and provide a possible mode of action for the anti-inflammatory effect of counter-irritation and acupuncture." Pinter E, Szolcsanyi J. Systemic anti-inflammatory effect induced by antidromic stimulation of the dorsal roots in the rat. *Neurosci Lett*. 1996;212(1):33-6

[474] Vasquez A. *Integrative Orthopedics: Second Edition*. Fort Worth, Texas; Integrative and Biological Medicine Research and Consulting, 2007 OptimalHealthResearch.com

[475] Vasquez A. *Integrative Rheumatology: Second Edition*. Fort Worth, Texas; Integrative and Biological Medicine Research and Consulting, 2007 OptimalHealthResearch.com

Special Communication

IN THE UNITED STATES DISTRICT COURT
FOR THE NORTHERN DISTRICT OF ILLINOIS
EASTERN DIVISION

CHESTER A. WILK, et al.,   )
)
                        Plaintiffs,   )
)
            v.   )   No. 76 C
)   3777
AMERICAN MEDICAL ASSOCIATION,   )
et al.,   )
)
                        Defendants.   )

PERMANENT INJUNCTION ORDER AGAINST AMA

Susan Getzendanner, District Judge

The court conducted a lengthy trial of this case in May and June of 1987 and on August 27, 1987, issued a 101 page opinion finding that the American Medical Association ("AMA") and its members participated in a conspiracy against chiropractors in violation of the nation's antitrust laws. Thereafter an opinion dated September 25, 1987 was substituted for the August 27, 1987 opinion. The question now before the court is the form of injunctive relief that the court will order.

See also p 83.

As part of the injunctive relief to be ordered by the court against the AMA, the AMA shall be required to send a copy of this Permanent Injunction Order to each of its current members. The members of the AMA are bound by the terms of the Permanent Injunction Order if they act in concert with the AMA to violate the terms of the order. Accordingly, it is important that the AMA members understand the order and the reasons why the order has been entered.

The AMA's Boycott and Conspiracy

In the early 1960s, the AMA decided to contain and eliminate chiropractic as a profession. In 1963 the AMA's Committee on Quackery was formed. The committee worked aggressively—both overtly and covertly—to eliminate chiropractic. One of the principal means used by the AMA to achieve its goal was to make it unethical for medical physicians to professionally associate with chiropractors. Under Principle 3 of the AMA's Principles of Medical Ethics, it was unethical for a physician to associate with an "unscientific practitioner," and in 1966 the AMA's House of Delegates passed a resolution calling chiropractic an unscientific cult. To complete the circle, in 1967 the AMA's Judicial Council issued an opinion under Principle 3 holding that it was unethical for a physician to associate professionally with chiropractors.

The AMA's purpose was to prevent medical physicians from referring patients to chiropractors and accepting referrals of patients from chiropractors, to prevent chiropractors from obtaining access to hospital diagnostic services and membership on hospital medical staffs, to prevent medical physicians from teaching at chiropractic colleges or engaging in any joint research, and to prevent any cooperation between the two groups in the delivery of health care services.

Published by order of Susan Getzendanner, US District Judge, Sept 25, 1987.

The AMA believed that the boycott worked—that chiropractic would have achieved greater gains in the absence of the boycott. Since no medical physician would want to be considered unethical by his peers, the success of the boycott is not surprising. However, chiropractic achieved licensing in all 50 states during the existence of the Committee on Quackery.

The Committee on Quackery was disbanded in 1975 and some of the committee's activities became publicly known. . Several lawsuits were filed by or on behalf of chiropractors and this case was filed in 1976.

Change in AMA's Position on Chiropractic

In 1977, the AMA began to change its position on chiropractic. The AMA's Judicial Council adopted new opinions under which medical physicians could refer patients to chiropractors, but there was still the proviso that the medical physician should be confident that the services to be provided on referral would be performed in accordance with accepted scientific standards. In 1979, the AMA's House of Delegates adopted Report UU which said that not everything that a chiropractor may do is without therapeutic value, but it stopped short of saying that such things were based on scientific standards. It was not until 1980 that the AMA revised its Principles of Medical Ethics to eliminate Principle 3. Until Principle 3 was formally eliminated, there was considerable ambiguity about the AMA's position. The ethics code adopted in 1980 provided that a medical physician "shall be free to choose whom to serve, with whom to associate, and the environment in which to provide medical services."

The AMA settled three chiropractic lawsuits by stipulating and agreeing that under the current opinions of the Judicial Council a physician may, without fear of discipline or sanction by the AMA, refer a patient to a duly licensed chiropractor when he believes that referral may benefit the patient. The AMA confirmed that a physician may also choose to accept or to decline patients sent to him by a duly licensed chiropractor. Finally, the AMA confirmed that a physician may teach at a chiropractic college or seminar. These settlements were entered into in 1978, 1980, and 1986.

The AMA's present position on chiropractic, as stated to the court, is that it is ethical for a medical physician to professionally associate with chiropractors provided the physician believes that such association is in the best interests of his patient. This position has not previously been communicated by the AMA to its members.

Antitrust Laws

Under the Sherman Act, every combination or conspiracy in restraint of trade is illegal. The court has held that the conduct of the AMA and its members constituted a conspiracy in restraint of trade based on the following facts: the purpose of the boycott was to eliminate chiropractic; chiropractors are in competition with some medical physicians; the boycott had substantial anti-competitive effects; there were no pro-competitive effects of the boycott; and the plaintiffs were injured as a result of the conduct. These facts add up to a violation of the Sherman Act.

In this case, however, the court allowed the defendants the opportunity to establish a "patient care defense" which has the following elements:

(1) that they genuinely entertained a concern for what they perceive as scientific method in the care of each person with whom they have entered into a doctor-patient relationship; (2) that this concern is objectively reasonable; (3) that this concern has been the dominant motivating factor in defendants' promulgation of Principle 3 and in the

conduct intended to implement it; and (4) that this concern for scientific method in patient care could not have been adequately satisfied in a manner less restrictive of competition.

The court concluded that the AMA had a genuine concern for scientific methods in patient care, and that this concern was the dominant factor in motivating the AMA's conduct. However, the AMA failed to establish that throughout the entire period of the boycott, from 1966 to 1980, this concern was objectively reasonable. The court reached that conclusion on the basis of extensive testimony from both witnesses for the plaintiffs and the AMA that some forms of chiropractic treatment are effective and the fact that the AMA recognized that chiropractic began to change in the early 1970s. Since the boycott was not formally over until Principle 3 was eliminated in 1980, the court found that the AMA was unable to establish that during the entire period of the conspiracy its position was objectively reasonable. Finally, the court ruled that the AMA's concern for scientific method in patient care could have been adequately satisfied in a manner less restrictive of competition and that a nationwide conspiracy to eliminate a licensed profession was not justified by the concern for scientific method. On the basis of these findings, the court concluded that the AMA had failed to establish the patient care defense.

None of the court's findings constituted a judicial endorsement of chiropractic. All of the parties to the case, including the plaintiffs and the AMA, agreed that chiropractic treatment of diseases such as diabetes, high blood pressure, cancer, heart disease and infectious disease is not proper, and that the historic theory of chiropractic, that there is a single cause and cure of disease is wrong. There was disagreement between the parties as to whether chiropractors should engage in diagnosis. There was evidence that the chiropractic theory of subluxations was unscientific, and evidence that some chiropractors engaged in unscientific practices. The court did not reach the question of whether chiropractic theory was in fact scientific. However, the evidence in the case was that some forms of chiropractic manipulation of the spine and joints was therapeutic. AMA witnesses, including the present Chairman of the Board of Trustees of the AMA, testified that some forms of treatment by chiropractors, including manipulation, can be therapeutic in the treatment of conditions such as back pain syndrome.

Need for Injunctive Relief

Although the conspiracy ended in 1980, there are lingering effects of the illegal boycott and conspiracy which require an injunction. Some medical physicians' individual decisions on whether or not to professionally associate with chiropractors are still affected by the boycott. The injury to chiropractors' reputations which resulted from the boycott has not been repaired. Chiropractors suffer current economic injury as a result of the boycott. The AMA has never affirmatively acknowledged that there are and should be no collective impediments to professional association and cooperation between chiropractors and medical physicians, except as provided by law. Instead, the AMA has consistently argued that its conduct has not violated the antitrust laws.

Most importantly, the court believes that it is important that the AMA members be made aware of the present AMA position that it is ethical for a medical physician to professionally associate with a chiropractor if the physician believes it is in the best interests of his patient, so that the lingering effects of the illegal group boycott against chiropractors finally can be dissipated.

Under the law, every medical physician, institution, and hospital has the right to make an individual decision as to whether or not that physician, institution, or hospital shall associate professionally with chiropractors. Individual choice by a medical physician voluntarily to associate professionally with chiropractors should be governed only by restrictions under state law, if any, and by the individual medical physician's personal judgment as to what is in the best interest of a patient or patients. Professional association includes referrals, consultations, group practice in partnerships, Health Maintenance Organizations, Preferred Provider Organizations, and other alternative health care delivery systems; the provision of treatment privileges and diagnostic services (including radiological and other laboratory facilities) in or through hospital facilities; association and cooperation in educational programs for students in chiropractic colleges; and cooperation in research, health care seminars, and continuing education programs.

An injunction is necessary to assure that the AMA does not interfere with the right of a physician, hospital, or other institution to make an individual decision on the question of professional association.

Form of Injunction

1. The AMA, its officers, agents and employees, and all persons who act in active concert with any of them and who receive actual notice of this order are hereby permanently enjoined from restricting, regulating or impeding, or aiding and abetting others from restricting, regulating or impeding, the freedom of any AMA member or any institution or hospital to make an individual decision as to whether or not that AMA member, institution, or hospital shall professionally associate with chiropractors, chiropractic students, or chiropractic institutions.

2. This Permanent Injunction does not and shall not be construed to restrict or otherwise interfere with the AMA's right to take positions on any issue, including chiropractic, and to express or publicize those positions, either alone or in conjunction with others. Nor does this Permanent Injunction restrict or otherwise interfere with the AMA's right to petition or testify before any public body on any legislative or regulatory measure or to join or cooperate with any other entity in so petitioning or testifying. The AMA's membership in a recognized accrediting association or society shall not constitute a violation of this Permanent Injunction.

3. The AMA is directed to send a copy of this order to each AMA member and employee, first class mail, postage prepaid, within thirty days of the entry of this order. In the alternative, the AMA shall provide the Clerk of the Court with mailing labels so that the court may send this order to AMA members and employees.

4. The AMA shall cause the publication of this order in JAMA and the indexing of the order under "Chiropractic" so that persons desiring to find the order in the future will be able to do so.

5. The AMA shall prepare a statement of the AMA's present position on chiropractic for inclusion in the current reports and opinions of the Judicial Council with an appropriate heading that refers to professional association between medical physicians and chiropractors, and indexed in the same manner that other reports and opinions are indexed. The court imposes no restrictions on the AMA's statement but only requires that it be consistent with the AMA's statements of its present position to the court.

6. The AMA shall file a report with the court evidencing compliance with this order on or before January 10, 1988.

It is so ordered.

Susan Getzendanner
United States District Judge

Naturopathic Medicine

"The work of the naturopathic physician is to elicit healing by helping patients to create or recreate conditions for health to exist within them. Health will occur where the conditions for health exist. Disease is the product of conditions which allow for it."

Jared Zeff, ND[476]

The diagram on this page is derived from the review by Zeff published in 1997 in *Journal of Naturopathic Medicine* entitled "The process of healing: a unifying theory of naturopathic medicine." By my interpretation, the diagram is important for at least three reasons.

First, whereas the allopathic profession describes the genesis of most diseases as *idiopathic* and therefore [somehow] exclusively serviceable by drugs and surgery, the naturopathic profession describes disease processes as *multifactorial* and *logical* and therefore treatable by the skilled discovery and treatment of the underlying causes. Such underlying causes, which nearly always occur as a plurality, may vary mildly or significantly even within a group of patients with the same diagnosis.

Second, the diagram shows that the development of disease and the restoration of health are both *processes*. The restoration and retention of health requires *intentionality* and *tenacity* in lieu of the simplistic *miracle medicines* and *passive treatments* proffered by the pharmaceutical industry. Generally, disease does not arrive from outside; it is the result of one or more internal imbalances. Chronic illness is generally the result of manifold internal imbalances that culminate in numerous physiologic insults which compromise essential functions to the point that one or more organ systems begin to fail; we as patients and doctors generally label this as some specific "disease" or other, and the general—often erroneous—assumption has been that each *specific disease* (i.e., label, …abstraction, …conceptual entity) requires a *specific treatment* rather than a generalized health-restorative approach. Health is restored through a progressive and stepwise program that addresses as many facets of the illness as possible while vigorously supporting optimal physiologic function.

Third, the fact that Zeff considered the discharge or "healing crisis" so important that it merited inclusion in this diagram shows, indirectly, the naturopathic emphasis on detoxification and the eradication of dysbiosis. Both in the treatment of toxic metal/chemical exposure and in the treatment of chronic infections, patients often go through an acute or subacute phase of feeling ill before experiencing a dramatic alleviation of symptoms; the fact that symptoms may temporarily "get worse before getting better" has been referred to as the "healing crisis." This can occur for at least three reasons. First, in the elimination of chemicals and metals from the body, they must first be released from the tissues; the transition from tissues to blood is similar to a subacute re-exposure which triggers symptoms of toxicity until the toxin is excreted via sweat, urine, bile, or breath. Similarly, improvement in nutritional status—a cornerstone of all naturopathic interventions—expedites/facilitates/restores physiologic processes that have been relatively dormant due to lack of enzymatic cofactors such as vitamins and minerals[477]; optimization of nutritional status provides an opportunity for these pathways (such as detoxification of stored xenobiotics) to function again at which time they must "catch up" on work that has not been performed during the time of nutritional deficiency. The activation of these pathways is an essential step toward health restoration but results in an initial upregulation of hepatic phase-1/oxidative biotransformation which often

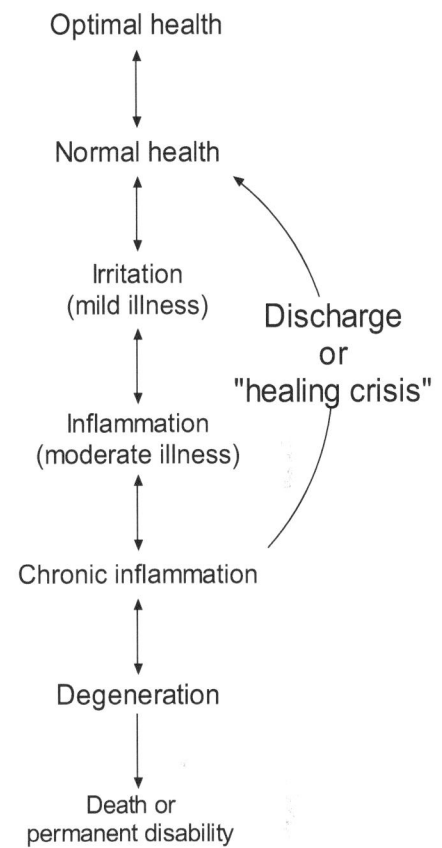

---

[476] Zeff JL. The process of healing: a unifying theory of naturopathic medicine. *Journal of Naturopathic Medicine* 1997; 7: 122-5
[477] Ames BN. The metabolic tune-up: metabolic harmony and disease prevention. *J Nutr*. 2003 May;133(5 Suppl 1):1544S-8S

results in the formation of reactive intermediates that temporarily impair physiologic processes and cause an initial exacerbation of symptoms. Third, whether through immunorestoration or the use of botanical/pharmacologic antimicrobial agents, the symptom-exacerbating "die off" reaction—classically called the Jarisch-Herxheimer reaction in the context of treating syphilis—is a result of increased (endo)toxin production/release by bacteria/microbes in response effective antimicrobial processes, whether physiologic or pharmacologic.

Modern naturopathic medicine has grown from deeply rooted European healing traditions reaching back several centuries. Naturopathic physicians have unwaveringly demonstrated respect, love, and appreciation for the healing powers of nature and the process of life itself.[478] Following their coursework in the basic biomedical sciences, naturopathic physicians are trained in urology, oncology, neurology, pediatrics, obstetrics and gynecology, urology, manual physical manipulation (including spinal manipulation), minor surgery, medical procedures, professional ethics, therapeutic diets, clinical and interventional nutrition, botanical medicines, psychological counseling, environmental medicine, and other modalities. Licensed naturopathic physicians commonly practice as generalists and family doctors.[479,480,481,482]

Naturopathic Principles, Concepts, & the *Vis Medicatrix Naturae*

"The healing power of nature is the inherent self-organizing and healing process of living systems… It is the naturopathic physician's role to support, facilitate and augment this process by identifying and removing obstacles to health and recovery, and by supporting the creation of a healthy internal and external environment."[483]

1. **First, Do No Harm (*Primum Non Nocere*)**: Naturopathic physicians use good judgment and compassion to ensure that the treatment does not cause harm to the patient. This contrasts with the effects of allopathic treatment, which collectively kill more than 180,000-220,000 patients per year, at least 493 American patients per day.[484]

2. **Identify and Treat the Causes (*Tolle Causam*)**: *"Illness does not occur without cause."* Naturopathic physicians focus on identifying and addressing the underlying deficiency, toxicity, impairment, or imbalance that is the cause of the health problem or disease.

3. **Treat the Whole Person**: *"The multifactorial nature of health and disease requires a personalized and comprehensive approach to diagnosis and treatment."* On some occasions the illness does take precedence over the person who has it—such in emergency situations like septic arthritis, acute ischemia, and pulmonary edema. In these cases, the situation must be managed appropriately, and these situations are not immediately amenable to long-term lifestyle changes—they require immediate treatment. However, the vast majority of cases in routine outpatient clinical practice will require detailed and bipartite attention to the facets of both **the disease process** and **the person who has the illness**. Our focus as naturopathic physicians on the individual patient is what sets our healing profession apart from others that focus exclusively on the disease and do not consider the manifold intricacies of the individual patient.

4. **The Healing Power of Nature: *Vis Medicatrix Naturae***: Naturopathic medicine recognizes an inherent self-healing process in the person that is ordered and intelligent. The body has many highly efficient mechanisms for sustaining and regaining health. These mechanisms have their specific and necessary components (e.g., nutrients) and means by which they can be impaired (e.g., xenobiotic

---

[478] Kirchfeld F, Boyle W. Nature Doctors: Pioneers in Naturopathic Medicine. Portland, Oregon; Medicina Biologica (Buckeye Naturopathic Press, East Palestine, Ohio), 1994

[479] Boon HS, Cherkin DC, Erro J, Sherman KJ, Milliman B, Booker J, Cramer EH, Smith MJ, Deyo RA, Eisenberg DM. Practice patterns of naturopathic physicians: results from a random survey of licensed practitioners in two US States. *BMC Complement Altern Med*. 2004;4(1):14

[480] Smith MJ, Logan AC. Naturopathy. *Med Clin North Am*. 2002 Jan;86(1):173-84

[481] Cherkin DC, Deyo RA, Sherman KJ, et al. Characteristics of visits to licensed acupuncturists, chiropractors, massage therapists, and naturopathic physicians. *J Am Board Fam Pract*. 2002 Nov-Dec;15(6):463-72

[482] Cherkin DC, Deyo RA, Sherman KJ, et al. Characteristics of licensed acupuncturists, chiropractors, massage therapists, and naturopathic physicians. *J Am Board Fam Pract*. 2002 Sep-Oct;15(5):378-90

[483] Quoted from the American Association of Naturopathic Physicians website http://aanp.net/Basics/h.naturo.philo.html on February 4, 2001. Other italicized quotes in this section are from the same source. This website has since been replaced by http://naturopathic.org/

[484] "Recent estimates suggest that each year more than 1 million patients are injured while in the hospital and approximately 180,000 die because of these injuries. Furthermore, drug-related morbidity and mortality are common and are estimated to cost more than $136 billion a year." Holland EG, Degruy FV. Drug-induced disorders. *Am Fam Physician*. 1997;56(7):1781-8, 1791-2

immunosuppression). Poor health and disease can result from impairment of these self-healing processes and biologic mechanisms, and thus the body's inherent, natural, self-healing mechanisms—the "healing power of nature"—can be diminished to the state of ineffectiveness or harm (e.g., autoimmunity). Recognizing that the body has this inherent goal of and movement toward self-healing, naturopathic physicians start by identifying and removing "obstacles to cure" rather than ignoring these factors and masking the manifestations of dysfunction with symptom-suppressing drugs.

5. <u>**Prevention**</u>: Healthy lifestyle, proper nutrition, and emotional hygiene go a long way toward preventing (and treating) most conditions. Specific conditions have specific risk factors and causes that have to be considered per patient and condition.

6. <u>**Doctor As Teacher (*Docere*)**</u>: Naturopathic physicians explain the situation and the proposed solution to the patient so that the patient is empowered with understanding and with the comfort of knowing what has happened, what is happening, and the proposed course of upcoming events. Naturopathic physicians strive to let their own lives serve as a models for our patients. This does not mean that naturopathic doctors have to feign perfection; the task is to live the best and most conscious life that we can, to be present with our emotions, qualities, and faults and to treat ourselves with respect and acceptance. We can exemplify health (rather than perfection) to our patients by being who we authentically are and by so doing we can facilitate their own acceptance of their current health situation, which is a prerequisite to self-initiated change.

> **"Physician, heal thyself.**
> Thus you help your patient, too.
> Let this be his best medicine that he beholds with his eyes: the doctor who heals himself."
>
> Nietzsche FW. <u>Thus Spoke Zarathustra (1892)</u>. [Kaufmann W, translator]. Viking Penguin: 1954, page 77

7. <u>**Re-Establish the Foundation for Health**</u>: An overview of this important naturopathic concept is provided throughout this chapter.

8. <u>**Removing "obstacles to cure"**</u>: *examples*

Obstacle to the optimization of health	*Example of possible intervention*
o Toxic exposures, medication side-effects	▪ Reduce drug use and dependency
o Toxic relationships, emotional obstacles, past events, unfulfilling occupation,	▪ Improve self-esteem, develop conflict resolution skills, determine life goals and values and a plan for their pursuit
o Social isolation: the typical American has only two friends no-one in whom to confide[485]	▪ Encourage social interaction
o Diet with excess fat, arachidonate, sugar, additives, colorants, and insufficiency of protein, fiber, phytonutrients, and health-promoting fatty acids: ALA, GLA, EPA, DHA, and oleic acid	▪ Diet improvement and nutritional supplementation
o Sedentary lifestyle, lack of exercise	▪ Encourage exercise
o Weight gain/loss as necessary for weight optimization	▪ Encourage self-valuing
o Epidemic exposure to mercury, lead, and xenobiotics	▪ Support detoxification process as a lifestyle

<u>**Hierarchy of Therapeutics**</u>: This naturopathic concept articulates the importance of addressing *the underlying cause* rather than simply focusing on *the presenting problem*, which is the *symptom of the cause*. Further, interventions are **prioritized**, *for example*:

- Patient-implemented *before* doctor-implemented.

---

[485] McPherson M, Smith-Lovin L, Brashears ME. Social Isolation in America: Changes in Core Discussion Networks over Two Decades. *American Sociological Review* 2006; 71: 353-75 http://www.asanet.org/galleries/default-file/June06ASRFeature.pdf

- Removal of harming agent *before* addition of a therapeutic agent: e.g., stop smoking *before* investing in respiratory therapy; implement healthy diet and exercise before higher-risk and higher-cost drugs for hypertension and hypercholesterolemia.
- Low-force interventions *before* high-force interventions.
- Diet *before* nutritional supplements; nutrients *before* botanicals; botanicals *before* drugs; modulatory drugs *before* suppressive/inhibitory drugs; integrative care *before* surgery.
- *See examples below.*

Hierarchy of Therapeutics (specifically sequential)	Example of possible intervention
1. <u>Reestablishing the foundation for health</u>	<ul><li>Mental/emotional/spiritual health</li><li>Meditation, freeze-frame, "time out"</li><li>Relaxation</li><li>Positive visualization, positive expectation, affirmation</li><li>Counseling, social contact, group work[486]</li><li>Family contact and resolution</li><li>Dietary intake and nutritional health which addresses the patient's biochemical individuality[487] and correction of deficiencies or excesses</li><li>Identification and elimination of food allergies and food sensitivities</li><li>Reduce toxin exposure, promote detoxification</li><li>Identification and elimination of exposure to gastrointestinal and inhalant xenobiotics</li><li>Remove or reduce specific "obstacles to cure"</li></ul>
2. <u>Stimulation of the "healing power of nature" and the "vital force"</u>	<ul><li>Constitutional hydrotherapy</li><li>Homeopathy</li><li>Exercise</li><li>Acupuncture, Spinal manipulation</li><li>Meditation, rest</li><li>Tai Chi, Qigong: "energy-cultivation"</li><li>Botanical adaptogens</li></ul>
3. <u>Tonification of weakened systems:</u>	<ul><li>Botanical medicines and other supplements to help restore normal tissue function</li><li>Spinal manipulation to address the primary somatovisceral dysfunction and/or secondary musculoskeletal disorders</li><li>Hormonal supplementation</li><li>Nutritional supplementation</li><li>Exercise</li><li>Physiotherapy</li></ul>
4. <u>Correction of structural integrity:</u>	<ul><li>Spinal manipulation, deep tissue massage, visceral manipulation, lymphatic pump to promote immune surveillance[488]</li><li>Stretching, balancing, muscle strengthening, and proprioceptive retraining</li><li>Surgery, as a last resort</li></ul>

---

[486] See http://www.mkp.org and www.WomanWithin.org for examples.
[487] Williams RJ. <u>Biochemical Individuality: The Basis for the Genetotrophic Concept</u>. Austin and London: University of Texas Press, 1956
[488] "Lymph flow in the thoracic duct increased from 1.57±0.20 mL·min-1 to a peak TDF of 4.80±1.73 mL·min-1 during abdominal pump, and from 1.20±0.41 mL·min-1 to 3.45±1.61 mL·min-1 during thoracic pump." Knott EM, Tune JD, Stoll ST, Downey HF. Increased lymphatic flow in the thoracic duct during manipulative intervention. *J Am Osteopath Assoc*. 2005 Oct;105(10):447-56 http://www.jaoa.org/cgi/content/full/105/10/447

Osteopathic Medicine

Osteopathic medicine and chiropractic are American-born healthcare professions and paradigms that started at nearly the same time in history and from many of the same foundational principles. Both professions were started in the late 1800's and early 1900's and were founded upon the philosophical premise that the body functioned as a whole and that therefore medicine in general and therapeutic interventions in particular needed to be comprehensive in scope and multifaceted in their application. Further, both professions emphasized the importance of structural integrity as a foundational component of health and thus embraced manual manipulative therapy and spinal manipulation.

From their common origins, subtle differences and chance historic events shaped and further separated these professions from each other. Osteopathy was founded by Andrew Taylor Still, a medical doctor who sought to reform what was then called the "Heroic" paradigm of medicine, which embraced bloodletting and the administration of leeches, purgatives, emetics, and poisons such as mercury as means for "rebalancing" what were perceived to be internal causes of disease, namely the "four humours" of the body which were thought to be blood, phlegm, black bile, and yellow bile. In part because of his training within and identification with the medical profession, Still sought to *reform* rather than *directly oppose* the "mainstream medicine" of his day; in contrast, chiropractic's founder Daniel David Palmer was more strongly opposed to the horrific medicine of his time and thus was more *revolutionary* than *evolutionary* in his approach to forging a new paradigm of health and healthcare. Still's willingness to align with the medical profession and the increasingly powerful and influential pharmaceutical industry unquestionably helped his fledgling profession survive the extinction that otherwise would have been swift at the hands of allopathic groups such as **the American Medical Association (AMA), which labeled osteopathic physicians as "cultists" and systematically restricted inclusion of the osteopathic profession into mainstream healthcare by proclamation in 1953 that "...all voluntary associations with osteopaths are unethical." When osteopathic resistance mounted, the AMA and its co-conspirators, who were later found guilty of violating the nation's antitrust laws by illegally suppressing competition and attempting to build a medical monopoly**[489], acquiesced and accepted osteopaths into its ranks—a strategy which the medical profession believed would eventually destroy the osteopathic profession by forcing it to resign its ideals and identity. In his review of osteopathic history, Gevitz[490] writes, **"...the M.D.'s gradually came to believe that the only way to destroy osteopathy was through the absorption of D.O.'s, much as the homeopaths and eclectics [naturopaths] had been swallowed up early in the century."** Even recently, the AMA has listed osteopathic medicine under "alternative medicine"[491] although several osteopathic medical colleges have consistently provided training that is superior to most "conventional" allopathic medical schools.[492] Today, osteopathic physicians practice in most ways similarly to allopaths—i.e., with unlimited scope of practice in all 50 states, full access to the use of drugs and surgery, and with a very pharmacosurgical paradigm of disease and healthcare. Osteopathic medicine is one of the fastest growing healthcare professions in America.

Osteopathic Manipulative Medicine:

Osteopathic manipulative medicine (OMM) is similar to and yet distinct from chiropractic manipulation; the naturopathic profession—true to its eclectic roots—incorporates techniques from all professions. In contrast to chiropractic, OMM terminology and therapeutics focus much more on soft tissues, and the osteopathic lesion—"somatic dysfunction"—is clearly originated from soft tissues in contrast to the chiropractic lesion—the "vertebral subluxation"—which obviously originates from spinal articulations. Whereas the chiropractic intent of correcting or "adjusting" the "subluxation" was historically to improve function of the nervous system, the osteopathic lesion is addressed to more fully improve not only function of the nervous system but also of the vascular, lymphatic, and myofascial systems, too.[493] With regard to the latter, the osteopathic profession has always emphasized the importance of fascia in the genesis of "somatic dysfunction." Indeed, fascia appears to play an

[489] Getzendanner S. Permanent injunction order against AMA. *JAMA*. 1988 Jan 1;259(1):81-2
[490] Gevitz N. The D.O.'s: Osteopathic Medicine in America. Johns Hopkins University Press; 1991; pages 100-103
[491] American Medical Association. Report 12 of the Council on Scientific Affairs (A-97) Full Text http://www.ama-assn.org/ama/pub/category/13638.html Accessed November 23, 2006
[492] Special report. America's best graduate schools. Schools of Medicine. The top schools: primary care. *US News World Rep*. 2004 Apr 12;136(12):74
[493] Williams N. Managing back pain in general practice--is osteopathy the new paradigm? *Br J Gen Pract*. 1997 Oct;47(423):653-5
http://www.pubmedcentral.nih.gov/articlerender.fcgi?tool=pubmed&pubmedid=9474832

important and dynamic (not passive) role in neuromusculoskeletal health, particularly as it is a major contributor to proprioception and may also have a more direct effect through the recently described ability of fascia to actively contract in a smooth-muscle-like manner.[494]

From this author's perspective, an unfortunate consequence of the broadness of osteopathic manipulative conceptualizations/techniques (i.e., vertebral, skeletal, vascular, lymphatic, myofascial,...) is the relative lack (compared to chiropractic) of modernization and sophistication and development of its terminology and training textbooks; two of the most widely used osteopathic texts—*Osteopathic Principles in Practice* (1994) by Kuchera and Kuchera[495], and *Outline of Osteopathic Manipulative Procedures* (2006) by Kimberly[496]—both leave very much to be desired with respect to their clarity, terminology, clinical applicability, and referencing to the scientific literature. *Manipulation of the Spine, Thorax and Pelvis: An Osteopathic Perspective* (2006) by Gibbons and Tehan[497] is much more accessible and clinically applicable; however the text focuses exclusively on high-velocity low-amplitude (HVLA) techniques and therefore does not provide sufficient background and training for students in the very techniques that distinguish osteopathic from chiropractic techniques, namely heightened attention to the myofascial dysfunction that (appropriately) underlies the osteopathic lesion.

Ironically, the very growth and "allopathicization" of the profession that has threatened the profession's adherence to its holistic tenets has caused a reflexive re-affirmation of these tenets, and the profession has responded with a well-funded and intentional directive to scientifically investigate the mechanisms and efficacy of osteopathic manipulative medicine.[498,499] Recent findings include improved function and reduced pain in patients treated with a comprehensive manipulative technique for the shoulder[500], as well as the significant efficacy of ankle manipulation for patients with recent ankle injuries.[501] Further, OMM treatment of patients medicated for depression was found to triple the effectiveness of drug monotherapy.[502] Other studies have shown benefit of OMM in the treatment of geriatric pneumonia[503], pediatric asthma[504], pediatric

> ## Osteopathic Interventions need to be Consistent with Osteopathic Philosophy
>
> "In contrast to the description of the osteopathic medical profession by the American Osteopathic Association, namely, "doctors of osteopathic medicine, or D.O.s, apply the philosophy of treating the whole person to the prevention, diagnosis and treatment of illness, disease and injury," [the authors of the article in question] essentially reviewed only pharmacologic treatment.
>
> …
>
> It is hoped that future reviews in this journal can include a more balanced survey of the literature, inclusive of non-pharmacologic and "holistic" interventions that are consistent with osteopathic philosophy."
>
> **Vasquez A.** Interventions need to be Consistent with Osteopathic Philosophy. [Letter] JAOA: Journal of the American Osteopathic Association 2006 Sep;106(9):528-9
> http://www.jaoa.org/cgi/content/full/106/9/528

---

[494] "...the existence of an active fascial contractility could have interesting implications for the understanding of musculoskeletal pathologies with an increased or decreased myofascial tonus. It may also offer new insights and a deeper understanding of treatments directed at fascia, such as manual myofascial release therapies or acupuncture." Schleip R, Klingler W, Lehmann-Horn F. Active fascial contractility: Fascia may be able to contract in a smooth muscle-like manner and thereby influence musculoskeletal dynamics. *Med Hypotheses.* 2005;65(2):273-7

[495] Kuchera WA, Kuchera ML. *Osteopathic Principles In Practice, revised second edition.* Kirksville, MO, KCOM Press; 1994

[496] Kimberly PE. *Outline of Osteopathic Manipulative Procedures. The Kimberly Manual 2006.* Kirksville College Osteopathic Medicine. Walsworth Publish. Co., Marceline, Mo

[497] Gibbons P, Tehan P. *Manipulation of the Spine, Thorax and Pelvis: An Osteopathic Perspective.* Churchill Livingstone; 2006. Isbn: 044310039X

[498] Wisnioski SW 3rd. "Circle Turns Round" to "Allopathic Osteopathy." *J Am Osteopath Assoc* 2006; 106: 423-4 http://www.jaoa.org/cgi/content/full/106/7/423

[499] Teitelbaum HS, Bunn WE 2nd, Brown SA, Burchett AW. Osteopathic medical education: renaissance or rhetoric? *J Am Osteopath Assoc.* 2003 Oct;103(10):489-90 http://www.jaoa.org/cgi/reprint/103/10/489

[500] The "seven stages of Spencer" is an organized technique of range-of-motion exercises and post-isometric stretching to improve functionality of the shoulder. This clinical trial showed improved shoulder function in a group of elderly patients treated with this technique. Knebl JA, Shores JH, Gamber RG, Gray WT, Herron KM. Improving functional ability in the elderly via the Spencer technique, an osteopathic manipulative treatment: a randomized, controlled trial. *J Am Osteopath Assoc.* 2002 Jul;102(7):387-96 http://www.jaoa.org/cgi/reprint/102/7/387 See also "CONCLUSION: Manipulative therapy for the shoulder girdle in addition to usual medical care accelerates recovery of shoulder symptoms." Bergman GJ, Winters JC, Groenier KH, Pool JJ, Meyboom-de Jong B, Postema K, van der Heijden GJ. Manipulative therapy in addition to usual medical care for patients with shoulder dysfunction and pain: a randomized, controlled trial. *Ann Intern Med.* 2004 Sep 21;141(6):432-9 http://www.annals.org/cgi/reprint/141/6/432.pdf

[501] This study shows the rapid onset and benefit of manipulative medicine for the treatment of acute ankle sprains: Eisenhart AW, Gaeta TJ, Yens DP. Osteopathic manipulative treatment in the emergency department for patients with acute ankle injuries. *J Am Osteopath Assoc.* 2003 Sep;103(9):417-21 http://www.jaoa.org/cgi/reprint/103/9/417

[502] This study impressively showed that musculoskeletal manipulation improved treatment effectiveness for depression from 33% to 100%. "After 8 weeks, 100% of the OMT treatment group and 33% of the control group tested normal by psychometric evaluation. ... The findings of this pilot study indicate that OMT may be a useful adjunctive treatment for alleviating depression in women." Plotkin BJ, Rodos JJ, Kappler R, Schrage M, Freydl K, Hasegawa S, Hennegan E, Hilchie-Schmidt C, Hines D, Iwata J, Mok C, Raffaelli D. Adjunctive osteopathic manipulative treatment in women with depression: a pilot study. *J Am Osteopath Assoc.* 2001 Sep;101(9):517-23 http://www.jaoa.org/cgi/reprint/101/9/517

[503] This study showed improved clinical outcomes and reduced antibiotic use in elderly patients with pneumonia when treated with manipulative medicine: "The treatment group had a significantly shorter duration of intravenous antibiotic treatment and a shorter hospital stay." Noll DR, Shores JH, Gamber RG, Herron KM, Swift J Jr. Benefits of osteopathic manipulative treatment for hospitalized elderly patients with pneumonia. *J Am Osteopath Assoc.* 2000 Dec;100(12):776-82 http://www.jaoa.org/cgi/reprint/100/12/776

[504] Osteopathic manipulation improved pulmonary function in pediatric patients with asthma: "With a confidence level of 95%, results for the OMT group showed a statistically significant improvement of 7 L per minute to 9 L per minute for peak expiratory flow rates. These results suggest that OMT has a therapeutic effect among this patient population." Guiney PA, Chou R, Vianna A, Lovenheim J. Effects of osteopathic manipulative treatment on pediatric patients with asthma: a randomized controlled trial. *J Am Osteopath Assoc.* 2005 Jan;105(1):7-12 http://www.jaoa.org/cgi/content/full/105/1/7

dysfunctional voiding[505], carpal tunnel syndrome[506], low-back pain[507], and recovery from cardiac bypass surgery.[508] Replication and validation of these studies—many of which are small or of nonrigorous design (e.g., open clinical trials with no control group)—is important to further define and establish the value of osteopathic manipulation in clinical care.

---

[505] "RESULTS: The treatment group exhibited greater improvement in DV symptoms than did the control group (Z=-2.63, p=0.008, Mann-Whitney U-test). Improved or resolution of vesicoureteral reflux and elimination of post-void urine residuals were more prominent in the treatment group." Nemett DR, Fivush BA, Mathews R, Camirand N, Eldridge MA, Finney K, Gerson AC. A randomized controlled trial of the effectiveness of osteopathy-based manual physical therapy in treating pediatric dysfunctional voiding. *J Pediatr Urol.* 2008 Apr;4(2):100-6

[506] Sucher BM, Hinrichs RN, Welcher RL, Quiroz LD, St Laurent BF, Morrison BJ. Manipulative treatment of carpal tunnel syndrome: biomechanical and osteopathic intervention to increase the length of the transverse carpal ligament: part 2. Effect of sex differences and manipulative "priming". *J Am Osteopath Assoc.* 2005 Mar;105(3):135-43. Erratum in: J Am Osteopath Assoc. 2005 May;105(5):238 http://www.jaoa.org/cgi/content/full/105/3/135

[507] "CONCLUSION: OMT significantly reduces low back pain. The level of pain reduction is greater than expected from placebo effects alone and persists for at least three months." Licciardone JC, Brimhall AK, King LN. Osteopathic manipulative treatment for low back pain: a systematic review and meta-analysis of randomized controlled trials. *BMC Musculoskelet Disord.* 2005 Aug 4;6:43 http://www.biomedcentral.com/1471-2474/6/43

[508] This study showed benefit from osteopathic manipulation administered immediately after coronary artery bypass graft surgery: "The observed changes in cardiac function and perfusion indicated that OMT had a beneficial effect on the recovery of patients after CABG surgery. The authors conclude that OMT has immediate, beneficial hemodynamic effects after CABG surgery when administered while the patient is sedated and pharmacologically paralyzed." O-Yurvati AH, Carnes MS, Clearfield MB, Stoll ST, McConathy WJ. Hemodynamic effects of osteopathic manipulative treatment immediately after coronary artery bypass graft surgery. *J Am Osteopath Assoc.* 2005 Oct;105(10):475-81 http://www.jaoa.org/cgi/content/full/105/10/475

Functional Medicine

Introduction: The purpose of this monograph is to provide healthcare professionals with an overview of the "functional medicine" assessment and management strategies that are applicable to painful neuromusculoskeletal disorders. A comprehensive description of functional medicine from the Institute for Functional Medicine (IFM) is provided later in this section, while a more comprehensive explication is provided in *The Textbook of Functional Medicine*.[509] In recognition of the diversity of this document's readership (inclusive of students, recent graduates, experienced professionals, academicians, and policymakers) and the pervasive deficiencies in musculoskeletal knowledge among healthcare providers[510,511,512,513,514,515], this monograph on pain will necessarily review some basic concepts; however, this document alone cannot replace professional training in musculoskeletal medicine nor does it include protocols for patient management and differential diagnosis for each of the neuromusculoskeletal problems seen in clinical practice. This text should be used in conjunction with the reader's professional training and other reference texts. Clinicians utilizing a functional medicine approach to patient care must be knowledgeable in the details of integrative physiology and nutritional biochemistry and must also posses the clinical acumen necessary to ensure safe and expedient patient care. These traits and skills are of particular necessity when a serious condition is presented. Life-threatening and limb-threatening neuromusculoskeletal problems are notorious for presenting under the guise of an apparently benign complaint such as fatigue, headache, or simple joint pain.

Since approximately 1 of every 7 (14% of total) visits to a primary healthcare provider is for the treatment of musculoskeletal pain or dysfunction[516], every healthcare provider needs to have: 1) knowledge of important concepts related to musculoskeletal medicine, 2) the ability to recognize urgent and emergency conditions, 3) the ability to competently perform orthopedic examination procedures and interpret laboratory assessments, and 4) the knowledge and ability to design and implement effective treatment plans and to coordinate patient management. While this monograph will be thorough in its review of topics discussed, like any other textbook it cannot contain every nuance and examination procedure that clinicians should have in their clinical toolkits. This text should be used in conjunction with the clinician's previous professional training, other textbooks, and best judgment for the delivery of personalized care for each individual patient, including those who present with similar or identical diagnoses. Supportive texts include *Current Medical Diagnosis and Treatment* edited by Tierney

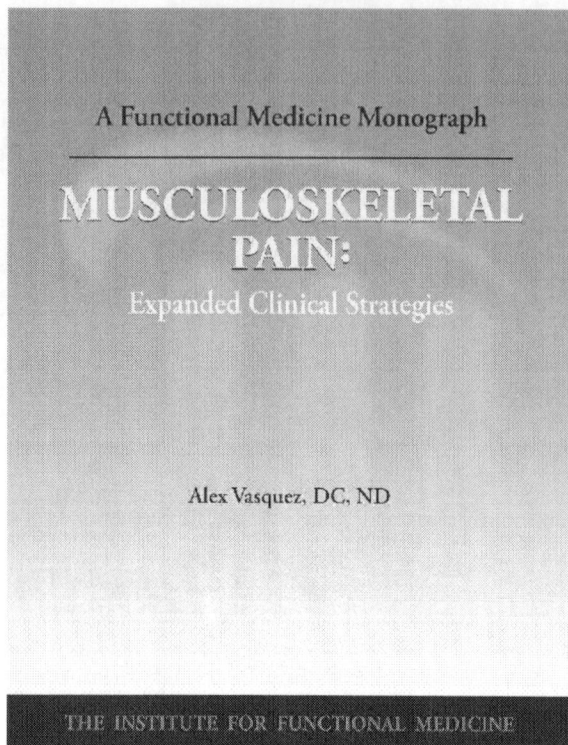

A Functional Medicine Monograph

MUSCULOSKELETAL PAIN:
Expanded Clinical Strategies

Alex Vasquez, DC, ND

THE INSTITUTE FOR FUNCTIONAL MEDICINE

---

[509] Jones DS (Editor-in-Chief). *Textbook of Functional Medicine*. Institute for Functional Medicine, Gig Harbor, WA 2005

[510] Freedman KB, Bernstein J. The adequacy of medical school education in musculoskeletal medicine. *J Bone Joint Surg Am.* 1998;80(10):1421-7

[511] Freedman KB, Bernstein J. Educational deficiencies in musculoskeletal medicine. *J Bone Joint Surg Am.* 2002;84-A(4):604-8

[512] Joy EA, Hala SV. Musculoskeletal Curricula in Medical Education: Filling In the Missing Pieces. *The Physician and Sportsmedicine.* 2004; 32: 42-45

[513] Matzkin E, Smith ME, Freccero CD, Richardson AB. Adequacy of education in musculoskeletal medicine. *J Bone Joint Surg Am.* 2005 Feb;87-A(2):310-4

[514] Schmale GA. More evidence of educational inadequacies in musculoskeletal medicine. *Clin Orthop Relat Res.* 2005 Aug;(437):251-9

[515] Stockard AR, Allen TW. Competence levels in musculoskeletal medicine: comparison of osteopathic and allopathic medical graduates. *J Am Osteopath Assoc.* 2006 Jun;106(6):350-5

[516] American College of Rheumatology Ad Hoc Committee on Clinical Guidelines. Guidelines for the initial evaluation of the adult patient with acute musculoskeletal symptoms. *Arthritis Rheum.* 1996 Jan;39(1):1-8 See also: **Vasquez A.** Musculoskeletal disorders and iron overload disease: comment on the American College of Rheumatology guidelines. *Arthritis Rheum* 1996;39: 1767-8

et al[517], *Orthopedic Physical Assessment* by Magee[518], and *Integrative Orthopedics* and *Integrative Rheumatology* by Vasquez.[519,520] Further, clinicians can note that this monograph is written primarily for routine outpatient management rather than emergency department management or "playing field" situations.

Musculoskeletal disorders are extremely prevalent and represent a major cause of human suffering, healthcare expenses, and lost productivity. Additionally, many standard medical interventions show high rates of inefficacy and iatrogenesis in addition to their high costs.[521,522,523] The vast majority of painful neuromusculoskeletal disorders can be alleviated and often effectively treated with nutritional interventions, but physicians trained only in standard medicine receive little to no training in nutrition and are therefore generally unable or unwilling to use these science-based interventions to help their patients.[524,525] Further, distain toward nutritional and other nonsurgical and nonpharmacologic interventions is represented in many standard medical textbooks despite proof of efficacy shown in replicable high-quality clinical trials published in top-tier medical journals. For example, despite the more than 800 articles documenting the role of nutritional interventions in the direct or adjunctive treatment of rheumatoid arthritis, the seventeenth edition of *The Merck Manual* published in 1999 wrote that, "Food and diet quackery is common and should be discouraged."[526] Combining these factors with the aforementioned pervasive lack of competence in musculoskeletal knowledge among healthcare providers (exceptions noted[527]), we see that patients with musculoskeletal disorders often face a series of difficult and insurmountable obstacles between their present condition of suffering and the relief that they seek and deserve. Clearly, the field of musculoskeletal medicine is in need of pervasive paradigm shifts in both physician training and patient management to improve patient care.

Background: Historically, prevailing views of disorders of pain and inflammation were conceptually similar to those of most other diseases and premodern accounts of life in general. Our clinical predecessors did the best they could to understand, describe, and treat the health problems with which their patients presented, and the paradigm from which these clinical entities were viewed and addressed was shaped by the social, religious, and scientific views and limitations of their time. Lacking a molecular and physiologic understanding of disease origination, and restrained by metaphysical and simplistic models of "cause and effect", premodern clinicians devised models for the understanding and treatment of disease that generally appear unsatisfactory today in light of the advances in our understanding in disparate yet interrelated fields such as psychoneuroimmunology, molecular biology, nutrigenomics, environmental medicine and toxicology. Despite these advances, we as a human society and as healthcare providers still carry many of these previous conceptualizations and misconceptualizations with us as we move forward toward a future wherein our views and interventions will be much more precise and "objective" in contrast to the generalized and phenomenalistic approaches that typified premodern medicine and which still permeate certain aspects of clinical care today. For example, we still use the term "stroke" to describe acute cerebrovascular insufficiency, although the term originated from the view that affected patients had been "struck" by the gods or fates perhaps as a form of punishment for some ethical or religious transgression. Even today, patients and clinicians commonly interpret disease as some form of punishment or as an extension of spiritual or intrapersonal shortcoming. Advancing science allows us to disassemble complex events that were previously experienced as *phenomena*, that is, as undecipherable and enigmatic events that overwhelmed comprehension. The **Functional Medicine Matrix** provides an extremely useful tool for helping clinicians grasp a multidimensional decipherable view of disease and its corresponding

[517] Tierney ML. McPhee SJ, Papadakis MA (eds). Current Medical Diagnosis and Treatment. New York: Lange Medical Books. Updated annually
[518] Magee DJ. Orthopedic Physical Assessment. Third edition. Philadelphia: WB Saunders, 1997. Newer editions have been published.
[519] Vasquez A. *Integrative Orthopedics: Second Edition*. Fort Worth, Texas; Integrative and Biological Medicine Research and Consulting, 2007 OptimalHealthResearch.com
[520] Vasquez A. *Integrative Rheumatology: Second Edition*. Fort Worth, Texas; Integrative and Biological Medicine Research and Consulting, 2007 OptimalHealthResearch.com
[521] Moseley JB, O'Malley K, Petersen NJ, Menke TJ, Brody BA, Kuykendall DH, Hollingsworth JC, Ashton CM, Wray NP. A controlled trial of arthroscopic surgery for osteoarthritis of the knee. *N Engl J Med* 2002 Jul 11;347(2):81-8
[522] Kolata G. A Knee Surgery for Arthritis Is Called Sham. *The New York Times*, July 11, 2002
[523] Rosner AL. Evidence-based clinical guidelines for the management of acute low-back pain: response to the guidelines prepared for the Australian Medical Health and Research Council. *J Manipulative Physiol Ther*. 2001;24(3):214-20
[524] Lo C. Integrating nutrition as a theme throughout the medical school curriculum. *Am J Clin Nutr*. 2000 Sep;72(3 Suppl):882S-9S
[525] Adams KM, Lindell KC, Kohlmeier M, Zeisel SH. Status of nutrition education in medical schools. *Am J Clin Nutr*. 2006 Apr;83(4):941S-944S
[526] Beers MH, Berkow R (eds). The Merck Manual. Seventeenth Edition. Whitehouse Station; Merck Research Laboratories: 1999, page 419
[527] Humphreys BK, Sulkowski A, McIntyre K, Kasiban M, Patrick AN. An examination of musculoskeletal cognitive competency in chiropractic interns. *J Manipulative Physiol Ther*. 2007;30(1):44-9

treatment which facilitates the achievement of higher clinical efficacy, improved patient outcomes, and more favorable safety and cost-effectiveness profiles.

Whereas the advancement of our scientific knowledge often leads us to discard previous models and interventions, occasionally modern science helps us to understand and revisit previous interventions that may have been prematurely or unduly discarded. For example, Hippocrates' admonition to "Let thy food be thy medicine, and thy medicine be thy food" experienced decades of devaluation when dietary, nutritional, and other natural interventions were misbranded as "quackery." On the contrary to these premature and unsubstantiated condemnations, simple natural interventions such as therapeutic fasting and augmentation of vitamin D3 status (via nutritional supplementation or exposure to ultraviolet-B radiation) have shown remarkable safety and efficacy in the mitigation of chronic hypertension, musculoskeletal pain, and autoimmunity.[528,529,530,531,532,533,534,535,536] Furthermore, the appropriate use of vitamin supplements helps prevent chronic disease by numerous mechanisms including modulation of gene transcription, enhancement of DNA repair and stability, and enhancement of metabolic efficiency.[537,538,539] This document will provide a representative survey of current research in the use of dietary, nutritional, and integrative therapeutics commonly utilized in the clinical management of disorders characterized by pain and inflammation.

State of the Evidence: The bulk of information in this monograph is derived from and referenced to peer-reviewed publications indexed in the database known as Medline/Pubmed provided by the U.S. National Library of Medicine and the National Institutes of Health. For the sake of practicality and publishability, not all statements carry citations, but the most important ones do; citations are always provided when referenced to a particular intervention of importance so that clinicians can access the primary source when refining their clinical decisions. A "blanket statement" to cover all the different assessments and interventions described herein would be necessarily inaccurate and therefore each intervention will be considered on the merits of its own rationale, safety, effectiveness, and cost-effectiveness. Again, however, these considerations must ultimately be viewed within the context of the individual patient's condition and the overall cohesion and comprehensiveness of the treatment plan.

While all clinicians can appreciate the importance of protocols and clinical practice guidelines, we must also perpetually ratify the preeminence of patient individuality and therefore the importance of tailoring treatment to the patient's unique combination of biochemical individuality, comorbid conditions, drug use, personal goals, and willingness to participate in a health-promoting lifestyle. Standardized protocols and practice guidelines are founded on the fallacy of disease homogeneity and the irrelevance of physiologic, psychosocial, and biochemical individuality. As the advancement of biomedical science provides the means for and underscores the importance of customized treatments for each patient, so too has the standard of care begun to shift in the direction of requiring the consideration of these variables before and during the implementation of treatment. Failure to utilize nutritional interventions when such interventions are clinically indicated is inconsistent with the delivery of quality healthcare and may be considered malpractice.[540,541,542,543]

A clinician who is unaware of the political forces that shape healthcare policy and research is analogous to a captain of an oceangoing ship not knowing how to use a compass, sextant, or coastline map. Medical science

[528] Goldhamer A, et al. Medically supervised water-only fasting in the treatment of hypertension. *J Manipulative Physiol Ther* 2001 Jun;24(5):335-9

[529] Goldhamer AC, et al. Medically supervised water-only fasting in the treatment of borderline hypertension. *J Altern Complement Med*. 2002 Oct;8(5):643-50

[530] Goldhamer AC. Initial cost of care results in medically supervised water-only fasting for treating high blood pressure and diabetes. *J Altern Complement Med*. 2002 Dec;8(6):696-7

[531] Krause R, Bühring M, Hopfenmüller W, Holick MF, Sharma AM. Ultraviolet B and blood pressure. *Lancet*. 1998 Aug 29;352(9129):709-10

[532] Pfeifer M, Begerow B, Minne HW, Nachtigall D, Hansen C. Effects of a short-term vitamin D(3) and calcium supplementation on blood pressure and parathyroid hormone levels in elderly women. *J Clin Endocrinol Metab*. 2001 Apr;86(4):1633-7

[533] McCarty MF. A preliminary fast may potentiate response to a subsequent low-salt, low-fat vegan diet in the management of hypertension - fasting as a strategy for breaking metabolic vicious cycles. *Med Hypotheses*. 2003 May;60(5):624-33

[534] Hyppönen E, Läärä E, Reunanen A, Järvelin MR, Virtanen SM. Intake of vitamin D and risk of type 1 diabetes: a birth-cohort study. *Lancet*. 2001 Nov 3;358(9292):1500-3

[535] Fuhrman J, Sarter B, Calabro DJ. Brief case reports of medically supervised, water-only fasting associated with remission of autoimmune disease. *Altern Ther Health Med*. 2002 Jul-Aug;8(4):112, 110-1

[536] Holick MF. Vitamin D deficiency: what a pain it is. *Mayo Clin Proc*. 2003 Dec;78(12):1457-9

[537] Fletcher RH, Fairfield KM. Vitamins for chronic disease prevention in adults: clinical applications. *JAMA*. 2002 Jun 19;287(23):3127-9

[538] Heaney RP. Long-latency deficiency disease: insights from calcium and vitamin D. *Am J Clin Nutr*. 2003 Nov;78(5):912-9

[539] Ames BN. The metabolic tune-up: metabolic harmony and disease prevention. *J Nutr*. 2003 May;133(5 Suppl 1):1544S-8S

[540] Heaney RP. Vitamin D, nutritional deficiency, and the medical paradigm. *J Clin Endocrinol Metab*. 2003 Nov;88(11):5107-8

[541] Fletcher RH, Fairfield KM. Vitamins for chronic disease prevention in adults: clinical applications. *JAMA*. 2002 Jun 19;287(23):3127-9

[542] Berg A. Sliding toward nutrition malpractice: time to reconsider and redeploy. *Am J Clin Nutr*. 1993 Jan;57(1):3-7

[543] Cobb DK, Warner D. Avoiding malpractice: the role of proper nutrition and wound management. *J Am Med Dir Assoc*. 2004 Jul-Aug;5(4 Sup):H11-6

and healthcare policy are influenced by a myriad of powerful private interests which are motivated by their own goals, at times different from the stated goals of medicine, which purports to hold paramount the patient's welfare. Scientific objectivity and the guiding ethical principles of informed consent, beneficence, autonomy, and non-malfeasance are subject to different interpretations depending upon the lens through which a dilemma is viewed. When this "dilemma" is the whole of healthcare, what first appears as order and structure now appears as the disarrayed tug-of-war between factions and private interests, with paradigmatic victory often being awarded to those with the best marketing campaigns and political influence with less importance given to safety, efficacy, and the economic burden to consumers.[544,545,546,547,548,549,550,551,552,553,554,555,556,557,558,559,560,561,562,563,564,565,566,567,568,569,570,571,572,573,574,575] To be ignorant of such considerations is to be blind to the nature of research, policy, and our own biased inclinations for and against particular paradigms, assessments, and interventions. Research articles and sources of authority must be approached with an artist's delicacy, and with a willingness to receive new information as worthy of preeminence over deeply rooted and well ensconced institutionalized fallacies.

<u>**Understanding the Multifaceted Nature of Disease Pathogenesis: The Functional Medicine Matrix as Paradigm and Clinical Tool**</u>: At its simplest and most practical level, the Functional Medicine Matrix is a teaching tool and clinical method that facilitates consideration of the different contributions of major intrinsic systems and

[544] Editorial. Drug-company influence on medical education in USA. *Lancet*. 2000 Sep 2;356(9232):781

[545] Horton R. Lotronex and the FDA: a fatal erosion of integrity. *Lancet*. 2001 May 19;357(9268):1544-5

[546] Editorial. Politics trumps science at the FDA. *Lancet*. 2005 Nov 26;366(9500):1827

[547] Topol EJ. Failing the public health--rofecoxib, Merck, and the FDA. *N Engl J Med*. 2004 Oct 21;351(17):1707-9

[548] Wolinsky H, Brune T. The Serpent on the Staff: The Unhealthy Politics of the American Medical Association. GP Putnam and Sons, New York, 1994

[549] Wilk CA. Medicine, Monopolies, and Malice: How the Medical Establishment Tried to Destroy Chiropractic. Garden City Park: Avery, 1996

[550] Carter JP. Racketeering in Medicine: The Suppression of Alternatives. Norfolk: Hampton Roads Pub; 1993

[551] National Alliance of Professional Psychology Providers. AMA Seeks To Control and Restrict Psychologist's Scope of Practice. http://www.nappp.org/scope.pdf Accessed November 25, 2006

[552] Daly R, American Psychiatric Association. AMA Forms Coalition to Thwart Non-M.D. Practice Expansion. *Psychiatric News* 2006 March; 41: 17

[553] Angell M. The Truth About the Drug Companies: How They Deceive Us and What to Do About it. Random House; August 2004

[554] Terrett AG. Misuse of the literature by medical authors in discussing spinal manipulative therapy injury. *J Manipulative Physiol Ther*. 1995 May;18(4):203-10

[555] Morley J, Rosner AL, Redwood D. A case study of misrepresentation of the scientific literature: recent reviews of chiropractic. *J Altern Complement Med*. 2001 Feb;7(1):65-78

[556] Wenban AB. Inappropriate use of the title 'chiropractor' and term 'chiropractic manipulation' in the peer-reviewed biomedical literature. *Chiropr Osteopat*. 2006 Aug 22;14:16

[557] Spivak JL. The Medical Trust Unmasked. Louis S. Siegfried Publishers; New York: 1961

[558] Trever W. In the Public Interest. Los Angeles; Scriptures Unlimited; 1972. This is probably the most authoritative documentation of the illegal actions of the AMA up to 1972; contains numerous photocopies of actual AMA documents and minutes of official meetings with overt intentionality of destroying Americans' healthcare options so that the AMA and related organizations would have a monopoly in healthcare.

[559] Getzendanner S. Permanent injunction order against AMA. *JAMA*. 1988 Jan 1;259(1):81-2

[560] "A national study released today reports 20 million American families — or one in seven families — faced hardships paying medical bills last year, which forced many to choose between getting medical attention or paying rent or buying food..." Freeman, Liz. 'Working poor' struggle to afford health care. *Naples Daily News*. Published in Naples, Florida and online at http://www.naplesnews.com/npdn/news/article/0,2071,NPDN_14940_3000546,00.html Accessed July 28, 2004

[561] "The USA's 5.8 million small companies... Health care costs are rising about 15% this year for those with fewer than 200 workers vs. 13.5% for those with 500 or more... But many small employers cite increases of 20% or more. That's made insurance the No. 1 small business problem..." Jim Hopkins. Health care tops taxes as small business cost drain. *USA TODAY*. http://www.usatoday.com/news/health/2003-04-20-small-business-costs_x.htm. Accessed July 28, 2004

[562] "Though the U.S. has slightly fewer doctors per capita than the typical developed nation, we have almost twice as many MRI machines and perform vastly more angioplasties. ...at least 31 percent of all the incremental income we'll earn between 1999 and 2010 will go to health care." Pat Regnier, *Money Magazine*. Healthcare myth: We spend too much. October 13, 2003: 11:29 AM EDT http://money.cnn.com/2003/10/08/pf/health_myths_1/ Accessed Monday, July 12, 2004

[563] "Although they spend more on health care than patients in any other industrialized nation, Americans receive the right treatment less than 60 percent of the time, resulting in unnecessary pain, expense and even death..." Ceci Connolly. U.S. Patients Spend More but Don't Get More, Study Finds: Even in Advantaged Areas, Americans Often Receive Inadequate Health Care. *Washington Post*, May 5, 2004; Page A15. On-line at http://www.washingtonpost.com/ac2/wp-dyn/A1875-2004May4 accessed on July 28, 2004

[564] McGlynn EA, Asch SM, Adams J, Keesey J, Hicks J, DeCristofaro A, Kerr EA. The quality of health care delivered to adults in the United States. *N Engl J Med*. 2003 Jun 26;348(26):2635-45

[565] Brennan TA, Leape LL, Laird NM, Hebert L, Localio AR, Lawthers AG, Newhouse JP, Weiler PC, Hiatt HH. Incidence of adverse events and negligence in hospitalized patients: results of the Harvard Medical Practice Study I. 1991. *Qual Saf Health Care*. 2004 Apr;13(2):145-51; discuss 151-2

[566] "Basically, you die earlier and spend more time disabled if you're an American rather than a member of most other advanced countries." Christopher Murray MD PhD, Director of World Health Organization's Global Program on Evidence for Health Policy http://www.who.int/inf-pr-2000/en/pr2000-life.html Accessed July 12, 2004

[567] Shi L. Health care spending, delivery, and outcome in developed countries: a cross-national comparison. *Am J Med Qual* 1997;12(2):83-93

[568] Holland EG, Degruy FV. Drug-induced disorders. *Am Fam Physician*. 1997 Nov 1;56(7):1781-8, 1791-2

[569] Brennan TA, Leape LL, Laird NM, Hebert L, Localio AR, Lawthers AG, Newhouse JP, Weiler PC, Hiatt HH. Incidence of adverse events and negligence in hospitalized patients: results of the Harvard Medical Practice Study I. 1991. *Qual Saf Health Care*. 2004 Apr;13(2):145-51; discuss 151-2

[570] Whitaker R. The case against antipsychotic drugs: a 50-year record of doing more harm than good. *Med Hypotheses*. 2004;62(1):5-13

[571] The relevance of these citations is to show that the misuse of horse estrogens in humans as "hormone replacement therapy" exemplified the application of a strong carcinogen to millions of unsuspecting women: Zhang F, Chen Y, Pisha E, Shen L, Xiong Y, van Breemen RB, Bolton JL. The major metabolite of equilin, 4-hydroxyequilin, autoxidizes to an o-quinone which converts to the potent cytotoxin 4-hydroxyequilenin-o-quinone. *Chem Res Toxicol*. 1999 Feb;12(2):204-13; Pisha E, Lui X, Constantinou AI, Bolton JL. Evidence that a metabolite of equine estrogens, 4-hydroxyequilenin, induces cellular transformation in vitro. *Chem Res Toxicol*. 2001;14(1):82-90; Zhang F, Swanson SM, van Breemen RB, Liu X, Yang Y, Gu C, Bolton JL. Equine estrogen metabolite 4-hydroxyequilenin induces DNA damage in the rat mammary tissues: formation of single-strand breaks, apurinic sites, stable adducts, and oxidized bases. *Chem Res Toxicol*. 2001 Dec;14(12):1654-9

[572] Newman NM, Ling RS. Acetabular bone destruction related to non-steroidal anti-inflammatory drugs. *Lancet*. 1985 Jul 6; 2(8445): 11-4

[573] "In 1983, 2876 people died from medication errors. ... By 1993, this number had risen to 7,391 - a 2.57-fold increase." Phillips DP, Christenfeld N, Glynn LM. Increase in US medication-error deaths between 1983 and 1993. *Lancet*. 1998 Feb 28;351(9103):643-4

[574] Smith R. Medical journals are an extension of the marketing arm of pharmaceutical companies. *PLoS Med*. 2005 May;2(5):e138

[575] van der Steen WJ, Ho VK. Drugs versus diets: disillusions with Dutch health care. *Acta Biotheor*. 2001;49(2):125-40

extrinsic influences that are at play in a given disease process or individual patient. When viewed as a diagram, the web of influences can be appreciated to reveal the interconnected nature of influences and body systems and how imbalance or disruption in one area can lead to problems in another. Once homeostatic reserves and compensatory mechanisms are depleted, the patient experiences progressively worsening health (which may be asymptomatic) and the eventual manifestation of clinical disease.

Over the course of many years and discussions and reconsiderations, the faculty at IFM has elucidated eight preeminent systems or loci ("core clinical imbalances") for clinicians to consider when working with any chronic health disorder. These will be listed and described below with particular consideration of the topic of this monograph, which is neuromusculoskeletal pain and inflammation. Interested readers are directed to IFM's monograph series on topics such as "Depression" and "The Role of Gastrointestinal Inflammation in Systemic Disease" to see how this model is applied to disease states in different organ systems.

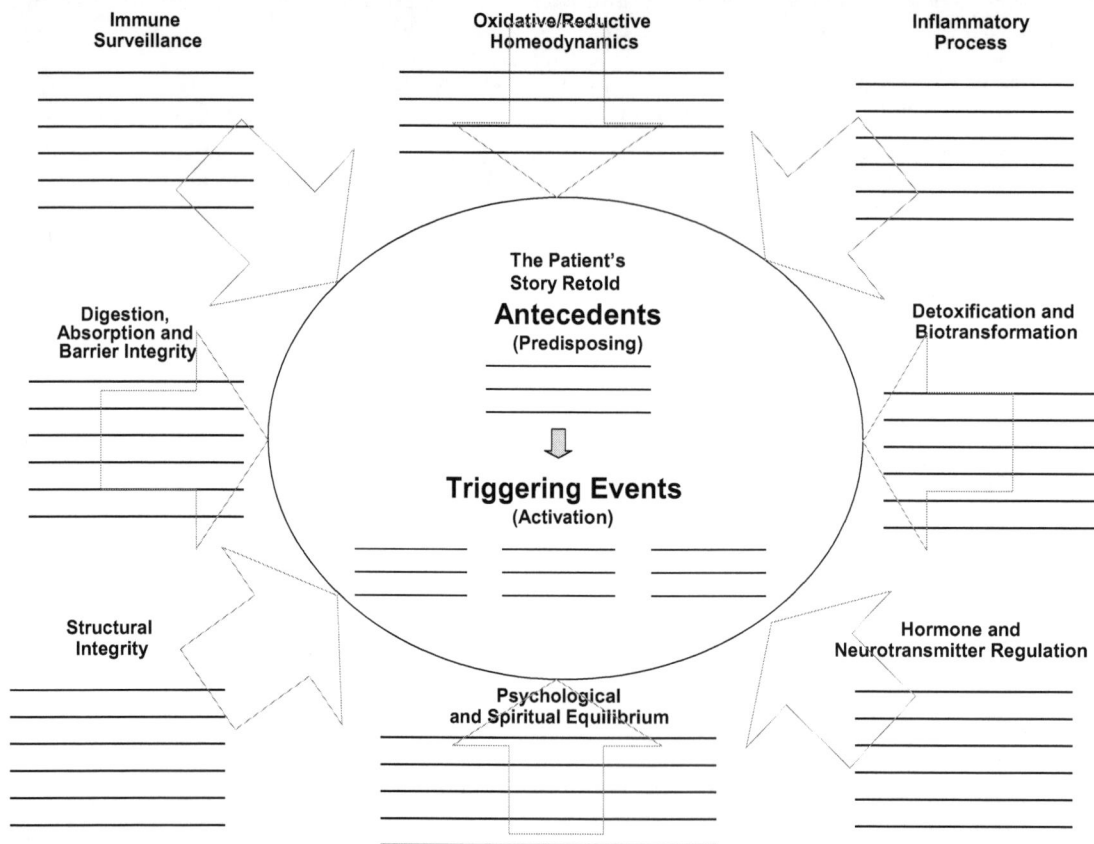

2008 rendering of The Functional Medicine Matrix: A concept, model, and clinical tool for evidence-based clinical care. Copyright Institute for Functional Medicine.

Exploring the Different Aspects of the Functional Medicine Matrix

1. Hormonal and neurotransmitter imbalances: While most clinicians are aware that neurotransmitters can either transmit pain signals or dampen their reception, many clinicians are not aware that neurotransmitter status is somewhat malleable and can be modulated with nutritional supplementation and botanical medicines. The examples that will be considered here are the tryptophan-serotonin-melatonin and the phenylalanine-tyrosine-dopamine-norepinephrine-epinephrine and enkephalin pathways.

   - Tryptophan and 5-hydroxytryptophan (5HTP) are prescription and nonprescription nutritional supplements that are the amino acid precursors for the formation of the neurotransmitter serotonin and, subsequently, the pineal hormone melatonin. Biochemically, these conversions are linear as follows: tryptophan → 5HTP → serotonin → melatonin. Tryptophan depletion and low levels of serotonin are consistently associated with depression, anxiety, exacerbation of eating disorders, and increased sensitivity to acute and chronic pain. Serotonergic pathways are impaired by chronic stress due to increased utilization of serotonin (e.g., serotonin-dependent cortisol release) and increased hepatic degradation of tryptophan by cortisol-stimulated tryptophan pyrrolase.[576] Therapeutically, supplementation with 5HTP augments serotonin and melatonin synthesis and has specific applicability in the alleviation of depression and pain syndromes such as fibromyalgia and headache, including migraine, tension headaches, and juvenile headaches.[577,578] Certainly part of the benefit from 5HTP supplementation is derived from the increased formation of melatonin, as the biological effects of melatonin extend beyond its sleep-promoting role to include powerful antioxidation, anti-infective immunostimulation[579], and preservation of mitochondrial function, a benefit which is of particular relevance to the treatment of fibromyalgia.[580]

- The conditionally essential fatty acids found in fish oil modulate serotonergic and adrenergic activity in the human brain[581], and given the role of serotonin and norepinephrine in the central processing of pain perception[582], a reasonable hypothesis holds that the pain-relieving activity of fish oil supplementation[583] is partly due to central modulation of pain perception and is not wholly due to modulation of eicosanoid production and inflammatory mediator transcription as previously believed.

- Vitamin D3 supplementation may also augment serotonergic activity[584], and this mechanism may partly explain the mood-enhancing and pain-relieving benefits of vitamin D3 supplementation. Attentive readers will note that this brief discussion has already begun to bridge the gaps between nutritional status, neurotransmitter synthesis, pain sensitivity, immune function, and mitochondrial bioenergetics.

- Supplementation with DL-phenylalanine (DLPA; racemic mixture of D- and L-forms of the amino acid phenylalanine derived from synthetic production) has long been used in the treatment of pain and depression.[585] The nutritional L-isomer is converted from phenylalanine to tyrosine to L-dopa to dopamine to norepinephrine and epinephrine. Augmentation of this pathway promotes resistance to fatigue, depression, and pain. The synthetic D-isomer augments pain-relieving enkephalin function by inhibiting enkephalin degradation by the enzyme carboxypeptidase A (enkephalinase); the resultant augmentation of enkephalin levels is generally believed to underlie the analgesic and mood-enhancing benefits of DLPA supplementation.

- Therapeutic massage is yet another means to modulate neurotransmitter synthesis for the alleviation of pain. In a study of patients with chronic back pain, massage increased serotonin and dopamine levels (measured in urine).[586]

Hormonal imbalances are particularly relevant to the discussion of chronic pain caused by inflammation characteristic of autoimmune diseases such as rheumatoid arthritis (RA). Often clinically subtle but nonetheless of extreme importance, these hormonal influences on painful inflammation are worthy of their own detailed discussion and thus will be reviewed later in this monograph in the context of the prototypic inflammatory disease RA. Generally speaking and with a few noted exceptions (such as Sjogren's syndrome), the research literature points to a specific pattern of hormonal imbalances among patients with autoimmunity, and this pattern is consistent with the proinflammatory and

[576] Sandyk R. Tryptophan availability and the susceptibility to stress in multiple sclerosis: a hypothesis. *Int J Neurosci*. 1996 Jul;86(1-2):47-53
[577] Turner EH, Loftis JM, Blackwell AD. Serotonin a la carte: supplementation with the serotonin precursor 5-hydroxytryptophan. *Pharmacol Ther*. 2006 Mar;109(3):325-38
[578] Birdsall TC. 5-Hydroxytryptophan: a clinically-effective serotonin precursor. *Altern Med Rev*. 1998 Aug;3(4):271-80
[579] Gitto E, Karbownik M, Reiter RJ, Tan DX, Cuzzocrea S, Chiurazzi P, Cordaro S, Corona G, Trimarchi G, Barberi I. Effects of melatonin treatment in septic newborns. *Pediatr Res*. 2001 Dec;50(6):756-60
[580] Acuna-Castroviejo D, Escames G, Reiter RJ. Melatonin therapy in fibromyalgia. *J Pineal Res*. 2006 Jan;40(1):98-9
[581] Hibbeln JR, Ferguson TA, Blasbalg TL. Omega-3 fatty acid deficiencies in neurodevelopment, aggression and autonomic dysregulation: opportunities for intervention. *Int Rev Psychiatry*. 2006 Apr;18(2):107-18
[582] Wise TN, Fishbain DA, Holder-Perkins V.Painful physical symptoms in depression: a clinical challenge. *Pain Med*. 2007 Sep;8 Suppl 2:S75-82
[583] Goldberg RJ, Katz J. A meta-analysis of the analgesic effects of omega-3 polyunsaturated fatty acid supplementation for inflammatory joint pain. *Pain*. 2007;129(1-2):210-23
[584] Lansdowne AT, Provost SC. Vitamin D3 enhances mood in healthy subjects during winter. *Psychopharmacology* (Berl). 1998 Feb;135(4):319-23
[585] Russell AL, McCarty MF. DL-phenylalanine markedly potentiates opiate analgesia - an example of nutrient/pharmaceutical up-regulation of the endogenous analgesia system. *Med Hypotheses*. 2000 Oct;55(4):283-8
[586] Hernandez-Reif M, Field T, Krasnegor J, Theakston H. Lower back pain is reduced and range of motion increased after massage therapy. *Int J Neurosci* 2001;106(3-4):131-45

immunodysregulatory effects of estrogens and prolactin and the anti-inflammatory and immunomodulatory effects of cortisol, dehydroepiandrosterone (DHEA), and testosterone. Patients with autoimmune neuromusculoskeletal inflammation generally display a complete or partial pattern of hormonal disturbances typified by elevated estrogen and prolactin and lowered testosterone, DHEA, and cortisol; appropriate therapeutic correction of these imbalances can safely result in disease amelioration. Rectification of endocrinologic imbalances ("orthoendocrinology") will be discussed in the section on RA and has been detailed with broader clinical applicability elsewhere by this author.[587]

2. <u>Oxidation-reduction imbalances and mitochondropathy</u>: Oxidative stress results from the chronic systemic inflammation seen in painful inflammatory disorders such as RA, and oxidative stress contributes to the perpetuation and exacerbation of inflammatory diseases via expedited tissue destruction and alterations in gene transcription and resultant enhancement of inflammatory mediator production.[588] Immune activation increases production of reactive oxygen species (ROS; "free radicals"), and oxidant stress increases activation of pro-inflammatory transcription factors (such as nuclear factor KappaB, NFkB) and also increases spontaneous oxidative modification of endogenous proteins such as cartilage matrix which then undergoes expedited degradation or immunologic attack; thus a vicious cycle of oxidation and inflammation exacerbates and perpetuates various inflammation-associated diseases, resulting in therapeutic recalcitrance and autonomous disease progression.[589,590] A rational clinical approach to breaking this vicious pathogenic cycle can include simultaneous antioxidation and immunomodulation, the former with diet optimization and nutritional supplementation and the latter with allergen avoidance, hormonal correction, xenobiotic detoxification, and specific phytonutritional modulation of pro-inflammatory pathways. Severe and acute inflammation can and often should be suppressed pharmacologically, but sole reliance on pharmacologic immunosuppression leaves the patient vulnerable to iatrogenic immunosuppression and the well-known increased risk for cardiovascular disease, infection, and clinical malignancy while failing to address the underlying biochemical and immunologic imbalances which lie at the bottom of all chronic inflammatory and autoimmune diseases. The contribution of mitochondrial dysfunction to chronic recurrent or persistent pain is most plainly demonstrated in migraine and fibromyalgia (discussed later in this monograph). An important characteristic of migraine is mitochondrial dysfunction, the severity of which correlates positively with the severity of the headache syndrome.[591] In fibromyalgia, numerous abnormalities in cellular bioenergetics are noted, which correlate clinically with the lowered lactate threshold, persistent muscle pain, reduced functional capacity, and the subjective fatigue that characterize the disorder.[592] Nutritional preservation and enhancement of mitochondrial function was termed "mitochondrial resuscitation" by Jeffrey Bland PhD in the 1990s, and clinical implementation of such an approach generally includes, in addition to diet and lifestyle modification, supplementation with coenzyme Q-10, niacin, riboflavin, thiamin, lipoic acid, magnesium, and other nutrients and botanical medicines which enhance production of adenosine triphosphate (ATP).[593]

3. <u>Detoxification and biotransformational imbalances</u>: As our environment becomes increasingly polluted and as researchers and clinicians mature and expand their appreciation and knowledge of the adverse effects of xenobiotics (toxic metals and chemicals), healthcare providers will need to attend to their patients' detoxification capacity and xenobiotic load as a component of the prevention and treatment of disease. By now, senior students and practicing clinicians should be aware of the association of xenobiotics in prototypic diseases such as Parkinson's disease[594,595], adult-onset diabetes mellitus[596,597,598,599],

[587] Vasquez A. *Integrative Rheumatology*. Fort Worth, Texas; Integrative & Biological Medicine Research & Consulting, 2007 OptimalHealthResearch.com
[588] Hitchon CA, El-Gabalawy HS. Oxidation in rheumatoid arthritis. *Arthritis Res Ther*. 2004;6(6):265-78
[589] Tak PP, Zvaifler NJ, Green DR, Firestein GS. Rheumatoid arthritis and p53: how oxidative stress might alter the course of inflammatory diseases. *Immunol Today*. 2000 Feb;21(2):78-82
[590] Kurien BT, Hensley K, Bachmann M, Scofield RH. Oxidatively modified autoantigens in autoimmune diseases. *Free Radic Biol Med*. 2006 Aug 15;41(4):549-56
[591] Lodi R, Kemp GJ, Montagna P, Pierangeli G, Cortelli P, Iotti S, Radda GK, Barbiroli B. Quantitative analysis of skeletal muscle bioenergetics and proton efflux in migraine and cluster headache. *J Neurol Sci*. 1997 Feb 27;146(1):73-80
[592] Park JH, Phothimat P, Oates CT, Hernanz-Schulman M, Olsen NJ. Use of P-31 magnetic resonance spectroscopy to detect metabolic abnormalities in muscles of patients with fibromyalgia. *Arthritis Rheum*. 1998 Mar;41(3):406-13
[593] Pieczenik SR, Neustadt J. Mitochondrial dysfunction and molecular pathways of disease. *Exp Mol Pathol*. 2007 Aug;83(1):84-92
[594] Corrigan FM, Wienburg CL, Shore RF, Daniel SE, Mann D. Organochlorine insecticides in substantia nigra in Parkinson's disease. *J Toxicol Environ Health A*. 2000 Feb 25;59(4):229-34
[595] Fleming L, Mann JB, Bean J, Briggle T, Sanchez-Ramos JR. Parkinson's disease and brain levels of organochlorine pesticides. *Ann Neurol*. 1994 Jul;36(1):100-3

and attention-deficit hyperactivity disorder.[600,601,602] The role of xenobiotic exposure and impaired detoxification in neuromusculoskeletal pain and inflammatory disorders is more subtle and is generally mediated through the resultant immunotoxicity that manifests as autoimmunity. Occasionally, clinicians will encounter patients with musculoskeletal symptomatology that defies standard diagnosis and treatment but which responds remarkably and permanently to empiric clinical detoxification treatment; such a case will be presented in the Case Reports later in this monograph. The numerous roles of xenobiotic exposure in the genesis and perpetuation of chronic health problems and the role of clinical detoxification in the treatment of such problems has been detailed elsewhere by Crinnion[603,604,605,606,607], Rea[608], Bland[609,610], Vasquez[611,612], and others.[613,614]

4. Immune imbalances: Immune imbalances have an obvious role in musculoskeletal inflammation when discussed in the context of autoimmune diseases such as rheumatoid arthritis, ankylosing spondylitis, and systemic lupus erythematosus. While the standard medical approach to this pathophysiology has focused almost exclusively on the pharmacologic suppression of resultant inflammation and tissue destruction, other disciplines such as naturopathic medicine and functional medicine have emphasized the importance of determining and addressing the underlying causes of such immune imbalance. While clinicians of all disciplines must appreciate the important role of pharmacologic immunosuppression in the treatment of inflammatory exacerbations as seen with giant cell arteritis or neuropsychiatric lupus, they should also appreciate that sole reliance on immunosuppression for long-term management of inflammatory disorders is destined to therapeutic failure insofar as it does not correct the underlying cause of the disease and creates dependency upon perpetual immunosuppression with its attendant costs (not uncommonly in the range of $20,000 - 50,000 per year) and adverse effects including infection and increased risk for cancer. Rather than presuming that immune dysfunction and the resultant inflammation and autoimmunity are results of spontaneous generation, astute clinicians seek to identify and correct the causes of these immune imbalances. By identifying and correcting the underlying causes of immune imbalance (when possible), clinicians can lessen or obviate the need for chronic polypharmaceutical treatment with anti-inflammatory and immunosuppressive agents. Vasquez[615] proposed that secondary immune imbalances (distinguished from primary congenital disorders) generally arise from one or more of five main problems: ❶ habitual consumption of a pro-inflammatory diet, ❷ food allergies and intolerances, ❸ microbial dysbiosis, including multifocal polydysbiosis, ❹ hormonal imbalances, and ❺ xenobiotic exposure and accumulation resulting in immunotoxicity via bystander activation and enhanced processing of autoantigens as well as haptenization and neoantigen formation. These influences may act singularly or when combined may be additive and synergistic. While

[596] Fujiyoshi PT, Michalek JE, Matsumura F. Molecular epidemiologic evidence for diabetogenic effects of dioxin exposure in U.S. Air force veterans of the Vietnam war. *Environ Health Perspect*, 2006 Nov;114(11):1677-83

[597] Lee DH, Lee IK, Song K, Steffes M, Toscano W, Baker BA, Jacobs DR Jr. A strong dose-response relation between serum concentrations of persistent organic pollutants and diabetes: results from the National Health and Examination Survey 1999-2002. *Diabetes Care* 2006 Jul;29(7):1638-44

[598] Lee DH, Lee IK, Jin SH, Steffes M, Jacobs DR Jr. Association between serum concentrations of persistent organic pollutants and insulin resistance among nondiabetic adults: results from the National Health and Nutrition Examination Survey 1999-2002. *Diabetes Care*, 2007 Mar;30(3):622-8

[599] Remillard RB, Bunce NJ. Linking dioxins to diabetes: epidemiology and biologic plausibility. *Environ Health Perspect*, 2002 Sep;110(9):853-8

[600] Rauh VA, Garfinkel R, Perera FP, Andrews HF, Hoepner L, Barr DB, Whitehead R, Tang D, Whyatt RW. Impact of prenatal chlorpyrifos exposure on neurodevelopment in the first 3 years of life among inner-city children. *Pediatrics*. 2006 Dec;118(6):e1845-59

[601] Cheuk DK, Wong V. Attention-deficit hyperactivity disorder and blood mercury level: a case-control study in Chinese children. *Neuropediatrics*. 2006 Aug;37(4):234-40

[602] Nigg JT, Knottnerus GM, Martel MM, Nikolas M, Cavanagh K, Karmaus W, Rappley MD. Low blood lead levels associated with clinically diagnosed attention-deficit/hyperactivity disorder and mediated by weak cognitive control. *Biol Psychiatry*. 2008 Feb 1;63(3):325-31

[603] Crinnion W. Results of a Decade of Naturopathic Treatment for Environmental Illnesses: A Review of Clinical Records. *J Naturopathic Medicine* vol. 7; 2, 21-27

[604] Crinnion WJ. Environmental medicine, part 1: the human burden of environmental toxins and their common health effects. *Altern Med Rev*. 2000 Feb;5(1):52-63

[605] Crinnion WJ. Environmental medicine, part 2 - health effects of and protection from ubiquitous airborne solvent exposure. *Altern Med Rev*. 2000 Apr;5(2):133-43

[606] Crinnion WJ. Environmental medicine, part 3: long-term effects of chronic low-dose mercury exposure. *Altern Med Rev*. 2000 Jun;5(3):209-23

[607] Crinnion WJ. Environmental medicine, part 4: pesticides - biologically persistent and ubiquitous toxins. *Altern Med Rev*. 2000 Oct;5(5):432-47

[608] Rea WJ, Pan Y, Johnson AR. Clearing of toxic volatile hydrocarbons from humans. *Bol Asoc Med P R*. 1991 Jul;83(7):321-4

[609] Bland JS, Barrager E, Reedy RG, Bland K. A Medical Food-Supplemented Detoxification Program in the Management of Chronic Health Problems. *Altern Ther Health Med*. 1995 Nov 1;1(5):62-71

[610] Minich DM, Bland JS. Acid-alkaline balance: role in chronic disease and detoxification. *Altern Ther Health Med*. 2007 Jul-Aug;13(4):62-5

[611] Vasquez A. *Integrative Rheumatology: Second Edition*. Fort Worth, Texas; Integrative and Biological Medicine Research and Consulting, 2007 OptimalHealthResearch.com

[612] Vasquez A. Diabetes: Are Toxins to Blame? *Naturopathy Digest* 2007; April

[613] Kilburn KH, Warsaw RH, Shields MG. Neurobehavioral dysfunction in firemen exposed to polychlorinated biphenyls (PCBs): possible improvement after detoxification. *Arch Environ Health*. 1989 Nov-Dec;44(6):345-50

[614] Cecchini M, LoPresti V. Drug residues store in the body following cessation of use: impacts on neuroendocrine balance and behavior--use of the Hubbard sauna regimen to remove toxins and restore health. *Med Hypotheses*. 2007;68(4):868-79

[615] **Vasquez A**. *Integrative Rheumatology: Second Edition*. Fort Worth, Texas; Integrative and Biological Medicine Research and Consulting, 2007 OptimalHealthResearch.com

it is beyond the scope of this monograph to detail each of these here, they will be sufficiently reviewed in later sections dealing with assessment and interventions as well as in the clinical focus subsections, particularly the section on rheumatoid arthritis.

5. Inflammatory imbalances: Inflammatory imbalances may be distinguished from immune imbalances insofar as inflammatory imbalances connote disorders of inflammatory mediator production in the absence of the immunodysfunction that typifies allergy, autoimmunity, or immunosuppression. Here again, long-term consumption of a pro-inflammatory diet[616] is a primary consideration because such a diet typically oversupplies inflammatory precursors such as arachidonate and undersupplies anti-inflammatory phytonutrients such as vitamin D, zinc, selenium, and the numerous phytochemicals that reduce activation of inflammatory pathways.[617,618,619,620] Three of the best examples of correctable inflammatory imbalances are those due to vitamin D deficiency, fatty acid imbalances, and overconsumption of simple sugars and saturated fats. Vitamin D deficiency is a widespread and serious health problem that spans nearly all geographic regions and socioeconomic strata with several important adverse effects. Vitamin D deficiency results in systemic inflammation[621] and chronic musculoskeletal pain[622] which both resolve quickly upon correction of the nutritional deficiency. Similarly and consistent with the Western/American pattern of dietary intake, overconsumption of alpha-linoleic acid and arachidonate along with underconsumption of alpha-linolenic acid (ALA), gamma-linolenic acid (GLA), eicosapentaenoic acid (EPA), docosahexaenoic acid (DHA), and oleic acid subtly yet powerfully shift nutrigenomic tendency and precursor availability in favor of enhanced systemic inflammation. Correction of this imbalance such as with reduced consumption of arachidonate and increased consumption of EPA and DHA has consistently proven to be of significant clinical value in the management of chronic inflammatory disorders.[623,624] Measurable increases in systemic inflammation and oxidative stress follow glucose challenge[625], consumption of saturated fatty acids as found in cream[626], and consumption of a "fast food" breakfast, which triggers the prototypic inflammatory activator NF-kappaB for enhanced production of inflammatory mediators.[627] This triad (vitamin D deficiency, fatty acid imbalance, and overconsumption of sugars and saturated fats) is typical of the Western/American pattern of dietary intake, and the molecular means and clinical consequences of such dietary choices is quite clear, evidenced by burgeoning epidemics of metabolic and inflammatory diseases.

6. Digestive, absorptive, and microbiological imbalances: The grouping of digestive and absorptive considerations suggests that the alimentary tract and its accessory organs of the liver, gall bladder and pancreas will be the focus of these core clinical imbalances, and the addition of microbiological imbalances should remind current clinicians that gastrointestinal dysbiosis is an important and frequent clinical consideration. Impaired digestion begins neither in the stomach nor in the mouth, but it stems rather from any socioeconomic milieu which deprives people of the means to prepare wholesome health-promoting meals and the time to consume those meals in a relaxed parasympathetic-dominant mode, preferably among good company, stimulating conversation, and appropriate ambiance. Poor dentition, xerostomia, hypochlorhydria, cholestasis or cholecystectomy, pancreatic insufficiency, mucosal atrophy,

[616] Seaman DR. The diet-induced proinflammatory state: a cause of chronic pain and other degenerative diseases? *J Manipulative Physiol Ther*. 2002 Mar-Apr;25(3):168-79

[617] **Vasquez A**. Reducing Pain and Inflammation Naturally. Part 1: New Insights into Fatty Acid Biochemistry and the Influence of Diet. *Nutritional Perspectives* 2004; October: 5, 7-10, 12, 14

[618] **Vasquez A**. Reducing Pain and Inflammation Naturally. Part 2: New Insights into Fatty Acid Supplementation and Its Effect on Eicosanoid Production and Genetic Expression. *Nutritional Perspectives* 2005; January: 5-16

[619] **Vasquez A**. Reducing pain and inflammation naturally - Part 3: Improving overall health while safely and effectively treating musculoskeletal pain. *Nutritional Perspectives* 2005; 28: 34-38, 40-42

[620] **Vasquez A**. Reducing pain and inflammation naturally - Part 4: Nutritional and Botanical Inhibition of NF-kappaB, the Major Intracellular Amplifier of the Inflammatory Cascade. A Practical Clinical Strategy Exemplifying Anti-Inflammatory Nutrigenomics. *Nutritional Perspectives* 2005;July: 5-12

[621] Timms PM, Mannan N, Hitman GA, Noonan K, Mills PG, Syndercombe-Court D, Aganna E, Price CP, Boucher BJ. Circulating MMP9, vitamin D and variation in the TIMP-1 response with VDR genotype: mechanisms for inflammatory damage in chronic disorders? *QJM*. 2002 Dec;95(12):787-96

[622] Al Faraj S, Al Mutairi K. Vitamin D deficiency and chronic low back pain in Saudi Arabia. *Spine*. 2003 Jan 15;28(2):177-9

[623] James MJ, Gibson RA, Cleland LG. Dietary polyunsaturated fatty acids and inflammatory mediator production. *Am J Clin Nutr*. 2000 Jan;71(1 Suppl):343S-8S

[624] James MJ, Proudman SM, Cleland LG. Dietary n-3 fats as adjunctive therapy in a prototypic inflammatory disease: issues and obstacles for use in rheumatoid arthritis. Prostaglandins *Leukot Essent Fatty Acids*. 2003 Jun;68(6):399-405

[625] Mohanty P, Hamouda W, Garg R, Aljada A, Ghanim H, Dandona P. Glucose challenge stimulates reactive oxygen species (ROS) generation by leucocytes. *J Clin Endocrinol Metab*. 2000 Aug;85(8):2970-3

[626] Mohanty P, Ghanim H, Hamouda W, Aljada A, Garg R, Dandona P. Both lipid and protein intakes stimulate increased generation of reactive oxygen species by polymorphonuclear leukocytes and mononuclear cells. *Am J Clin Nutr*. 2002 Apr;75(4):767-72

[627] Aljada A, Mohanty P, Ghanim H, Abdo T, Tripathy D, Chaudhuri A, Dandona P. Increase in intranuclear nuclear factor kappaB and decrease in inhibitor kappaB in mononuclear cells after a mixed meal: evidence for a proinflammatory effect. *Am J Clin Nutr*. 2004 Apr;79(4):682-90

altered gut motility, and bacterial overgrowth of the small bowel are important and common contributors to impaired digestion and absorption; clinicians should consider these frequently and implement treatment with a low threshold for intervention. The relevance of these problems to pain and the musculoskeletal system is generally that of malnutrition and its macro- and micronutrient consequences. Sunlight-deprived individuals must rely on dietary sources of vitamin D, which are hardly adequate for the prevention of overt deficiency; any impairment in digestion, emulsification, or absorption of this fat-soluble vitamin can readily lead to hypovitaminosis D and its resultant musculoskeletal consequences of osteomalacia and unremitting pain.[628] Consumption of foods to which the individual is sensitized ("food allergies") can trigger migraine and other chronic headaches[629,630] as well as generalized musculoskeletal pain and arthritis.[631,632,633] Avoidance of the offending foods often results in amelioration or complete remission of the painful syndrome at low cost and high efficacy without reliance on expensive or potentially harmful or addictive pain-relieving drugs. Occasionally, gluten enteropathy (celiac disease) presents with arthritic pain and chronic synovitis; the pain and inflammation remit on a gluten-free diet.[634] Alterations in intestinal microbial balance or an individual's unique response to endogenous bacteria (i.e., dysbiosis) can lead to systemic inflammation, arthritis, vasculitis, and musculoskeletal pain; clinical nuances and molecular mechanisms of gastrointestinal dysbiosis will be surveyed later in this monograph based on a previous review by Vasquez.[635] Clinicians should appreciate that dysbiosis can occur at sites other than the gastrointestinal tract, most importantly the nasopharynx and genitourinary tracts. Eradication of the occult infection or mucosal colonization often results in marked reductions in systemic inflammation and its clinical complications. Interested readers are directed to the excellent review by Noah[636] on the relevance of dysbiosis and its treatment relative to psoriasis; additional citations and clinical applications will be discussed later in this monograph.

7. <u>Structural imbalances from cellular membrane function to the musculoskeletal system</u>: Molecular structural imbalances lie at the heart of the concept of "biochemical individuality" originated by Roger J. Williams[637] in 1956, and this concept was soon thereafter expanded into the theory and practice of "orthomolecular medicine" pioneered by Linus Pauling and colleagues.[638,639] Pauling is considered by many authorities to be the original source of the concept of molecular medicine because he coined the phrase "molecular disease" after his team's discovery in 1949 that sickle cell anemia resulted from a single amino acid substitution that caused physical deformation of the hemoglobin molecule in hypoxic conditions.[640] (One of Pauling's students, Jeffery Bland, continued this legacy with the organization of "functional medicine" which now lives on as the Institute for Functional Medicine.[641]) Single nucleotide polymorphisms (SNP; pronounced "snip") are DNA sequence variations that can result in amino acid substitutions that render the final protein (e.g., structural protein or enzyme) abnormal in structure and therefore function. This aberrancy may or may not cause clinical disease (depending on the severity and importance of the variation), and consequences of the dysfunction may be occult, subtle, or obvious. One of the most powerful and effective means for treating diseases resultant from SNPs that result in enzyme defects is the use of high-dose vitamin supplementation, and this forms the scientific basis for "mega-vitamin therapy" as elegantly and authoritatively reviewed by Bruce Ames, et al.[642] SNP-induced

[628] Basha B, Rao DS, Han ZH, Parfitt AM. Osteomalacia due to vitamin D depletion: a neglected consequence of intestinal malabsorption. *Am J Med.* 2000 Mar;108(4):296-300

[629] Grant EC. Food allergies and migraine. *Lancet.* 1979 May 5;1(8123):966-9

[630] Millichap JG, Yee MM. The diet factor in pediatric and adolescent migraine. *Pediatr Neurol.* 2003 Jan;28(1):9-15

[631] van de Laar MA, Aalbers M, Bruins FG, et al. Food intolerance in rheumatoid arthritis. II. Clinical and histological aspects. *Ann Rheum Dis.* 1992 ;51(3):303-6

[632] Golding DN. Is there an allergic synovitis? *J R Soc Med.* 1990 May;83(5):312-4

[633] Hvatum M, Kanerud L, Hällgren R, Brandtzaeg P. The gut-joint axis: cross reactive food antibodies in rheumatoid arthritis. *Gut.* 2006 Sep;55:1240-7

[634] Bourne JT, Kumar P, Huskisson EC, Mageed R, Unsworth DJ, Wojtulewski JA. Arthritis and coeliac disease. *Ann Rheum Dis.* 1985 Sep;44(9):592-8

[635] **Vasquez A**. Reducing Pain and Inflammation Naturally. Part 6: Nutritional and Botanical Treatments Against "Silent Infections" and Gastrointestinal Dysbiosis, Commonly Overlooked Causes of Neuromusculoskeletal Inflammation and Chronic Health Problems. *Nutr Perspect* 2006; Jan: 5-21

[636] Noah PW. The role of microorganisms in psoriasis. *Semin Dermatol.* 1990 Dec;9(4):269-76

[637] Williams RJ. <u>Biochemical Individuality : The Basis for the Genetotrophic Concept</u>. Austin and London: University of Texas Press, 1956. Page x

[638] Pauling L. On the Orthomolecular Environment of the Mind: Orthomolecular Theory. In: Williams RJ, Kalita DK. <u>A Physician's Handbook on Orthomolecular Medicine</u>. New Cannan; Keats Publishing: 1977. Page 76

[639] Pauling L, Robinson AB, Teranishi R, Cary P. Quantitative analysis of urine vapor and breath by gas-liquid partition chromatography. *Proc Natl Acad Sci* 1971 Oct;68:2374-6

[640] Pauling L, Itano HA, Singer SJ, Wells IC. Sickle cell anemia, a molecular disease. *Science.* 1949 Nov 25;110(2865):543-8

[641] Bland JS. Jeffrey S. Bland, PhD, FACN, CNS: functional medicine pioneer. *Altern Ther Health Med.* 2004 Sep-Oct;10(5):74-81

[642] Ames BN, Elson-Schwab I, Silver EA. High-dose vitamin therapy stimulates variant enzymes with decreased coenzyme binding affinity (increased K(m)): relevance to genetic disease and polymorphisms. *Am J Clin Nutr.* 2002 Apr;75(4):616-58

alterations in enzyme structure reduce affinity for vitamin-derived coenzyme binding; this reduced affinity can be "overpowered" by administration of high doses of the required vitamin cofactor to increase tissue concentrations of the nutrient to promote binding of the enzyme with its ligand for the performance of enzymatic function. Thus, the scientific rationale for nutritional therapy is derived in part from the recognition that altered enzymatic function due to altered enzyme structure can often be corrected by administration of supradietary doses of nutrients. Relatedly, the structure and function of cell membranes is determined by their composition, which is influenced by dietary intake of fatty acids, and which influences production prostaglandins and leukotrienes. This is an important aspect of the scientific rationale for the use of specific fatty acid supplements in the prevention and treatment of painful inflammatory musculoskeletal disease. Cell membrane structure and function can also be altered by systemic oxidative stress; the concomitant alterations in intracellular ions (e.g., calcium) and receptor function along with activation of transcription factors such as NF-kappaB contribute to widespread physiologic impairment which creates a vicious cycle of inflammation, metabolic disturbance, and additional free radical generation.[643,644] Somatic dysfunction, musculoskeletal disorders, and inefficient biomechanics contribute to pain, increased production of inflammatory mediators, and the expedited degeneration of tissues such as collagen and cartilage matrix. Physicians trained in clinical biomechanics and physical medicine appreciate the subtle nuances of musculoskeletal structure-function relationships and address these problems directly with physical and manual means rather than ignoring the physical problem and only treating its biochemical sequelae. While biomechanics, palpatory diagnosis, and manual therapeutics takes years of diligent study for the achievement of proficiency, some of these concepts will be reviewed later in this monograph, particularly in the section on chronic low back pain.

8. Psychological and Spiritual Equilibrium: The connections between physical pain and psychoemotional status and events is worthy of thorough discussion and not merely for the sake of improving upon outdated clinical practices which have typically marginalized these ethereal considerations or considered them only long enough to substantiate psychopharmaceutical intervention. A survey of the literature makes clear the interconnected nature of pain, inflammation, psychoemotional stress, depression, social isolation, and nutritional status; due to space limitations in this monograph, a brief overview must necessarily suffice for the exemplification of representative concepts. Stressful and depressive life events promote the development, persistence, and exacerbation of disorders of pain and inflammation through nutritional, hormonal, immunologic, oxidative, and microbiologic mechanisms. Stated most simply, the perception of stressful events and the resultant neurohormonal cascade results in expedited metabolic utilization and increased urinary excretion of nutrients (e.g., tryptophan , and zinc, magnesium, retinol, respectively) which sum to effect nutritional imbalances and depletion, particularly when the stress response is severe and prolonged.[645,646,647] Specific to the consideration of pain, the depletion of tryptophan (and thus serotonin and melatonin) leaves the patient vulnerable to increased pain from lack of antinociceptive serotonin and to increased inflammation due to impaired endogenous production of anti-inflammatory cortisol, the adrenal release of which requires serotonin-dependent stimulation.[648] Severe stress, inflammation, and drugs used to suppress immune-mediated tissue damage (e.g., cyclosporine) increase urinary excretion of magnesium[649], and the eventual magnesium depletion renders the patient more vulnerable to hyperalgesia, depression, and other central nervous system and psychiatric disorders.[650,651] Furthermore, experimental and clinical data have shown that magnesium deficiency leads to a systemic pro-inflammatory state associated with oxidative stress and increased levels of the

[643] Evans JL, Maddux BA, Goldfine ID. The molecular basis for oxidative stress-induced insulin resistance. *Antioxid Redox Signal*. 2005 Jul-Aug;7(7-8):1040-52

[644] Joseph JA, Denisova N, Fisher D, Shukitt-Hale B, Bickford P, Prior R, Cao G. Membrane and receptor modifications of oxidative stress vulnerability in aging. Nutritional considerations. *Ann N Y Acad Sci*. 1998 Nov 20;854:268-76

[645] Stephensen CB, Alvarez JO, Kohatsu J, Hardmeier R, Kennedy JI Jr, Gammon RB Jr. Vitamin A is excreted in the urine during acute infection. *Am J Clin Nutr*. 1994 Sep;60(3):388-92

[646] Ingenbleek Y, Bernstein L. The stressful condition as a nutritionally dependent adaptive dichotomy. *Nutrition*. 1999 Apr;15(4):305-20

[647] Henrotte JG, Plouin PF, Lévy-Leboyer C, Moser G, Sidoroff-Girault N, Franck G, Santarromana M, Pineau M. Blood and urinary magnesium, zinc, calcium, free fatty acids, and catecholamines in type A and type B subjects. *J Am Coll Nutr*. 1985;4(2):165-72

[648] Sandyk R. Tryptophan availability and the susceptibility to stress in multiple sclerosis: a hypothesis. *Int J Neurosci*. 1996 Jul;86(1-2):47-53

[649] DiPalma JR. Magnesium replacement therapy. *Am Fam Physician*. 1990 Jul;42(1):173-6

[650] Murck H. Magnesium and affective disorders. *Nutr Neurosci*. 2002 Dec;5(6):375-89

[651] Hashizume N, Mori M. An analysis of hypermagnesemia and hypomagnesemia. *Jpn J Med*. 1990 Jul-Aug;29(4):368-72

nociceptive and proinflammatory neurotransmitter substance P.[652] Stress increases secretion of prolactin, a hormone which plays an important pathogenic role in chronic inflammation and autoimmunity.[653,654] An abundance of experimental and clinical research supports the model that chronic psychoemotional stress reduces mucosal immunity, increases intestinal permeability, and allows for increased intestinal colonization by microbes that then stimulate immune responses that cross-react with musculoskeletal tissues and result in the clinical manifestation of autoimmunity and painful rheumatic syndromes which appear clinically as variants of acute and chronic reactive arthritis (formerly Reiter' syndrome[655]) in susceptible patients.[656,657,658,659,660,661,662,663] Very interestingly, certain intestinal bacteria can sense when their human host is stressed, and they take advantage of the situation by becoming more virulent whereas previously these same bacteria may have been incapable of causing disease.[664,665] Psychoemotional stress also reduces mucosal immunity and increases colonization in locations other than the gastrointestinal tract. Microbial colonization of the genitourinary tract ("genitourinary dysbiosis"[666]) appears highly relevant in the genesis and perpetuation of rheumatoid arthritis.[667,668,669,670] Stressful life events also lower testosterone in men and the resultant lack of hormonal immunomodulation can increase the frequency and severity of exacerbations of rheumatoid arthritis[671]; resultant inflammation further suppresses testosterone production and bioavailability[672] leading to a self-perpetuating cycle of hypogonadism and inflammation. Thus, by numerous routes and mechanisms, psychoemotional stress increases the prevalence, persistence, and severity of musculoskeletal inflammation and pain.

Psychiatric codiagnoses are common among patients with painful neuromusculoskeletal disorders, and when the prevailing medical logic cannot solve the musculoskeletal riddle, the disorder is often ascribed to its accompanying mental disorder. The "appropriate" treatment from this perspective is the prescription of psychoactive drugs, generally of the "antidepressant" class. Science-based explanations are needed to expand clinicians' consideration of new possibilities which may someday prevail over commonplace suppositions that leave both clinician and patient trapped within a paradigm of futilely cyclical reasoning and its resultant simplistic symptom-targeting interventions. The following subsections provide alternatives to the "idiopathic pain is caused by its associated depression and both should be treated with antidepressant drugs" hypothesis.

a. <u>Pain, inflammation, and mental depression are final common pathways for nutritional deficiencies and imbalances</u>: As a scientific community we now know that the epidemic problem

[652] Weglicki W, Quamme G, Tucker K, Haigney M, Resnick L. Potassium, magnesium, and electrolyte imbalance and complications in disease management. *Clin Exp Hypertens.* 2005 Jan;27(1):95-112

[653] Imrich R. The role of neuroendocrine system in the pathogenesis of rheumatic diseases (minireview). *Endocr Regul.* 2002 Jun;36(2):95-106

[654] Orbach H, Shoenfeld Y. Hyperprolactinemia and autoimmune diseases. Autoimmun Rev. 2007 Sep;6(8):537-42

[655] Panush RS, Wallace DJ, Dorff RE, Engleman EP. Retraction of the suggestion to use the term "Reiter's syndrome" sixty-five years later: the legacy of Reiter, a war criminal, should not be eponymic honor but rather condemnation. *Arthritis Rheum.* 2007 Feb;56(2):693-4

[656] Tlaskalová-Hogenová H, Stepánková R, Hudcovic T, Tucková L, Cukrowska B, Lodinová-Zádníková R, Kozáková H, Rossmann P, Bártová J, Sokol D, Funda DP, Borovská D, Reháková Z, Sinkora J, Hofman J, Drastich P, Kokesová A. Commensal bacteria (normal microflora), mucosal immunity and chronic inflammatory and autoimmune diseases. *Immunol Lett.* 2004 May 15;93(2-3):97-108

[657] Collins SM. Stress and the Gastrointestinal Tract IV. Modulation of intestinal inflammation by stress: basic mechanisms and clinical relevance. *Am J Physiol Gastrointest Liver Physiol.* 2001 Mar;280(3):G315-8

[658] Hart A, Kamm MA. Review article: mechanisms of initiation and perpetuation of gut inflammation by stress. *Aliment Pharmacol Ther.* 2002 Dec;16(12):2017-28

[659] Farhadi A, Fields JZ, Keshavarzian A. Mucosal mast cells are pivotal elements in inflammatory bowel disease that connect the dots: stress, intestinal hyperpermeability and inflammation. *World J Gastroenterol.* 2007 Jun 14;13(22):3027-30

[660] Yang PC, Jury J, Söderholm JD, Sherman PM, McKay DM, Perdue MH. Chronic psychological stress in rats induces intestinal sensitization to luminal antigens. *Am J Pathol.* 2006 Jan;168(1):104-14

[661] Rashid T, Ebringer A. Ankylosing spondylitis is linked to Klebsiella--the evidence. *Clin Rheumatol.* 2007 Jun;26(6):858-64

[662] Vasquez A. *Integrative Rheumatology.* Fort Worth, Texas; Integrative and Biological Medicine Research and Consulting, 2007 OptimalHealthResearch.com

[663] Samarkos M, Vaiopoulos G. The role of infections in the pathogenesis of autoimmune diseases. *Curr Drug Targets Inflamm Allergy.* 2005 Feb;4(1):99-103

[664] Alverdy J, Holbrook C, Rocha F, Seiden L, Wu RL, Musch M, Chang E, Ohman D, Suh S. Gut-derived sepsis occurs when the right pathogen with the right virulence genes meets the right host: evidence for in vivo virulence expression in Pseudomonas aeruginosa. *Ann Surg.* 2000 Oct;232(4):480-9

[665] Wu L, Holbrook C, Zaborina O, Ploplys E, Rocha F, Pelham D, Chang E, Musch M, Alverdy J. Pseudomonas aeruginosa expresses a lethal virulence determinant, the PA-I lectin/adhesin, in the intestinal tract of a stressed host: the role of epithelia cell contact and molecules of the Quorum Sensing Signaling System. *Ann Surg.* 2003;238(5):754-64

[666] **Vasquez A**. *Integrative Rheumatology: Second Edition.* Fort Worth, Texas; Integrative and Biological Medicine Research and Consulting, 2007 OptimalHealthResearch.com

[667] Ebringer A, Rashid T. Rheumatoid arthritis is an autoimmune disease triggered by Proteus urinary tract infection. *Clin Dev Immunol.* 2006 Mar;13(1):41-8

[668] Erlacher L, Wintersberger W, Menschik M, Benke-Studnicka A, Machold K, Stanek G, Söltz-Szöts J, Smolen J, Graninger W. Reactive arthritis: urogenital swab culture is the only useful diagnostic method for the detection of the arthritogenic infection in extra-articularly asymptomatic patients with undifferentiated oligoarthritis. *Br J Rheumatol.* 1995 Sep;34(9):838-42

[669] Rashid T, Ebringer A. Rheumatoid arthritis is linked to Proteus--the evidence. *Clin Rheumatol.* 2007 Jul;26(7):1036-43

[670] Ebringer A, Rashid T, Wilson C. Rheumatoid arthritis: proposal for the use of anti-microbial therapy in early cases. *Scand J Rheumatol.* 2003;32:2-11

[671] James WH. Further evidence that low androgen values are a cause of rheumatoid arthritis: the response of rheumatoid arthritis to seriously stressful life events. *Ann Rheum Dis* 1997;56:566

[672] Karagiannis A, Harsoulis F. Gonadal dysfunction in systemic diseases. *Eur J Endocrinol.* 2005 Apr;152(4):501-13

of vitamin D deficiency leads to both musculoskeletal pain[673] as well as depression[674], and that supplementation with physiologic doses of vitamin D results in an enhanced sense of well-being[675] and high-efficacy alleviation of musculoskeletal pain and depression while providing other major collateral benefits.[676] Since the existence of vitamin D deficiency is more probable than that of antidepressant deficiency, the appropriate intervention for the former is more scientific and rational than that of the latter. Relatedly, research in various fields has shown that Western/American lifestyle and diet patterns diverge radically from human physiologic expectations and human nutritional requirements.[677] With regard to fatty acid intake and the resultant effects on inflammation and neurotransmission, modernized diets are a "set up" for musculoskeletal pain and mental depression, which frequently occur concomitantly and which are both alleviated by corrective fatty acid intervention such as fish oil supplementation as a source of EPA and DHA.[678,679] Correction of fatty acid imbalance is therefore more rational in the comanagement of pain and depression than is sole reliance on antidepressant and anti-inflammatory drugs; the latter have their place in treatment but neither addresses the primary cause of the problem and both drug classes have important adverse effects and significant cost in contrast to the safety, affordability, and collateral benefits derived from fatty acid supplementation. Also relevant to this discussion of chronic pain triggered and perpetuated by nutritional imbalances are the pro-inflammatory nature of the Western/American diet[680] and the pain-sensitizing effects of epidemic magnesium deficiency.[681] Therefore, correction of nutritional deficiencies and optimization of nutritional status might supersede the prescription of drugs in patients with concomitant depression and pain.

b. Pain, inflammation, and depression are final common pathways of physical inactivity: Exercising muscle elaborates cytokines ("myokines") with anti-inflammatory activity; a sedentary lifestyle fails to stimulate this endogenous anti-inflammation and is therefore relatively pro-inflammatory.[682] Further, exercise has antidepressant benefits mediated by positive influences on neurotransmission, growth factor elaboration, endocrinologic function, self-image, and social contact.[683] Patients with musculoskeletal pain should be encouraged to exercise to the extent possible given the individual's capacity and type of injury and/or degree of disability. Thus, a prescription for exercise might supersede the prescription of drugs in patients with concomitant depression and pain. Exercise prescriptions must consider frequency, duration, intensity, variety, safety, enjoyment, accountability and objective measures of compliance and progress, as well as appropriate combinations of components which emphasize aerobic fitness, strengthening, flexibility, muscle balancing, and coordination.

c. Pain and depression are final common pathways of inflammation: Several pro-inflammatory cytokines are psychoactive and cause depression, social withdrawal, impaired cognition, and sickness behavior.[684] As an alternative to the use of antidepressant drugs, correction of the underlying inflammatory disorder by natural, pharmacologic, or integrative means may subsequently promote restoration of normal affect and cognitive function.

---

[673] Plotnikoff GA, Quigley JM. Prevalence of severe hypovitaminosis D in patients with persistent, nonspecific musculoskeletal pain. *Mayo Clin Proc.* 2003 Dec;78(12):1463-70

[674] Wilkins CH, Sheline YI, Roe CM, Birge SJ, Morris JC. Vitamin D deficiency is associated with low mood and worse cognitive performance in older adults. *Am J Geriatr Psychiatry.* 2006 Dec;14(12):1032-40

[675] Vieth R, Kimball S, Hu A, Walfish PG. Randomized comparison of the effects of the vitamin D3 adequate intake versus 100 mcg (4000 IU) per day on biochemical responses and the wellbeing of patients. *Nutr J.* 2004 Jul 19;3:8

[676] **Vasquez A**, Manso G, Cannell J. The clinical importance of vitamin D (cholecalciferol): a paradigm shift with implications for all healthcare providers. *Altern Ther Health Med.* 2004 Sep-Oct;10(5):28-36

[677] O'Keefe JH Jr, Cordain L. Cardiovascular disease resulting from a diet and lifestyle at odds with our Paleolithic genome: how to become a 21st-century hunter-gatherer. *Mayo Clin Proc.* 2004 Jan;79(1):101-8

[678] Kiecolt-Glaser JK, Belury MA, Porter K, Beversdorf DQ, Lemeshow S, Glaser R. Depressive symptoms, omega-6:omega-3 fatty acids, and inflammation in older adults. *Psychosom Med.* 2007 Apr;69(3):217-24

[679] Simopoulos AP. Omega-3 fatty acids in inflammation and autoimmune diseases. *J Am Coll Nutr.* 2002 Dec;21(6):495-505

[680] Aljada A, Mohanty P, Ghanim H, Abdo T, Tripathy D, Chaudhuri A, Dandona P. Increase in intranuclear nuclear factor kappaB and decrease in inhibitor kappaB in mononuclear cells after a mixed meal: evidence for a proinflammatory effect. *Am J Clin Nutr.* 2004 Apr;79(4):682-90

[681] Park JH, Niermann KJ, Olsen N. Evidence for metabolic abnormalities in the muscles of patients with fibromyalgia. *Curr Rheumatol Rep.* 2000 Apr;2(2):131-40

[682] Petersen AM, Pedersen BK. The anti-inflammatory effect of exercise. *J Appl Physiol.* 2005 Apr;98(4):1154-62

[683] Cotman CW, Berchtold NC, Christie LA. Exercise builds brain health: key roles of growth factor cascades and inflammation. *Trends Neurosci.* 2007 Sep;30(9):464-72

[684] Wilson CJ, Finch CE, Cohen HJ. Cytokines and cognition--the case for a head-to-toe inflammatory paradigm. *J Am Geriatr Soc.* 2002 Dec;50(12):2041-56

d. <u>Pain, inflammation, and mental depression are final common pathways for hormonal deficiencies and imbalances</u>: Deficiencies of thyroid hormones, estrogen (insufficiency or excess), testosterone, cortisol, and DHEA can cause depression and impaired neuroemotional status. Hormonal aberrations are common in patients with chronic musculoskeletal pain, particularly of the inflammatory and autoimmune types. Clinical trials have shown that administration of thyroid hormones, testosterone, DHEA, cortisol and suppression prolactin can each provide anti-inflammatory, analgesic, and antidepressant benefits among appropriately selected patients. Thus, identification and correction of hormonal imbalances might supersede the prescription of antidepressant drugs in patients with concomitant depression, inflammation, and pain.

Our cultural and scientific advancements in the knowledge of how the brain and mind function have been paradoxically paralleled by social trends showing increasing depression and social isolation; the typical American has only two friends and no one in whom to confide.[685] In the United States, violent injuries are epidemic, and the level of firearm morbidity and mortality in the US is far higher than anywhere else in the industrialized world.[686] This does to some extent beg the question of the value of "scientific knowledge" of the brain and mind within a social structure that is increasingly violent and fragmented. Further, the mental depression resultant from pandemic social isolation would be better served by physicians' admonition for increased social contact than by the continued overuse of drugs which inhibit neurotransmitter reuptake.

<u>Conclusion</u>: The clinical employment of the functional medicine approach to chronic disease management and health promotion rests upon a foundation of competent patient management and then extends to consider the well documented contributions of the causative *core clinical imbalances* that have allowed the genesis and perpetuation of the problem(s) under consideration. The attainment of wellness, the success of preventive medicine, and the optimization of socioemotional health cannot be attained by pharmacological suppression of the manifestations of dysfunction that result from nutritional and neuroendocrine imbalances, xenobiotic accumulation, sedentary lifestyles, social isolation, and mucosal microbial colonization. Rather, these problems are addressed directly, and these and other causative considerations must remain foremost in the mind of the physician committed to the successful, ethical, and cost-effective long-term prevention and management of chronic health disturbances, particularly those characterized by inflammation and pain.

---

[685] McPherson M, Smith-Lovin L, Brashears ME. Social Isolation in America: Changes in Core Discussion Networks over Two Decades. *American Sociological Review* 2006; 71: 353-75
[686] Preventing firearm violence: a public health imperative. *American College of Physicians. Ann Intern Med.* 1995 Feb 15;122(4):311-3

Functional medicine is a science-based field of health care that is grounded in the following principles:

- **Biochemical individuality** describes the importance of individual variations in metabolic function that derive from genetic and environmental differences among individuals.
- **Patient-centered** medicine emphasizes "patient care" rather than "disease care," following Sir William Osler's admonition that "It is more important to know what patient has the disease than to know what disease the patient has."
- **Dynamic balance** of internal and external factors.
- **Web-like interconnections** of physiological factors – an abundance of research now supports the view that the human body functions as an orchestrated network of interconnected systems, rather than individual systems functioning autonomously and without effect on each other. For example, we now know that immunological dysfunctions can promote cardiovascular disease, that dietary imbalances can cause hormonal disturbances, and that environmental exposures can precipitate neurologic syndromes such as Parkinson's disease.
- **Health as a positive vitality** – not merely the absence of disease.
- **Promotion of organ reserve** as the means to enhance health span.

Functional medicine is anchored by an examination of the core clinical imbalances that underlie various disease conditions. Those imbalances arise as **environmental inputs** such as diet, nutrients (including air and water), exercise, and trauma **are processed** by one's body, mind, and spirit through a unique set of genetic predispositions, attitudes, and beliefs. The **fundamental physiological** processes include communication, both outside and inside the cell; bioenergetics, or the transformation of food into energy; replication, repair, and maintenance of structural integrity, from the cellular to the whole body level; elimination of waste; protection and defense; and transport and circulation. The **core clinical imbalances** that arise from malfunctions within this complex system include:

- **Hormonal and neurotransmitter imbalances**
- **Oxidation-reduction imbalances and mitochondropathy**
- **Detoxification and biotransformational imbalances**
- **Immune imbalances**
- **Inflammatory imbalances**
- **Digestive, absorptive, and microbiological imbalances**
- **Structural imbalances** from cellular membrane function to the musculoskeletal system

Imbalances such as these are the precursors to the signs and symptoms by which we detect and label (diagnose) organ system disease. Improving balance – in the patient's environmental inputs and in the body's fundamental physiological processes – is the precursor to restoring health and it involves much more than treating the symptoms. Functional medicine is dedicated to improving the management of complex, chronic disease by intervening at multiple levels to address these core clinical imbalances and to restore each patient's functionality and health. Functional medicine is not a unique and separate body of knowledge. It is grounded in scientific principles and information widely available in medicine today, combining research from various disciplines into highly detailed yet clinically relevant models of disease pathogenesis and effective clinical management.

Functional medicine emphasizes a definable and teachable **process** of integrating multiple knowledge bases within a pragmatic intellectual matrix that focuses on functionality at many levels, rather than a single treatment for a single diagnosis. Functional medicine uses the patient's story as a key tool for integrating diagnosis, signs and symptoms, and evidence of clinical imbalances into a comprehensive approach to improve both the patient's environmental inputs and his or her physiological function. It is a clinician's discipline, and it directly addresses the need to transform the practice of primary care.

Newsletter & Updates

Be alerted to new integrative clinical research and updates to this textbook by registering for the free newsletter, sent 4-6 times per year. Subscribe via
www.OptimalHealthResearch.com/newsletter.html

Also, check for updates to all books at **http://optimalhealthresearch.com/updates**.html

Index for this section:

Dysregulated Inflammation and Immune Activation *as the Cause of* Inflammation, Allergy, and Autoimmunity:
Nutritional & Functional Medicine Approaches

Overview of Concepts, Research, and Foundational Interventions for Diabetes Type-2, Hypertension, Allergy, Asthma, and Autoimmunity such as Rheumatoid Arthritis and Psoriasis

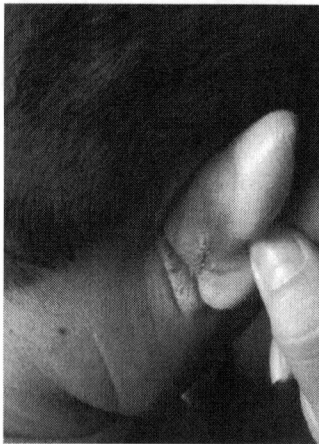

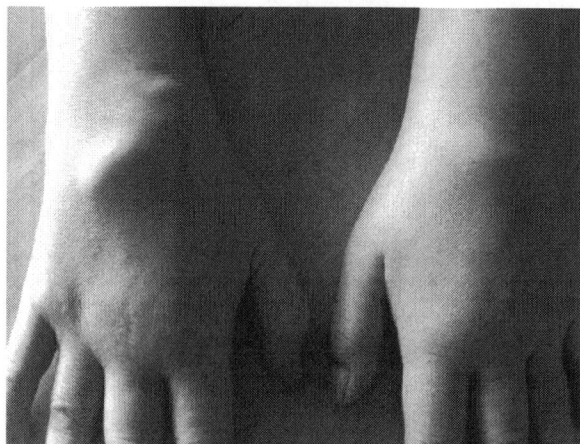

▸ **Alex Vasquez, D.C., N.D., D.O.**

Dr Vasquez: Introduction

▹ Education:

 ▹ **Doctor of Chiropractic**, University of Western States (March 1996) Portland, Oregon

 ▹ **Doctor of Naturopathic Medicine**, Bastyr University (September 1999) Seattle, Washington

 ▹ **Doctor of Osteopathic Medicine**, University of North Texas Health Science Center (May 2010) Fort Worth, Texas

 ▹ Read thousands of articles/books; thousands of hours of post-graduate training in seminars, clinics, hospitals; many years of experience with thousands of patients

▹ Publications and presentations:

 ▹ International lecturer to physicians and clinicians on integrative/functional medicine

 ▹ Several textbooks for doctors and health science students

 ▹ Approximately 100 articles and letters in professional magazines and peer-reviewed journals

▹ Current professional activities:

 ▹ Associate/adjunct/affiliate faculty for several universities and post-graduate institutions

 ▹ Compiling research, conducting research, authoring books and articles

 ▹ Healthcare product design

 ▹ International seminars and presentations

 ▹ Private practice of naturopathic medicine specializing in difficult and complex cases of autoimmune/inflammatory diseases in Portland, Oregon

Dr Vasquez: Articles (~100)

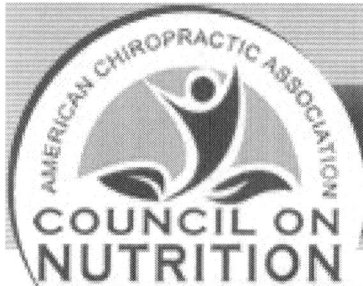

Dr Vasquez: Books

INTEGRATIVE ORTHOPEDICS

INTEGRATIVE RHEUMATOLOGY

A Functional Medicine Monograph

MUSCULOSKELETAL PAIN:

CHIROPRACTIC AND NATUROPATHIC
MASTERY OF COMMON CLINICAL DISORDERS

INTEGRATIVE MEDICINE AND
FUNCTIONAL MEDICINE FOR
CHRONIC HYPERTENSION:

INTEGRATIVE CHIROPRACTIC
MANAGEMENT OF
HIGH BLOOD PRESSURE
AND CHRONIC HYPERTENSION

MIGRAINE HEADACHES,
HYPOTHYROIDISM, AND
FIBROMYALGIA:
ASSESSMENTS AND THERAPEUTIC APPROACHES
USING INTEGRATIVE CHIROPRACTIC, NATUROPATHIC,
OSTEOPATHIC, AND FUNCTIONAL MEDICINE

Published books

1. Integrative Orthopedics ('04,'07,'12)
2. Integrative Rheumatology ('04,'07,'12pending)
3. Musculoskeletal Pain ('08, published by IFM)
4. Chiropractic and Naturopathic Mastery of Common Clinical Disorders ('09)
5. Integrative Medicine and Functional Medicine for Chronic Hypertension ('10)
6. Integrative Chiropractic Management of High Blood Pressure & Chronic Hypertension ('10,'11)
7. Migraine Headaches, Hypothyroidism, and Fibromyalgia ('12)

Upcoming books

▸ Fibromyalgia in a Nutshell (Jun'12)
▸ Textbook of Functional Immunology and Nutritional Immunomodulation (Aug'12)
▸ Psoriasis and Psoriatic Arthritis (Sept'12)

Audio Files

▶ <u>**Audio files, Mp3 downloads, Podcasts**</u>:

  ▷ <u>Paris, France</u>: approximately 6 hours of recordings.

  ▷ <u>Belgium and Holland</u>: several hours of recordings over several days in several cities.

  ▷ <u>Vancouver, Washington USA</u>: 2 hours on diabetes mellitus and hypertension.

  ▷ <u>Blaine, Washington just south of British Columbia, Canada</u>: 90 minutes on the updated protocol.

▶ <u>**And a growing list of audios and videos**</u>:

OptimalHealthResearch.com

OptimalHealthResearch.com/action

InternationalCMEonline.com

…USA, Spain, Colombia, France, Belgium, Holland, Canada, England…

Notices

<u>Affiliations</u>: Dr Vasquez's presentation is not necessarily endorsed by nor representative of any of his affiliations (i.e., intellectual freedom).

  ▹ Director of the Medical Board of Advisors, Biotics Research Corporation

  ▹ Adjunct Professor of Pharmacology, University of Western States

  ▹ Program Director, UWS Master of Science in Nutrition & Functional Medicine

  ▹ Adjunct Faculty, Master of Science Advanced Clinical Practice, NUHS

  ▹ Adjunct Faculty (Immune Advanced Practice Module: "The Many Faces of Immune Dysregulation and Chronic Inflammation: Chronic Infections, Atopy, and Autoimmune Disorders"), Institute for Functional Medicine

<u>Disclaimer</u>: The information in these presentations is accurate but not applicable to all patients at all times and does not substitute for a clinician's professional judgment in patient care. Opinions and perspectives presented here are those of Dr Vasquez and not necessarily shared by his affiliations. Doses mentioned are for adults.

<u>Copyright</u>: Except for quotations and images obtained elsewhere, the material and contents of these presentations are copyrighted by Dr Alex Vasquez and have often been excerpted from his books which are also copyrighted. Any unauthorized use of this material—including photocopying—is prohibited.

Goals: Personal and practical

▸ My main personal goal is to outline a "new" way to manage disorders of inflammation-allergy-autoimmunity beyond both 1) ineffective unscientific treatments, and 2) drug-based treatments that do little other than suppress the end manifestations of immune-metabolic physiologic disturbance.

▸ Achieving this goal:

= better success for you as professionals,

= the delivery of true **authentic healthcare** (rather than perpetuation of **our current system of diseasecare**)

= better care for our shared human society,

= progress for humanity ☺

Goals

1. <u>Identification</u>: To review the **seven most important modifiable factors that mediate immune dysfunction**, which are the cause(s) of *or major modifiable contributor(s)* to chronic **inflammation, allergy, and autoimmune disease**.

2. <u>Recitation</u>: For clinicians-practitioners to be able to **list these factors from memory** (declarative knowledge) so that they can explain these factors to their clients/patients.

3. <u>Explanation and implementation</u>: For clinicians-practitioners to be able to **explain the mechanisms and interventions for each of these 7 factors**.

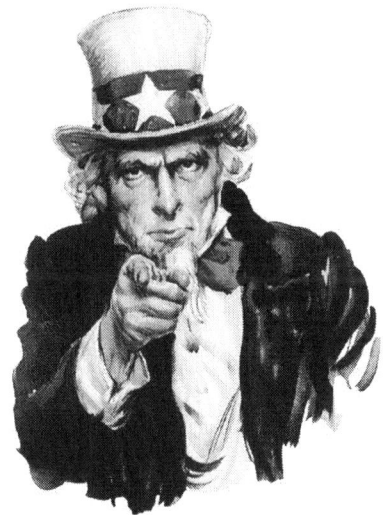

This means you.

Perspectives and Promises

1. **I am well-known for having a lot of information in my presentations; I will try to make this accessible and easy to understand.**

    ▸ These new presentations are the most efficient presentations I've ever made. Even if you've been doing nutritional/functional medicine for several years, I think that you will still learn some new tools. I will try to be efficient and say less than usual when we must allow for translations.

2. **In this new presentation, I give the <u>information in a pattern</u> that will help make sense of the information.**

    ▸ Intentional redundancy exists; you also have in your notes some slides that we will not cover in the lecture; these are for you to review later.

3. **I can promise you that by the end of the day, all of this will make sense and that you will have an easy-to-remember protocol that you can use safely and effectively in your practice.**

Medical education—nutritionally deficient, drug dependent

J. Clin. Gastroenterol. 2009 Jul;43(6):559-64
How much do gastroenterology fellows know about nutrition?
Raman M, Violato C, Coderre S.

Original Research

What Do Resident Physicians Know about Nutrition?
An Evaluation of Attitudes, Self-Perceived Proficiency
and Knowledge

Analysis of questions asked by family doctors regarding
patient care

John W Ely, Jerome A Osheroff, Mark H Ebell, George R Bergus, Barcey T Levy, M Lee Chambliss, Eric R Evans

Abstract

WEB-LIKE INTERCONNECTIONS OF PHYSIOLOGICAL FACTORS

Alex Vasquez, DC, ND

Editor's Note: This article is reprinted with permission from The Textbook of Functional Medicine (copyright © 2005 Institute for Functional Medicine; all rights reserved). The following is the second portion of the textbook's Chapter 10, "Web-like Interconnections, The Complex Human Organism." The first half of Chapter 10 ran in IMCD's last issue of February-March 2006, p. 40-42. For more information as to purchase the textbook, contact The Institute for Functional Medicine, PO Box 1697, Gig Harbor, WA 98335; 1-800-228-0622; or visit its website, www.functionalmedicine.org

Introduction
Understanding the scientific basis and clinical applications of functional medicine and a "whole patient" approach to health care requires that clinicians fully appreciate the interconnectedness of organ system histology with biochemical and physiological processes. Simplistic models of health and disease developed decades ago may no longer be accurate or clinically useful insofar as they fail to reflect the more recently discovered complex and multifaceted interrelationships (Figure 10.2 uses the functional medicine matrix to depict some of this complexity.) Numerous mechanisms mediate these interrelationships, including, but not limited to, those that can be described as biochemical, hormonal, neurological, immunological, piezoelectric, and physical or mechanical. Ultimately, we are forced to dissolve the artificial intellectual boundaries we have created between organ systems and expand our appreciation of individual molecules, cellular messengers, and the physiologic mechanisms that mediate intercellular communication and coordinate interorgan function.

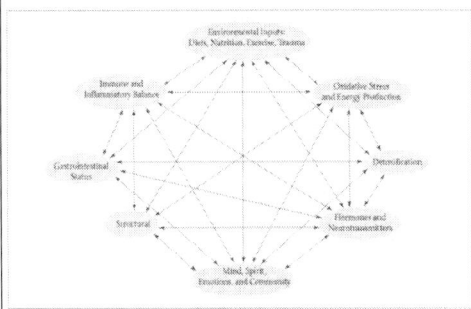

1. The tragic irony is that the vast majority of medical doctors—and therefore the largest component of the healthcare delivery system in the world—are untrained in nutrition and therefore incapable/ incompetent to deliver nutrition assessment and treatment to their patients. Raman. *J Clin Gastroenterol.* 2009 Jul; Vetter. *J Am Coll Nutr* 2008 Apr

2. Thus, not surprisingly, medical doctors practice in a way that focuses on 1) the diagnosis, and 2) the drug(s) for the diagnosis. Ely. *BMJ 1999* Aug

3. The medical profession generally lacks appreciation of how body systems work interactively and interdependently. Vasquez. *Integrative Med.* 2006 Apr

4. **Diagnosis and drugs are the emphasis of medical practice without consideration of the nutritional needs of the patient and without an appreciation of how the body works together as an integrated whole;** this fails to address the *reality* of most diseases and therefore keeps most patients dependent on drugs for the masking of metabolic imbalances better treated with nutritional interventions.

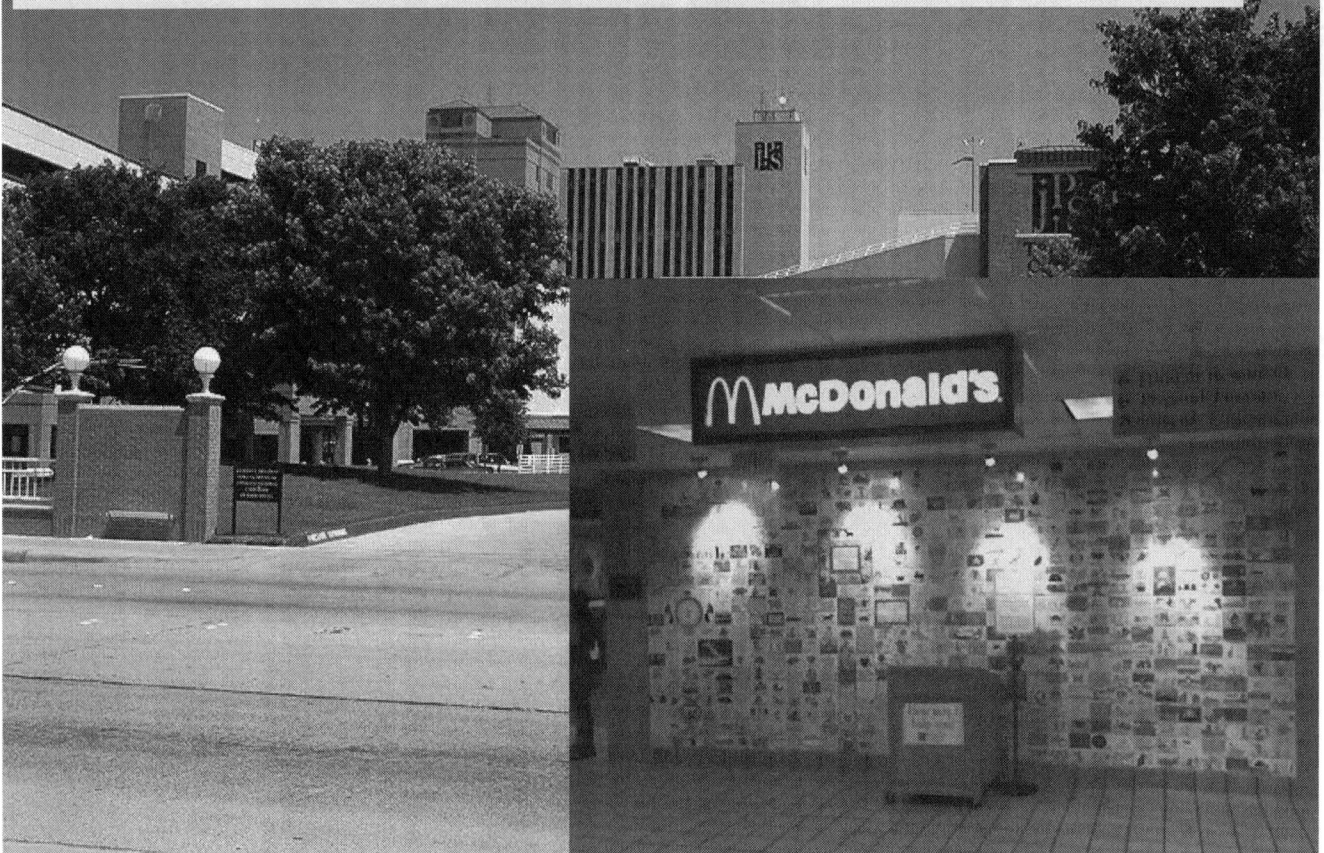

Our training hospital served McDonald's fast food on the first floor near the main entrance; also, we would feed post-CABG pts pancakes and sausage (should this be considered malpractice?)

USA Hospital food, "Family Medicine", soda, fried food

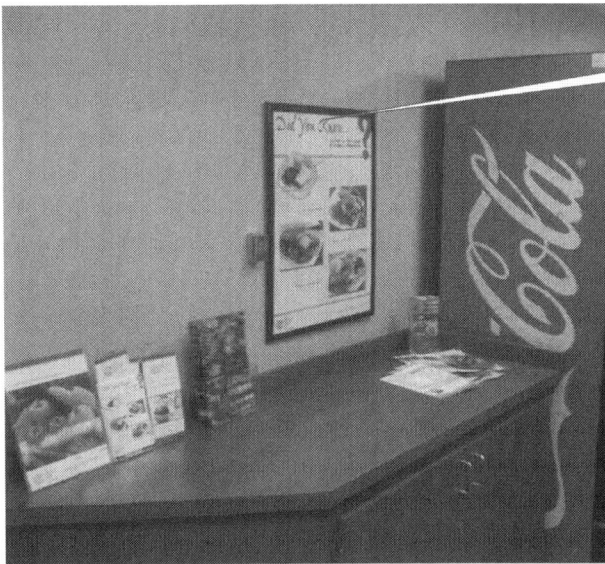

Posters advocating vegetables

Sugar, water, artificial colors and flavors, high-fructose corn syrup

All foods are fried in (wheat-egg-milk) batter; vegetables are steamed into tasteless mush.

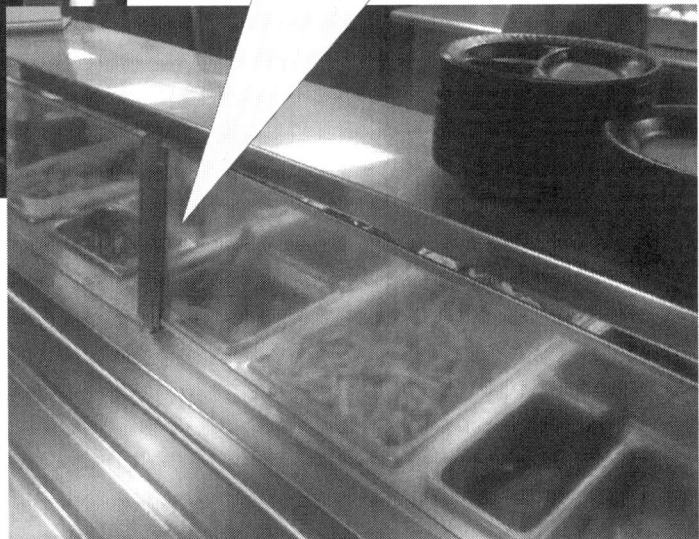

Products being sold here are: 1) Fried foods, simple carbohydrates, fructose, mercury, common antigens, advanced glycation end products (AGEs), and 2) confusion, contradiction, hypocrisy—let's be honest (about dishonesty).

Hospital Food in South America (Bogota, Colombia)

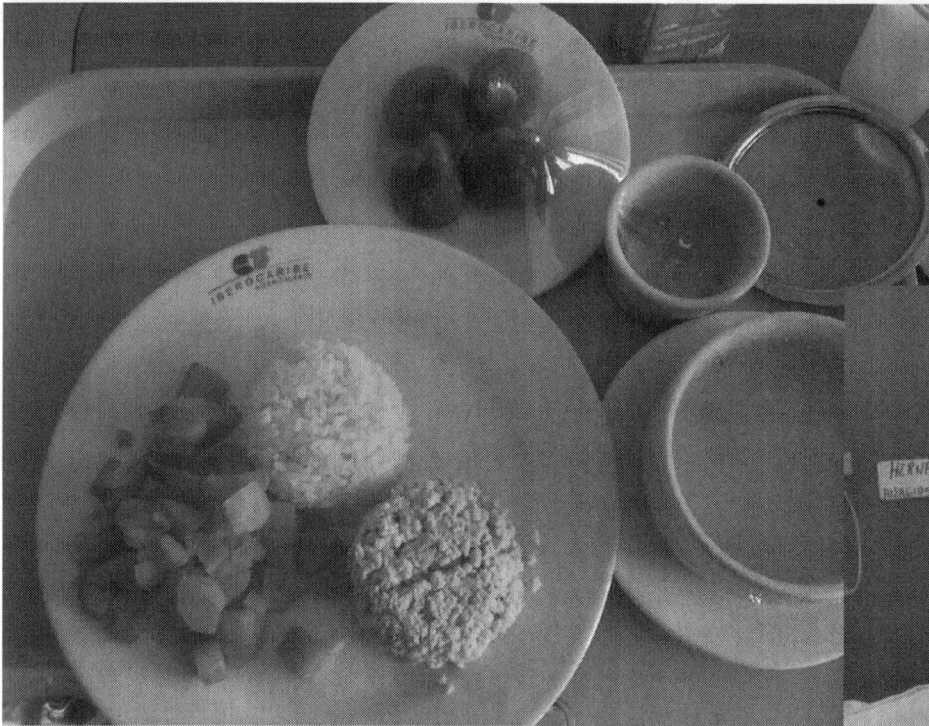

Thus, the chief products being sold here are: 1) low-antigen protein, carbs, phytonutrients, fiber, accessory nutrients, and 2) integrity, consistency—honesty

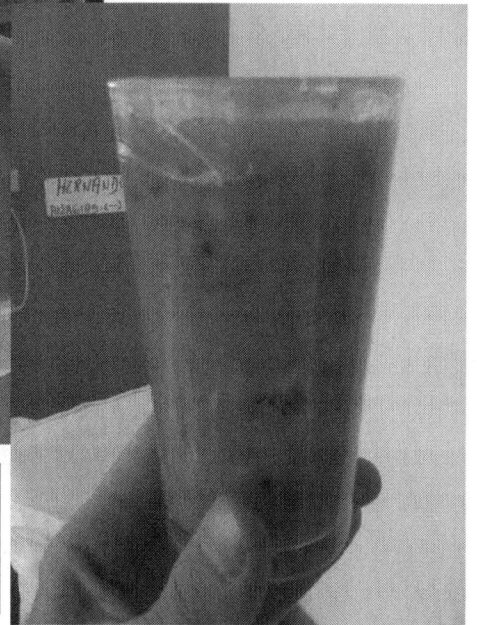

Evidence-Based Healthcare: Balancing Details & Practicality

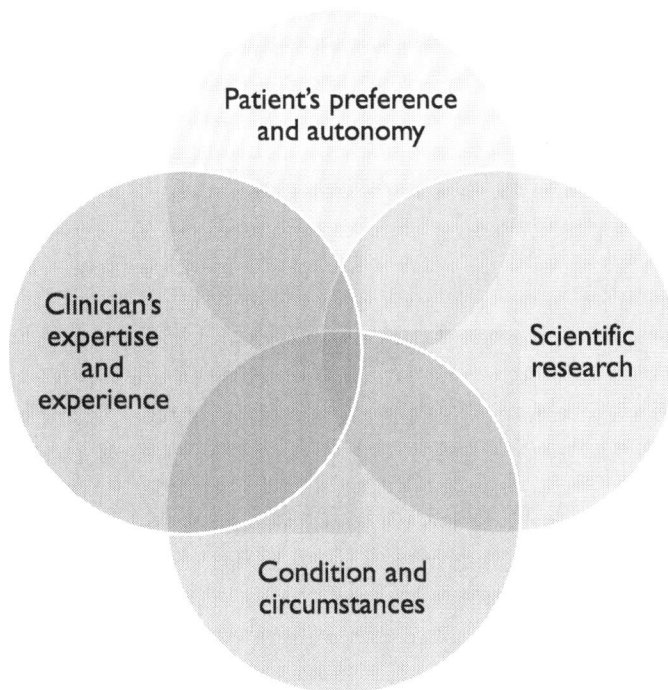

Patient's preference
and autonomy

Clinician's
expertise
and
experience

Scientific
research

Condition and
circumstances

Geyman. *J Am Board Fam Pract.* 1998 Jan
Haynes, Devereaux, Guyatt. *Evid Based Med* 2002;7

▶ This presentation will attempt to blend each of the 4 main components of evidence-based healthcare into a **rational system of clinical intervention.**

▷ Too much focus on molecules and research = not enough practical application to help patients.

▷ Too much focus on practical applications = failure to understand the scientific basis of treatments and the underlying rationale.

▷ Too much reliance on published research = failure to make progress in the present moment.

What we must learn *here* <u>today</u> in order to manage chronic inflammatory disorders:

WEB-LIKE INTERCONNECTIONS OF PHYSIOLOGICAL FACTORS

Alex Vasquez, DC, ND

Editor's Note: This article is reprinted with permission from The Textbook of Functional Medicine (copyright © 2005 Institute for Functional Medicine; all rights reserved). The following is the second portion of the textbook's Chapter 10, "Web-like Interconnections: The Complex Human Organism." The first half of Chapter 10 ran in IMCJ's last issue of February-March 2006, p. 40-42. For more information or to purchase the textbook, contact The Institute for Functional Medicine, PO Box 1697, Gig Harbor, WA 98335; 1-800-228-0622; or visit its website, www.functionalmedicine.org.

Introduction

Understanding the scientific basis and clinical applications of functional medicine and a "whole patient" approach to health care requires that clinicians fully appreciate the interconnectedness of organ system function with biochemical and physiological processes. Simplistic models of health and disease developed decades ago may no longer be accurate or clinically useful insofar as they fail to reflect the more recently discovered complex and multifaceted interrelationships. (Figure 10.2 uses the functional medicine matrix to depict some of this complexity.) Numerous mechanisms mediate these interrelationships, including, but not limited to, those that can be described as biochemical, hormonal, neurological, immunological, piezoelectric, and physical or mechanical. Ultimately, we are forced to dissolve the artificial intellectual boundaries we have created between organ systems and expand our appreciation of individual molecules, cellular messengers, and the physiologic mechanisms that mediate intercellular communication and coordinate interorgan function.

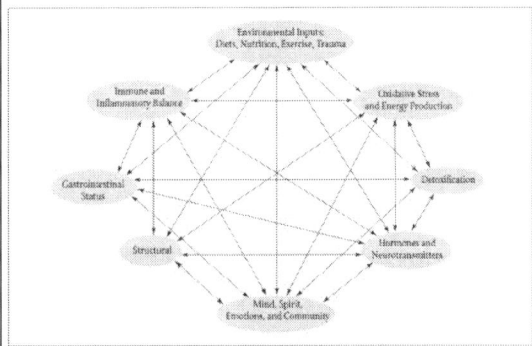

Vasquez. *Integrative Med.* 2006 Apr

1. **<u>Diseases are complex and understandable</u>:** We will look at the components of each disease.

2. **<u>We can understand the complexity of complex diseases, and we can apply scientific methods to patient assessment</u>:** We will focus on *understanding* and *providing effective treatment* based on that understanding.

3. **<u>Symptom-suppressing drugs are NOT the best answer—these patients need a multifaceted approach</u>:** We will review and understand each of the 7 major causes of chronic inflammation and immune dysfunction. For many of you, this will be an entirely new approach; so please be willing to accept new information and apply this to your patient care.

Causes of Inflammation-Immune-Metabolic Imbalance:

1. Food, Diet

2. Infection, Dysbiosis

3. Nutritional Immunomodulation

4. Dysfunctional mitochondria

5. Stress, Emotions, Psychology, Sociology

6. Endocrine, Hormones

7. Xenobiotics, Toxins

Today, we have a massive task in front of us:

▸ Our task is to learn a new approach to clinical diseases.

▸ **This requires much new information to be integrated into a model that we can use clinically with patients.**

▸ This presentation is entirely new. It had to be redesigned from the start in order to accommodate the new information, and the new paradigm.

▸ In order to present this large amount of information in a short amount of time, I have had to be very efficient with references and words; please review this information after the seminar in order to learn it at a deeper level.

Inflammatory disorders can only be understood in their totality

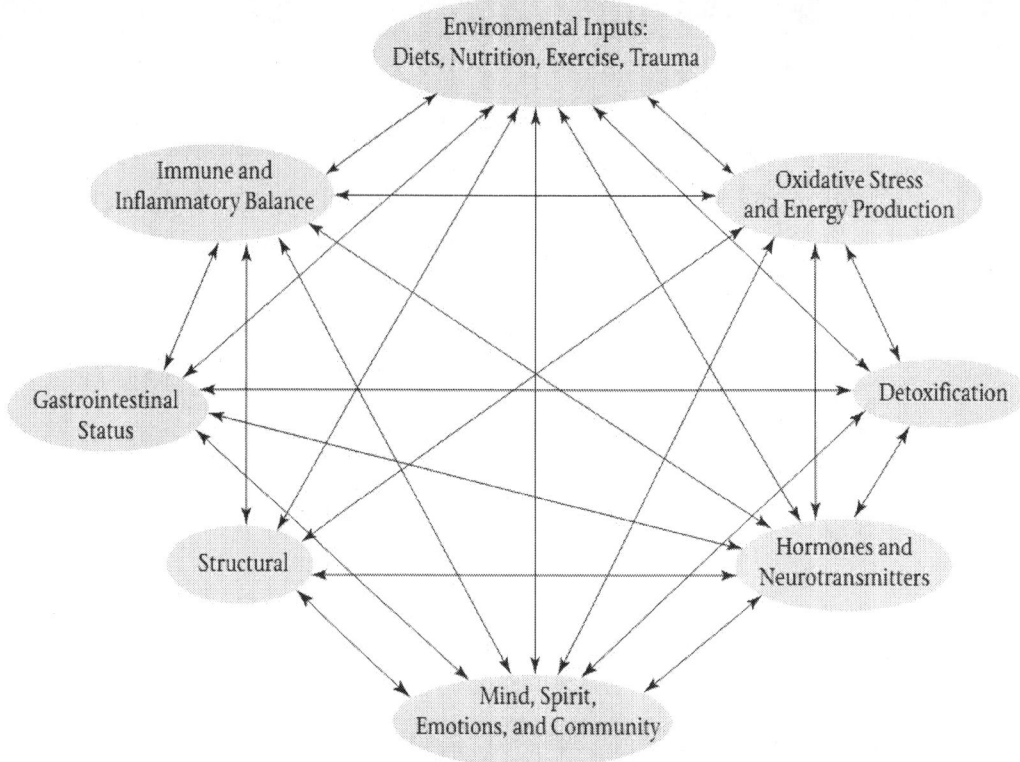

Functional Medicine Matrix illustrated by Alex Vasquez (2003): The "Matrix" provides a illustration of the interdependency of physiologic factors and organ systems; this version was published in <u>Textbook of Functional Medicine</u> and as Vasquez, *Integrative Medicine,* 2006

Protocol applications

This new protocol has a very broad range of clinical applications. This is because it corrects the underlying physiologic imbalances that are the "common themes" that result in clinical dis-orders, such as:

▸ Hypertension, Diabetes mellitus, Metabolic syndrome,

▸ Allergies, asthma, eczema,

▸ Autoimmune disorders including but not limited to rheumatoid arthritis, psoriasis, ankylosing spondylitis, systemic lupus erythematosus,

▸ Depression, attention-deficit hyperactivity,

▸ Alzheimer's disease and Parkinson's disease,

Protocol applications

Always start with good clinical care: *Competent care starts with an open-minded, compassionate, information-seeking excellence-aspiring clinician.*

- Subjective: history of presenting complaints; patient's concerns,

- Objective: physical exam, lab tests: always assess renal function and other basic biochemical parameters; more complex cases require evaluation of more sensitive markers of metabolic and immune imbalance, imaging, biopsy, procedures—as necessary,

- Assessment: reach an **assessment** of the entire constellation of patient's situation; **diagnosis** and appropriate management of each true disease and concern,

- Plan: informed consent (PARBQ): procedures, alternatives, risks, benefits, questions answered; treatments; follow-up, rescheduling, referral, co-management.

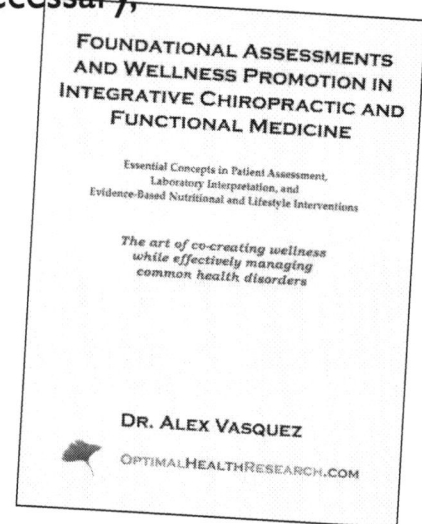

FOUNDATIONAL ASSESSMENTS AND WELLNESS PROMOTION IN INTEGRATIVE CHIROPRACTIC AND FUNCTIONAL MEDICINE

Essential Concepts in Patient Assessment,
Laboratory Interpretation, and
Evidence-Based Nutritional and Lifestyle Interventions

*The art of co-creating wellness
while effectively managing
common health disorders*

DR. ALEX VASQUEZ

OPTIMALHEALTHRESEARCH.COM

What are the common themes among obesity, hypertension, diabetes mellitus, metabolic syndrome, allergy-asthma, and autoimmunity?

0. Genetic predisposition—exploited by drug companies who want to justify patients' endless helplessness and doctors' endless prescriptions
1. Carbohydrate excess, food allergies, nutritional deficiencies and imbalances, positive response to skillful nutritional intervention
2. Microbe-induced inflammation
3. The need to induce anti-inflammatory benefits from T-regulatory cells and less inflammation from Th1, Th2, Th17.
4. Mitochondrial dysfunction
5. Stress, Psychology, Sociology, Lifestyle/exercise/sleep
6. Hormonal imbalances
7. Xenobiotic exposure, toxin accumulation

Main topics for now

▸ **Disorders of Immune Dysfunction:**

  ▸ **Presentations: Chronic Inflammation, Allergy, Autoimmunity**

  ▸ **Standard Medical Evaluations**

  ▸ **Examples of Common Medical Treatments**

▸ Causes of Immune Dysfunction—An Integrated Model:

  ▸ 7 major modifiable components of immune dysfunction will be presented, validated, and discussed with relevance for their clinical evaluations and interventions.

▸ Disorders of Immune Dysfunction—Interventions:

  1. Chronic Inflammation: Cardiovascular Disease, Diabetes Mellitus Type-2, and Other Common Inflammatory Syndromes

  2. Allergy: Asthma, Eczema,

  3. Autoimmunity: Rheumatoid arthritis, Psoriasis, Spondylitis, IBD

Immune Dysfunction: Presentations
1) Chronic Inflammation, Allergy, Autoimmunity

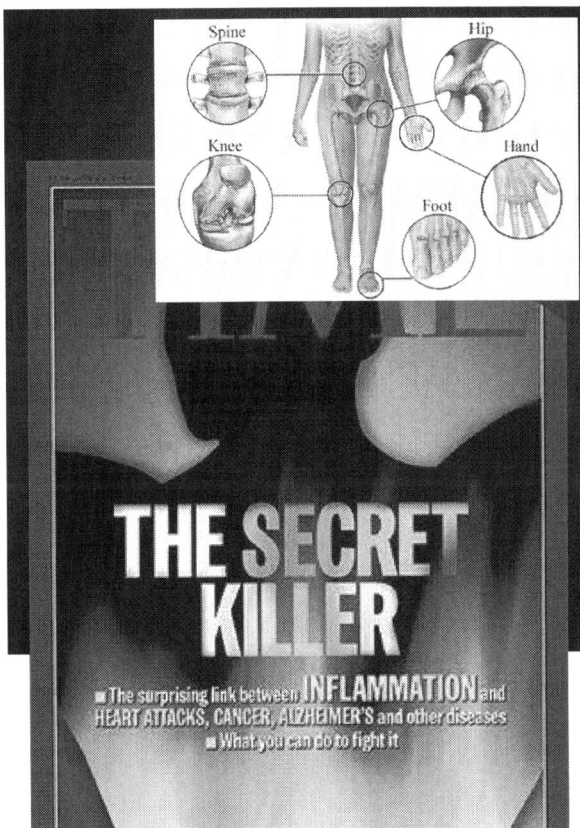

1. Cardiovascular disease,
2. Hypertension,
3. Diabetes Mellitus Type-2,
4. Metabolic Syndrome:
   - Standard medical evaluation: limited physical exam, blood pressure, lipids, glucose, CRP
   - Standard medical treatment: drugs to lower hypertension, lipids, glucose: *"treating the numbers; treat the manifestation of the problem—not the problem"*
   - Comments: fails to address aspects of the disease that can be treated effectively; leaves patients in a downward spiral of poor health.

"ABCD" of hypertension treatment Cornerstones of "medical" management

- **ACEi**: -pril, renoprotective, teratogenic, hyperkalemia risk, angioedema risk due to preserved bradykinin, cough,

- **ARB**: -sartan, angiotensin-2 receptor blocker, renoprotective, hyperkalemia risk, no cough or vasodilation due to bradykinin, losartan is uricousuric,

- **Alpha-2 agonist**: (clonopin) tricks the CNS into thinking it is in a hypercatecholamine state so that SNS output is reduced; used for acute/severe HTN,

- **Alpha-1 blocker**: -osin, high risk of syncope, also treates BPH, (eg, prazosin)

- **Beta-blocker**: aten**olol** and labet**olol** are the prototypes; also used for some migraines and anxiety; avoid abrupt discontinuation.

- **Calcium-channel blocker**: dihydropyridine class are peripheral vasodilators; many nutritional nondrug means exist for modulating intracellular calcium.

- **Diuretics**: **thiazide** diuretics are first-line outpt tx even though they worsen DM2-MetSyn and promote mineral depletion; Lasix isn't really used for chronic HTN except with fluid overload.

- **Direct vasodilators**: Hydralazine IV is commonly used in acute settings and is safe for PG pts. Other drugs in class: nitroprusside,

While effective at lowering blood pressure numbers, none of these drugs provides hope of actually curing the disease "primary hypertension" by addressing the underlying problems.

DM2-MetSyn: Drug Treatments Cornerstones of "medical" management

1. **Metformin**: Promoted as initial pharmacologic management due to benefits (reduction of HgbA1c by 2% max; reduction in mortality) and safety (less hypoglycemia); reduces hepatic gluconeogenesis and increases peripheral insulin sensitivity. *Causes B-12 deficiency, often misdiagnosed and mistreated as diabetic neuropathy, also depression, fatigue.*

2. **Sulfonylurea drugs—glyburide, glipizide, glimepiride**: Stimulate pancreatic insulin production and improve peripheral insulin sensitivity. These drugs increase morbidity and mortality in diabetic patients in a dose-response relationship despite reductions in glucose; they also increase death post angioplasty for MI. *CMAJ—Canadian Med Association Journal* 2006 Jan; *J Am Coll Cardiol.* 1999 Jan

3. **Thiazolidinedione drugs—pioglitazone and rosiglitazone**: Improve peripheral insulin sensitivity; reduction of HgbA1c by 1.5% max

4. **Dipeptidyl peptidase 4 (DPP-4) inhibitors**: sitagliptin/Januvia; reduce glucagon and thereby increases insulin secretion, slows gastric emptying.

5. **Insulin**: Basal/bolus insulin lowers glucose; some evidence shows that insulin directly promotes atherogenesis; possible "anti-inflammatory" effects of insulin are difficult to distinguish from glucose-lowering effects, since hyperglycemia is directly pro-inflammatory. Insulin promotes macrophage foam cell formation. *Lab Invest.* 2012 Apr

6. **Essentially all DM2 patients will also get a "statin" and an ACEi**

   While effective at lowering blood glucose numbers, none of these drugs provides hope of actually curing the disease by addressing the underlying problem(s).

45. **Which of the following drugs used to treat diabetes mellitus type-2 provides patients an opportunity for authentic cure of their disease:**
    A. Metformin
    B. Sulfonylureas
    C. TZD drugs
    D. Insulin
    E. None of the above.

UWS Pharmacology • Spring 2012 • Dr Alex Vasquez • Midterm exam page 9

1. <u>Asthma</u>:
2. <u>Allergic rhinitis/conjunctivitis</u>:
3. <u>Eczema, atopic dermatitis</u>:
   ▹ <u>Standard medical evaluation</u>: limited physical exam, blood oxygen, spirometry; maybe allergy tests via skin or blood.
   ▹ <u>Standard medical treatment</u>: antihistamines, bronchodilators (beta-agonists), steroids/prednisone, leukotriene blockers (montelukast/zafirlukast), anticholinergics (ipratropium), **"immunoparalytic agents" (AV)**: cyclosporin/ciclosporin and tacrolimus block intracellular signaling, (hydroxychloroquine impairs lysosomes and TLR9, cholchicine blocks microtubules and migration as a "mitotic poison")... Drug/suppress the manifestations of immune dysfunction, but never address the problem directly.
   ▹ <u>Comments</u>:, standard medical management of allergy fails to address the underlying causes of immune dysfunction, thereby leaving patients dependent on medications, many of which have high costs and serious adverse effects.

Immune Dysfunction: Presentations
Chronic Inflammation, Allergy, 3) Autoimmunity

"<u>Autoimmune diseases are the third leading cause </u>of morbidity and mortality in the industrialized world, <u>surpassed only by cancer and heart disease.</u>"

Ann Rheum Dis. 2007 Sep

Immune Dysfunction: Presentations
Chronic Inflammation, Allergy, 3) Autoimmunity

1. <u>Rheumatoid arthritis (RA)</u>: "idiopathic"

2. <u>Psoriasis</u>: "idiopathic"

3. <u>Other autoimmune syndromes</u>:

   ▸ <u>Standard medical evaluation</u>: clinical evaluation with serum testing for RF, CCP, ESR/CRP, ANA and other routine tests to determine the type—*not the causes*—of the immune dysfunction.

   ▸ <u>Standard medical treatment</u>: NSAIDs, prednisone, methotrexate, sulfasalazine, hydroxychloroquine, "biologics", stem cell transplant; bowel removal for IBD.

   ▸ <u>Comments</u>: None of these drugs addresses the underlying problems—immune activation, inflammation dysregulation.

Drug/medical management of musculoskeletal pain and inflammation: sequence of medicalization

1. ASA, NSAIDs, and APAP,
2. Prednisone
3. Methotrexate
4. Sulfasalazine
5. Hydroxychloroquine
6. "Biologics"—TNFa inhibitors
7. Stem cell transplant

None of the drugs 'traditionally' used against autoimmune diseases provides any hope of actually curing the disease(s).

None of these drugs (perhaps except sulfasalazine) addresses the underlying causative factors that trigger and perpetuate chronic inflammation and autoimmunity.

Prince *et al. Arthritis Research & Therapy* 2012, **14**:R68
http://arthritis-research.com/content/14/2/R68

arthritis
research&therapy

RESEARCH ARTICLE

Sustained rheumatoid arthritis remission is uncommon in clinical practice

Femke HM Prince[*], Vivian P Bykerk, Nancy A Shadick, Bing Lu, Jing Cui, Michelle Frits, Christine K Iannaccone, Michael E Weinblatt and Daniel H Solomon

Abstract

Introduction: Remission is an important goal of therapy in rheumatoid arthritis (RA), but data on duration of remission are lacking. Our objective was to describe the duration of remission in RA, assessed by different criteria.

Methods: We evaluated patients from the Brigham and Women's Rheumatoid Arthritis Sequential Study (BRASS) not in remission at baseline with at least 2 years of follow-up. Remission was assessed according to the Disease Activity Score 28-C-reactive protein (DAS28-CRP4), Simplified Disease Activity Index (SDAI), and Clinical Disease Activity Index (CDAI) scores, and the recently proposed American College of Rheumatology (ACR)/European League against Rheumatism (EULAR) criteria for remission. Analyses were performed by using Kaplan-Meier survival curves.

Results: We identified 871 subjects with ≥2 years of follow-up. Of these subjects, 394 were in remission at one or more time-points and not in remission at baseline, according to at least one of the following criteria: DAS28-CRP < 2.6 (n = 309), DAS28-CRP < 2.3 (n = 275), SDAI (n = 168), CDAI (n = 170), and 2010 ACR/EULAR (n = 158). The median age for the 394 subjects at entrance to BRASS was 56 years; median disease duration was 8 years; 81% were female patients; and 72% were seropositive. Survival analysis performed separately for each remission criterion demonstrated that < 50% of subjects remained in remission 1 year later. Median remission survival time was 1 year. Kaplan-Meier curves of the various remission criteria did not significantly differ (P = 0.29 according to the log-rank test).

Conclusions: This study shows that in clinical practice, a minority of RA patients are in sustained remission.

Medical schools teach students and doctors that 1) most diseases are complex and "idiopathic", and 2) drugs are the answer.

Analysis of questions asked by family doctors regarding patient care

"three most common [question taxonomies]"

1. "What is the cause of symptom X?"
2. "What is the dose of drug X?"
3. "How should I manage disease or finding X?"

"Answers to most questions (702, 64%) were not immediately pursued, but, of those pursued, most (318, 80%) were answered. Doctors spent an average of less than 2 minutes pursuing an answer, and they used readily available print and human resources. Only two questions led to a formal literature search." Ely et al. *BMJ*. 1999 Aug

What we learn in medical school:

1. Nearly all diseases are complex and idiopathic—some mixture of genetics and "unknown environmental factors."

2. We can apply scientific methods to patient assessment and treatment…but this will almost always result in the use of drugs and/or surgery/procedures.

3. Symptom-suppressing with pharmacologic monotherapy ("silver bullet") or polypharmacy is the goal—not simply the means.

Medical schools teach students and doctors that 1) most diseases are complex and "idiopathic", and 2) drugs are the answer.

Diabetes type-2	Hypertension	Allergy	Pain & Inflammation
1. Metformin	1. ACEi	1. Antihistamines	1. NSAIDs
2. Sulfonylureas	2. ARB	2. Bronchodilators (beta-agonists)	2. Prednisone/steroids
3. TZDs	3. Alpha-2 agonist	3. Steroids	3. Methotrexate
4. Dipeptidyl peptidase (DPP) 4 inhibitors	4. Alpha-1 blocker	4. Leukotriene blockers	4. Sulfasalazine
5. Insulin	5. Beta-blocker	5. Anticholinergics (ipratropium)	5. Hydroxychloroquine
6. Statin	6. Calcium-channel blocker	6. "immunoparalytic agents" (AV): ciclosporin, tacrolimus, hydroxychloroquine, cholchicine "mitotic poison"	6. "Biologics"—notice the misuse of language in labeling these drugs*
7. ACEi	**7. Diuretics**		7. Opioids
	8. Vasodilators		8. "Antidepressants" and antiseizure drugs
			9. Anti-neuropathic drugs for GABA receptors

Cornerstones of "medical" management

*Marketing antiTNF drugs as "biologics" was brilliant for promoting sales because doing so gives the impression that these drugs are "logical for life" despite the major risks for cancer, infection, and bankruptcy for the patients taking these drugs.

Give them (more) drugs

America, the medicated

We buy more medicine than any other country, a trend that threatens our health and wealth

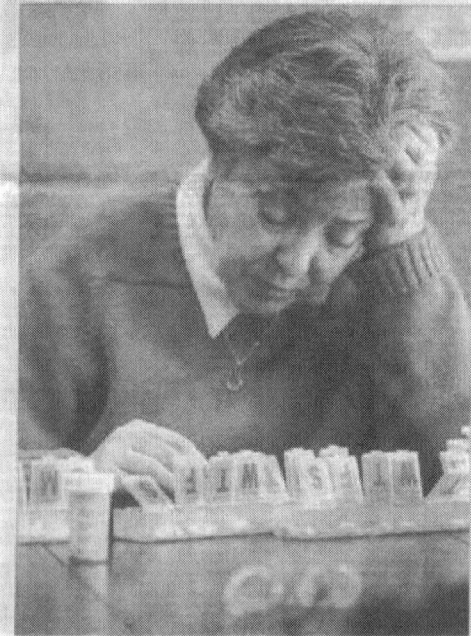

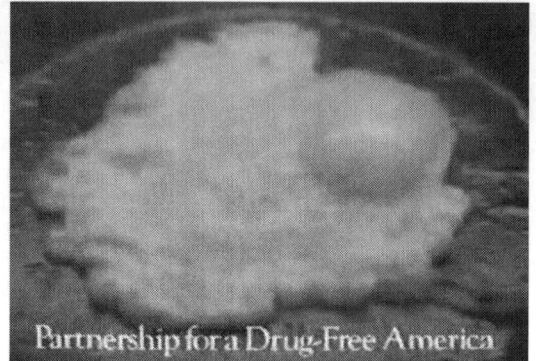

Partnership for a Drug-Free America

Americans are the most drugged society in human existence: This is accepted and considered OK as long as the drugs come from corporations. "Natural" treatments from nature are generally viewed by the allopathic medical profession as suspect ("alternative" and "unproven"), illegal (cannabis: analgesic, anxiolytic, antinausea) if not evil.

▶ "Recent estimates suggest that each year more than 1 million patients are injured while in the hospital and approximately 180,000 die because of these injuries. Furthermore, drug-related morbidity and mortality are common and are estimated to cost more than $136 billion a year." Holland, Degruy. Am Fam Physician. 1997 Nov

We can—*must*—address the causes of immune dysfunction and inflammatory imbalance:

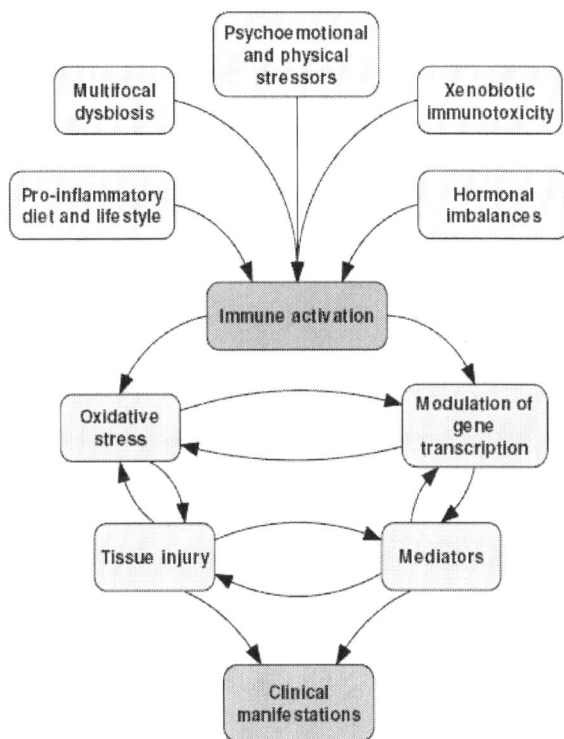

Vasquez A. *Integrative Rheumatology. Second Edition.*

What we will review today:

1. **Diseases are complex and understandable:**

2. **We can apply scientific methods to patient assessment and treatment (even if this means NOT relying on drugs) to correct the underlying imbalances that cause the disease and its manifestations.**

3. **Symptom-suppressing drugs are NOT the best answer— these patients need a multifaceted approach:**

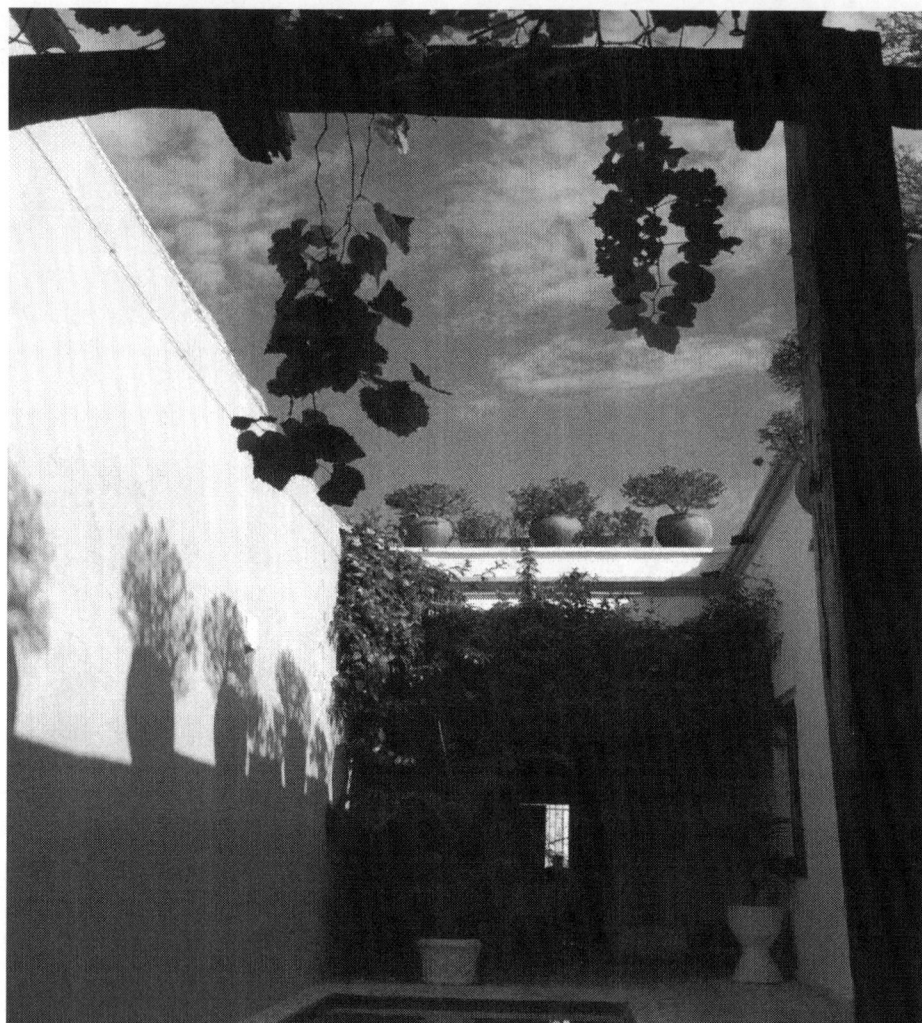

Time for a brief rest:
Santa Marta, Colombia
2012

Dysregulated Inflammation and Immune Activation *as the Cause of* Inflammation, Allergy, and Autoimmunity:
Nutritional & Functional Medicine Approaches

▸ **Part 1**: Introduction
The Seven Most Important Mechanisms/Triggers for Chronic Inflammation & Immune Dysfunction

▸ **Alex Vasquez, D.C., N.D., D.O.**

Immune Dysfunction: 7 Main Modifiable Factors

- **Non-modifiable mechanisms:**
  - ▸ "Genes" in the form of DNA

> Note that the standard medical evaluation fails to consider these important modifiable components.

- **Modifiable mechanisms:**
  1. **Diet**: Pro-inflammatory *versus* anti-inflammatory diets,
  2. **Dysbiosis**: Multifocal polydysbiosis,
  3. **Nutritional immunomodulation**: Therapeutic modulation of immunocyte phenotype via epigenetic mechanisms,
  4. **Mitochondrial dysfunction**: Proinflammatory effects of dysfunctional mitochondria,
  5. **Psychoneuroimmunology**: Stress, paradigms and immune disorders,
  6. **Hormonal imbalance**: Dysendocrinology, orthoendocrinology,
  7. **Xenobiotic immunotoxicity**: Chemical and toxic metal exposures.

Immune Dysfunction: Mechanisms

▸ *How can we remember all of that?*

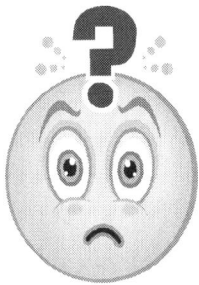

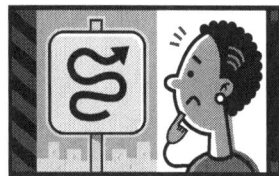

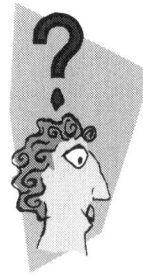

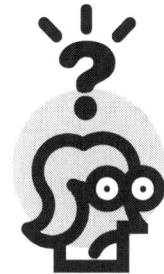

▸ I have a simple memory aid for you!

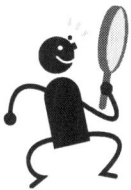

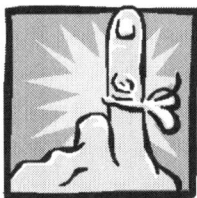

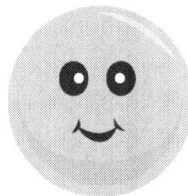

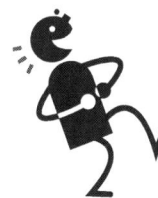

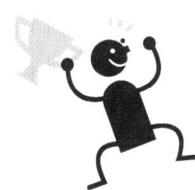

Nutrition & FxMed for chronic immune-inflammatory disorders

Causes of Inflammation-Immune-Metabolic Imbalance:

1. Food, Diet

2. Infection, Dysbiosis

3. Nutritional Immunomodulation

4. Dysfunctional mitochondria

5. Stress, Emotions, Psychology, Sociology

6. Endocrine, Hormones

7. Xenobiotics, Toxins

<u>Let's memorize these</u>
1. Food
2. Infection
3. Nutrition
4. Dysfunctional mitochondria
5. Stress
6. Endocrine
7. Xenobiotics

Nutrition & FxMed for chronic immune-inflammatory disorders

Causes of Inflammation-
Immune-Metabolic
Imbalan

1. Foo

2. Infe

3. Nu
   Imr

4. Dy
   mit

5. Str
   Psychology, Sociology,
   Lifestyle

6. Endocrine
   Hormone

7. Xenobiotics, Toxins

Let's memorize these
1. Food and Lifestyle
2. Infection
3. Nutrition
4. Dysfunctional mitochondria
5. Stress, pSychology, Lifestyle
6. Endocrine
7. Xenobiotics/Toxins

These are the 7 main modifiable factors in the cause and control of chronic inflammatory disorders.

(Each of these could take 2 hours [2 days] to explore.)

Notice that these 7 factors can be remembered by the acronym:

F.I.N.D. S.E.Xenobiotics or F.I.N.D. S.E.Toxins

Nutrition & FxMed for chronic immune-inflammatory disorders

Causes of Inflammation-Immune-Metabolic Imbalance:

1. Food, Lifestyle

2. Infection, Dysbiosis

3. Nutritional Immunomodulation

4. Dysfunctional mitochondria

5. Stress, Emotions, Psychology, Sociology, Lifestyle

6. Endocrine, Hormones

7. Xenobiotics, Toxins

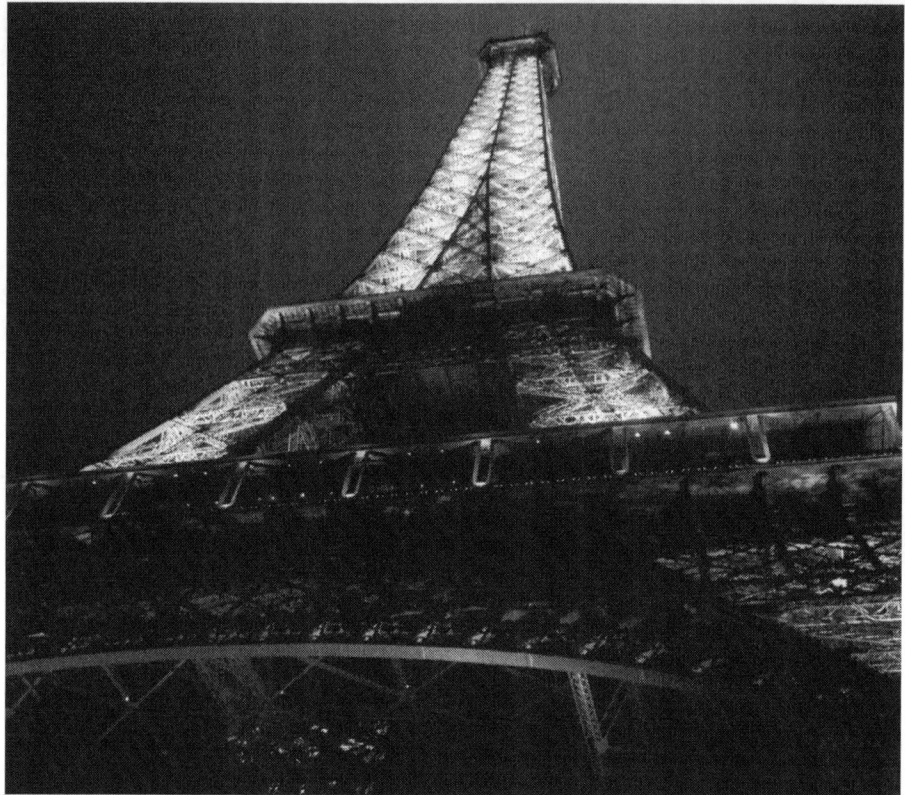

Notice that these 7 factors can be remembered by the acronym: **F.I.N.D. S.E.X.**
♥ First presented in Paris in 2012 ♥

Clinical protocol

▸ **Subjective**—patient's concerns and complaints

▸ **Objective**—clinical findings

▸ **Assessment**—diagnoses

▸ **Plan**—treatments, tests, referral, follow-up

1. Food and lifestyle
2. Infection and dysbiosis
3. Nutritional immunomodulation
4. Dysfunctional mitochondria
5. Stress, Sociology-psychology, Lifestyle
6. Endocrine/hormones
7. Toxins/Xenobiotics

Nutrition & FxMed for chronic immune-inflammatory disorders

1. Food & lifestyle

2. Infection, Dysbiosis

3. Nutritional Immunomodulation

4. Dysfunctional mitochondria

5. Stress, Psychology, Sociology, Lifestyle

6. Endocrine, Hormones

7. Xenobiotics, Toxins

Format of the slides

▸ Most slides have an index or "table of contents" (*table of progress*) in the side panel.

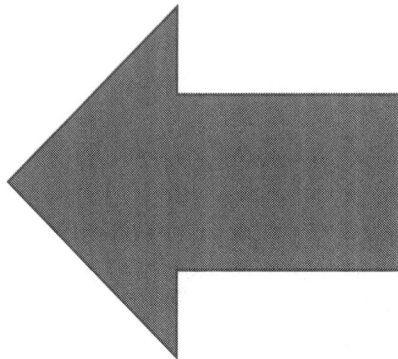

Causes of Inflammation-Immune-Metabolic Imbalance:

1. Food, Diet

2. Infection, Dysbiosis

3. Nutritional Immunomodulation

4. Dysfunctional mitochondria

5. Stress, Emotions, Psychology, Sociology

6. Endocrine, Hormones

7. Xenobiotics, Toxins

← **Common to each problem**: What we are going to notice is that every clinical disorder characterized by chronic inflammation, allergy, and/or autoimmunity has treatable contributors within each of these 7 categories.

▸ **Why isn't genetics specifically mentioned?** Because we are focusing on areas where we can take *action*. Although we cannot change the DNA, we *can* change genetic expression, transcription factors, and epigenetic mechanisms such as DNA methylation and histone methylation and acetylation.

▸ **Oxidative stress and free radicals are important; why aren't these specifically mentioned?** Oxidative balance is an epiphenomenon related to other factors such as dietary intake, nutritional supplementation, mitochondrial function, infections, and toxin exposure.

▸ We will briefly detail each of these 7 mechanisms now, then apply additional details to each inflammation-immune problem discussed.

Food, Diet

1. Food-induced inflammation

2. Oxidative stress

3. Immune suppression

4. Phytonutrient deficiency

5. Sugar/insulin excess

6. GI dysbiosis & the need for probiotics

7. Deficiencies of vitamins, minerals, ALA, GLA, EPA, DHA

8. Allergens

Important concepts:

▸ Diet (food intake) affects immune function and inflammatory balance in ways that are clinically and pathologically significant.

▸ Most patients should consume an Anti-Inflammatory Diet (AID) best described as the "5-Part Supplemented Paleo-Mediterranean Diet" (5-SPMD)

Clinical assessments:

▸ Impaired renal function predisposes to hyperkalemia; this diet is high in potassium.

Therapeutic implementation:

▸ The Supplemented Paleo-Mediterranean Diet. *Nutritional Perspectives* 2011 January

http://optimalhealthresearch.com/reprints/series/vasquez_2011_five-part_protocol_revisited.pdf

The Solution: 5-Part Nutrition Protocol

1. **Paleo-Mediterranean Diet**: fruits, vegetables, nuts, seeds, berries, high-quality protein; allergy avoidance.

2. **Multivitamin/multimineral**: high potency broad-spectrum

3. **Vitamin D3**: 2,000 – **4,000** – 10,000 IU/d to optimize serum levels

4. **Combination fatty acid supplementation**: ALA, GLA, EPA, DHA, Oleic acid

5. **Probiotics**: especially with allergies, IBS, and/or antibiotics

Vasquez A. Five-Part Nutritional Wellness Protocol That Produces Consistently Positive Results. *Nutritional Wellness* 2005 Sept
http://optimalhealthresearch.com/protocol.html

Revisiting the Five-Part Nutritional Wellness Protocol: The Supplemented Paleo-Mediterranean Diet

Alex Vasquez, DC, ND, DO

ABSTRACT: This article reviews the five-part nutritional protocol that incorporates a health-promoting nutrient-dense diet and essential supplementation with vitamins/minerals, specific fatty acids, probiotics, and physiologic doses of vitamin D3. This foundational nutritional protocol has proven benefits for disease treatment, disease prevention, and health maintenance and restoration. Additional treatments such as botanical medicines, additional nutritional supplements, and pharmaceutical drugs can be used atop this foundational protocol to further optimize clinical effectiveness. The rationale for this five-part protocol is presented, and consideration is given to adding iodine-iodide as the sixth component of the protocol.

INTRODUCTION:

In 2004 and 2005 I first published a "five-part nutrition protocol"[1, 2] that provides the foundational treatment plan for a wide range of health disorders. This protocol served and continues to serve as the foundation upon which other treatments are commonly added, and without which those other treatments are likely to fail, or attain suboptimal results at best.[3] Now as then, I will share with you what I consider a basic foundational protocol for wellness promotion and disease treatment. I have used this protocol in my own self-care for many years and have used it in the treatment of a wide range of health-disease conditions in clinical practice.

REVIEW:

This nutritional protocol is validated by biochemistry, physiology, experimental research, peer-reviewed human trials, and the clinical application of common sense. It is the most nutrient-dense diet available, satisfying nutritional needs and thereby optimizing metabolic processes while promoting satiety and weight loss/optimization. Nutrients are required in the proper amounts, forms, and approximate ratios for critical and innumerable physiologic functions; if nutrients are lacking, the body cannot function *normally*, let alone *optimally*. Impaired function results in subjective and objective manifestations of what is eventually labeled as "disease." Thus, a powerful and effective alternative to treating diseases with drugs is to re-establish normal/optimal physiologic function by replenishing the body with essential ("orthoend... ... ... ronmental toxins, and by reestablishing the optimal miccobial milieu, especially the eradication of (multifocal)

term management their problems, all clinicians should agree that everyone needs a foundational nutrition plan because nutrients—not drugs—are universally required for life and health. This five-part nutrition protocol is briefly outlined below; a much more detailed substantiation of the underlying science and clinical application of this protocol was recently published in a review of more than 650 pages and approximately 3,500 citations.[5]

1. Health-promoting Paleo-Mediterranean diet: Following an extensive review of the research literature, I developed what I call the "supplemented Paleo-Mediterranean diet." In essence, this diet plan combines the best of the Mediterranean diet with the best of the Paleolithic diet, the latter of which has been best distilled by Dr. Loren Cordain in his book "The Paleo Diet"[6] and his numerous scientific articles.[7, 8, 9] The Paleolithic diet is superior to the Mediterranean diet in nutrient density for promoting satiety, weight loss, and improvements/normalization in overall metabolic function.[10, 11] This diet places emphasis on fruits, vegetables, nuts, seeds, and berries that meet the body's needs for fiber, carbohydrates, and most importantly, the 8,000+ phytonutrients that have additive and synergistic health effects[12]—including immunomodulating, antioxidant, anti-inflammatory, and anti-cancer benefits. High-quality protein sources such as fish, poultry, eggs, and grass-fed meats are emphasized. Slightly modifying Cor... ... ...whey ...n and ...ood-enhancing (due to the high tryptophan content)

The Pro-inflammatory Lifestyle (most people)

1. **High-sugar foods**: Immunosuppression + oxidative stress for 4 hours
2. **High-fat foods**: Especially arachidonic acid, linoleic acid, and saturated fats
3. **Fatty acid imbalances**: Insufficiencies of ALA, EPA, DHA, GLA, with excesses of saturated fat, arachidonate, linoleic acid, and trans-fats
4. **Vitamin and mineral deficiencies**, especially magnesium and vitamin D.
5. **Allergens**: molecular mimicry, immune-complexes,
6. **Insufficient phytonutrients**: Anti-inflammatory benefits, antioxidants, fiber, nutrigenomic benefits (e.g., salicylate, phytate)
7. **Insufficiency of fiber**: Fiber is "decoy" for bacterial adhesion; lack of fiber = constipation and increased intraluminal pressure; reduced mucosal repair = increased bacterial translocation
8. **Foods that promote bacterial overgrowth of the small bowel**: Sucrose, wheat, potatoes, lactose/dairy
9. **Dysbiosis**: GI is most appreciated, but sinorespiratory and GU are problems
10. **Insufficient exercise**: 1) Adipose is pro-inflammatory and pro-estrogenic, 2) exercising muscle reduces inflammation (myokines) and 3) improves insulin sensitivity for a secondary anti-inflammatory benefit
11. **Xenobiotic/toxin accumulation**: Underdiagnosed pandemic
12. **Emotional stress and toxic relationships**: Promote inflammation, impair wound healing, and promote mucosal immunosuppression which facilitates dysbiosis

Western lifestyle = inflammation

Disease-promoting:

- Physical inactivity and sedentary lifestyle
- Insufficient sleep
- Obesity
- Frequent exposure to chemicals, drugs, pollution, exhaust, tobacco smoke
- Daily consumption of processed and artificial foods
- Insufficient (common) or excessive (rare) protein
- Diet high in simple carbohydrates and sugars
- Use of disease-promoting beverages such as cola, artificially colored/flavored/sweetened drinks, and hard liquor
- Increased intake of linoleic acid (vegetable oils) and arachidonic acid (beef, liver, pork, lamb and most farm-raised land animals)
- Low intake of vitamins and minerals
- Excess iron and insufficient vitamin D
- Dysbiosis: intestinal overgrowth of yeast, parasites, and harmful bacteria
- Use of synthetic chemical drugs to suppress symptoms of poor health
- Reactive healthcare that only responds to problems after they have developed
- Dysfunctional relationships that enable and foster illness, dependency and isolation
- Work environments that promote isolation, pressure, perfectionism and which disapprove of creativity, personal time, and flexibility

Health-promoting:

- Frequent exercise and physical activity
- Plenty of sleep
- Maintaining ideal body weight
- Avoiding exposure to chemicals, drugs, pollution, exhaust, tobacco smoke
- Daily consumption of fruits and vegetables
- Ideal protein intake for body size, physical activity, and health status
- Diet high in fiber and complex carbohydrates
- Use of health-promoting beverages such as green tea, fruit/vegetable juices, water, and light consumption of beer or red wine
- Increased intake of ALA, EPA, DHA, GLA, and oleic acid
- Multi-vitamin and multi-mineral supplementation
- Optimal vitamin D and iron status
- Beneficial gastrointestinal flora
- Natural and phytonutraceutical interventions to promote optimal health
- Pro-active healthcare
- Healthy and supportive relationships that foster responsibility, independence, interdependence, health and feelings of being wanted and cared for
- Work environments that promote collaboration and creativity and which appreciate personal time and allow for schedule flexibility

Wellness lifestyle = anti-inflammation

Copyright: Vasquez A. Integrative Rheumatology and Integrative Orthopedics. www.OptimalHealthResearch.com

Food, Diet

1. Food-induced inflammation

2. Oxidative stress

3. Immune suppression

4. Phytonutrient deficiency

5. Sugar/insulin excess

6. GI dysbiosis & the need for probiotics

7. Deficiencies of vitamins, minerals, ALA, GLA, EPA, DHA

8. Allergens

Important concepts:

▸ Diet (food intake) affects immune function and inflammatory balance in ways that are clinically and pathologically significant.

▸ Most patients should consume an Anti-Inflammatory Diet (AID) best described as the "5-Part Supplemented Paleo-Mediterranean Diet" (5-SPMD)

Clinical assessments:

▸ Impaired renal function predisposes to hyperkalemia; this diet is high in potassium.

Therapeutic implementation:

▸ The Supplemented Paleo-Mediterranean Diet. *Nutritional Perspectives* 2011 January

http://optimalhealthresearch.com/reprints/series/vasquez_2011_five-part_protocol_revisited.pdf

Unhealthy food fuels inflammation

THE DIET-INDUCED PROINFLAMMATORY STATE: A CAUSE OF CHRONIC PAIN AND OTHER DEGENERATIVE DISEASES?

David R. Seaman, DC[a]

Results: The typical American diet is deficient in fruits and vegetables and contains excessive amounts of meat, refined grain products, and dessert foods. Such a diet can have numerous adverse biochemical effects, all of which create a proinflammatory state and predispose the body to degenerative diseases. It appears that an inadequate intake of fruits and vegetables can result in a suboptimal intake of antioxidants and phytochemicals and an imbalanced intake of essential fatty acids. Through different mechanisms, each nutritional alteration can promote inflammation and disease.

Conclusion: We can no longer view different diseases as distinct biochemical entities. Nearly all degenerative diseases have the same underlying biochemical etiology, that is, a diet-induced proinflammatory state. Although specific diseases may require specific treatments, such as adjustments for hypomobile joints, β-blockers for hypertension, and chemotherapy for cancer, the treatment program must also include nutritional protocols to reduce the proinflammatory state. (J Manipulative Physiol Ther 2002; 25:168-79)

Food, Diet

1. Food-induced inflammation

2. Oxidative stress

3. Immune suppression

4. Phytonutrient deficiency

5. Sugar/insulin excess

6. GI dysbiosis & the need for probiotics

7. Deficiencies of vitamins, minerals, ALA, GLA, EPA, DHA

8. Allergens

"Unhealthy diet" = proinflammatory diet

1. <u>Grains, especially wheat</u>: wheat is highly allergenic and contains subfractions that have direct pro-inflammatory effects; baked wheat contains pro-inflammatory glycosylated amino acids via the "Maillard reaction"; grains in general and wheat in particular are difficult to digest and thereby provide fermentable carbohydrate to intestinal bacteria, promoting bacterial overgrowth of the small intestines which is pro-inflammatory.

2. <u>Simple carbohydrates</u>: Simple sugars cause 2-4 hours of increased inflammation coupled with immune suppression.

3. <u>Lack of fruits, vegetables, nuts, seeds, berries = lack of fiber and phytonutrients</u>: causes constipation/toxicity, deficiency of antioxidants and antiinflammatory agents.

4. <u>Insufficient protein</u>: impairs healing and detoxification.

5. <u>Excess n-6 fatty acids</u>: promotes inflammation and cancer.

Healthy diet = anti-inflammatory effects

1. **Composition**: primarily of fruits, vegetables, nuts, seeds, berries, and lean protein.

2. High in phytonutrients: 8,000 compounds that generally have antioxidant and antiinflammatory benefits.

3. Fiber to promote laxation: important to cleanse the bowels to avoid GI dysbiosis and to remove toxins.

4. Low-carbohydrate (CHO) intake: avoids immune suppression and oxidative stress from simple CHO intake; lowers insulin levels and Na retention

5. Nutrient-dense: promotes satiation and supports metabolic needs and physiologic expectations,

6. Promotes alkalinization: potassium citrate promotes optimal urine pH of 7.5 to enhance mineral retention, lower cortisol, eliminate toxins, and increase endorphin analgesia.

7. Sufficient protein and n-3 fatty acids:

8. Physiologic amounts of vitamin D3:

Nutrition & FxMed for chronic immune-inflammatory disorders

Food, Diet

1. Food-induced inflammation

2. Oxidative stress

3. Immune suppression

4. Phytonutrient deficiency

5. Sugar/insulin excess

6. GI dysbiosis & the need for probiotics

7. Deficiencies of vitamins, minerals, ALA, GLA, EPA, DHA

8. Allergens

Dietary patterns

1. <u>SAD—Standard American Diet, Western diet</u>: Perfect "set-up" for chronic disease, depression, inflammation, pain, acidosis.

2. <u>Vegetarian</u>: Beneficial if properly designed and supplemented (eg, B12, carnitine, DHA).

3. <u>Vegan</u>: More challenging than vegetarian.

4. <u>Paleo</u>: Optimal nutrient density, phytonutrient spectrum, alkalinization—best option.

5. <u>Mediterranean</u>: Let's enjoy some olive oil, red wine, and dark chocolate but avoid the potatoes, pasta and other wheat-based pro-inflammatory and SIBO-promoting foods.

6. <u>Hypoallergenic, oligoantigenic</u>: Per patient.

7. <u>Low-carb, Atkins, ketogenic diet</u>: Excellent for diabetes mellitus, hypertension, mitochondrial dysfunction. "Low-carb Paleo" is excellent.

Unhealthy food = inflammation

▸ A single meal of <u>egg and sausage muffin sandwiches with 2 hash browns</u> caused an **increase of 150% for NF-kappaB** (from ~190 to ~510 AUC) for approximately **2 hours** and was associated with increases in oxidative stress and the inflammatory marker **CRP**.

  ▸ Hospital food = inflammation = additional treatment with anti-inflammatory drugs, known to have multiple adverse effects, including CKD, ARF, gastric ulceration, DM, infxn, PPI/H2agonsts,

Aljada, *Am J Clin Nutr*, 2004

Increase in intranuclear nuclear factor κB and decrease in inhibitor κB in mononuclear cells after a mixed meal: evidence for a proinflammatory effect[1-3]

Ahmad Aljada, Priya Mohanty, Husam Ghanim, Toufic Abdo, Devjit Tripathy, Ajay Chaudhuri, and Paresh Dandona

ABSTRACT
Background: In view of the stimulatory effect of glucose on reactive oxygen species (ROS) generation, we investigated the possibility that a mixed meal stimulates ROS generation and possibly induces concomitant proinflammatory changes.
Objective: The objective was to determine whether the intake of a 900-kcal mixed meal induces an increase in ROS generation by leukocytes and an inflammatory response at the cellular level.
Design: Nine normal-weight subjects were given a 900-kcal mixed [...] and 9 normal-weight subjects were given [...] at 0, 1, 2, and 3 h.

(PMNLs) at 2 h, whereas cream (lipid) produces a peak at 1 h. The peak increase in ROS generation is the greatest with glucose, whereas it is the least with casein (protein). On the other hand, cream intake causes a prolonged increase in lipid peroxidation. Consistent with these observations, we also showed that a 48-h fast results in a marked decrease in ROS generation by leukocytes and oxidative damage of amino acids (3). Thus, we suggest that nutritional intake may be the major modulator of ROS generation. Indeed, we showed recently that the state of obesity reflecting chronic hypernutrition is associated with marked oxidative stress, as reflected in an increase in indexes of lipid [...] oxidative damage of

Sugar (simple carbohydrates) = oxidative stress and antioxidant depletion

▸ **"Glucose challenge stimulates reactive oxygen species (ROS) generation by leucocytes."**

▸ 14 normal subjects,

▸ following ingestion of 75 g (300 kcal) glucose,

▸ **ROS generation increased**: 240% of normal by polymorphonuclear leucocytes (PMNL) and mononuclear cells (MNC),

▸ **Antioxidant depletion**: alpha-Tocopherol levels decreased significantly at 1 h, 2 h, 3 h.

Mohanty. *J Clin Endocrinol Metab.* 2000 Aug

<u>Sugar (simple carbohydrates) = immune suppression</u>

▶ "Oral 100-g (400 kcal) portions of carbohydrate from glucose, fructose, sucrose, honey, or orange juice all **significantly decreased the capacity of neutrophils to engulf bacteria** ... The greatest effects occurred between 1 and 2 hr postprandial, but the values were still significantly below the fasting control values **5 hr after feeding**."

Sanchez. *Am J Clin Nutr.* 1973 Nov

Nutrition & FxMed for
chronic immune-
inflammatory disorders

Many/most phytonutrients have antioxidant and antiinflammatory activities that are synergistic and—in total—clinically significant

- Diets low in fruits, vegetables, nuts, seeds, berries are low in phytonutrients.
- "We propose that the additive and synergistic effects of phytochemicals in fruit and vegetables are responsible for their potent antioxidant and anticancer activities, and that the benefit of a diet rich in fruit and vegetables is attributed to the complex mixture of phytochemicals present in whole foods."

Liu. *Am J Clin Nutr.* 2003 Sep

Health benefits of fruit and vegetables are from additive and synergistic combinations of phytochemicals[1–4]

Rui Hai Liu

ABSTRACT   Cardiovascular disease and cancer are ranked as the first and second leading causes of death in the United States and in most industrialized countries. Regular consumption ... associated with reduced risks of cancer,

and vegetables in the diet (5). The value of adding citrus fruit, carotene-rich fruit and vegetables, and cruciferous vegetables to the diet for reducing the risk of cancer was specifically highlighted. In 1989, a National Academy of Sciences report on diet and health recommended consuming 5 or more servings of fruit ... risk of both cancer and heart

Nutrition & FxMed for chronic immune-inflammatory disorders

Food, Diet

1. Food-induced inflammation

2. Oxidative stress

3. Immune suppression

4. Phytonutrient deficiency

5. Sugar/insulin excess

6. GI dysbiosis & the need for probiotics

7. Deficiencies of vitamins, minerals, ALA, GLA, EPA, DHA

8. Allergens

Excess dietary carbohydrate is the *most common* cause of:

1. <u>Chronic hyperglycemia, type-2 diabetes mellitus</u>: immune suppression, oxidative stress, antioxidant depletion, protein glycosylation (nerve/eye, vascular, and kidney damage),

2. <u>Chronic hyperinsulinemia</u>: promotes dyslipidemia via stimulation of HMG-CoA reductase, promotes atherogenesis,

3. <u>Chronic hypertension, metabolic syndrome</u>: insulin promotes sodium and water retention thus leading to hypertension,

4. <u>Proinflammatory and pro-oxidative state</u>:

5. <u>Mitochondrial dysfunction</u>: synergistic with nutritional deficiencies

<u>**Food, Diet**</u>

1. Food-induced inflammation

2. Oxidative stress

3. Immune suppression

4. **Phytonutrient deficiency**

5. Sugar/insulin excess

6. GI dysbiosis & the need for probiotics

7. Deficiencies of vitamins, minerals, ALA, GLA, EPA, DHA

8. Allergens

Reasons to avoid wheat

1. <u>Nutrient-poor</u>: wheat is very low in nutrients compared with fruits and especially vegetables.

2. <u>Phytonutrient-poor</u>: wheat is very low in health-promoting phytonutrients when compared to fruits (e.g., antioxidant flavonoids) and vegetables (I3C, DIM).

3. <u>Celiac disease is common</u>: about 1 per 150 people.

4. <u>Wheat allergy is common</u>: acne, skin rashes, migraine headache....

5. <u>Triggers very odd problems, such as "gluten ataxia" and "dermatitis herpetiformis"</u>: commonly misdiagnosed as other problems.

6. <u>Circulating immune complexes (CIC)</u>: The are formed even in health people; CIC cause vasculitis, nephritis, arthritis, dermatitis... inflammation!

7. <u>High fermentation = promotes bacterial overgrowth of the small bowel</u>: see my work on dysbiosis, fibromyalgia; also IBS and RLS.

8. <u>Inherently proinflammatory</u>: Gliadin stimulates human monocytes to production of IL-8 and TNF-alpha through a mechanism involving NF-kappaB. *FEBS Lett.* 2004 Jul

Wheat = inflammation

In this context, it is important to note that a low CHO diet offers further possibilities to target inflammation through omission or inclusion of certain foods. Usually, CHO restriction is not only limited to avoiding sugar and other high-GI foods, but also to a reduced intake of grains. Grains can induce inflammation in susceptible individuals due to their content of omega-6 fatty acids, lectins and gluten [159,160]. In particular gluten might play a key role in the pathogenesis of auto-immune and inflammatory disorders and some malignant diseases. In the small intestine, gluten triggers the release of zonulin, a protein that regulates the tight junctions between epithelial cells and therefore intestinal, but also blood-brain barrier function. Recent evi-

Klement, Kämmerer. *Nutrition & Metabolism* 2011, 8:75

nutritionandmetabolism.com/content/8/1/75

Open access

Nutrition & FxMed for chronic immune-inflammatory disorders

Food, Diet

1. Food-induced inflammation

2. Oxidative stress

3. Immune suppression

4. Phytonutrient deficiency

5. Sugar/insulin excess

6. GI dysbiosis & the need for probiotics

7. Deficiencies of vitamins, minerals, ALA, GLA, EPA, DHA

8. Allergens

Low-carbohydrate diets reduce inflammation (which was obviously caused/triggered by excess dietary carbohydrate)

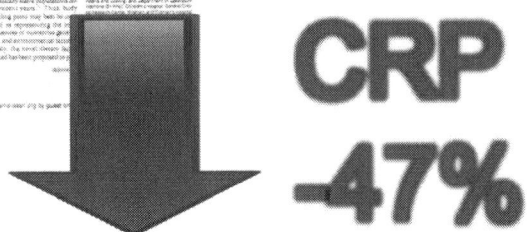

protein or high-density lipoprotein cholesterol with weight loss. C-reactive protein declined by nearly 50% with weight loss in the low–glycemic load group but remained essentially unchanged in the low-fat group ($P = .03$ for

Pereira, *JAMA*, 2004

Nutrition & FxMed for chronic immune-inflammatory disorders

Food, Diet

1. Food-induced inflammation

2. Oxidative stress

3. Immune suppression

4. Phytonutrient deficiency

5. Sugar/insulin excess

6. GI dysbiosis & the need for probiotics

7. Deficiencies of vitamins, minerals, ALA, GLA, EPA, DHA

8. Allergens

Unhealthy high-carbohydrate diets promote inflammation via several mechanisms, including gastrointestinal dysbiosis (bacterial overgrowth)

▸ Unhealthy diets with components such as **wheat**/grains, **sugar, and potatoes** promote inflammation via several mechanisms including promotion of **gastrointestinal dysbiosis and small intestine bacterial overgrowth (SIBO).**

▸ Proof of this concept is data showing that change to a **plant-based diet evokes clinical improvements in patients** with inflammatory diseases (RA) that correlate with and appear to be dependent on **favorable alterations in gastrointestinal flora—quality, quantity, and activity.**

Wheat = fermentation, dysbiosis, and small intestinal bacterial overgrowth (SIBO)

‣ We conclude that the malabsorbed fraction of wheat bread was dependent on the amount ingested, the composition of the meal, and individual gastrointestinal handling. Fermentation of wheat bran resulted in a very low breath-hydrogen response compared with lactulose or wheat bread. Addition of 11 g butter to the bread seemed to increase the malabsorbed fraction of the starch, an effect that was abolished when the amount of butter was increased to 26 g." Olesen, *Am J Clin Nutr* 1997;66

‣ "...hydrogen response was increased by all breads." Hallfrisch, *J Am Coll Nutr.* 1999

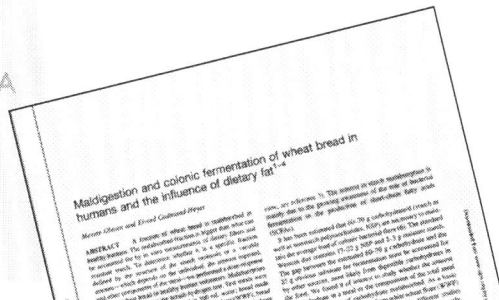

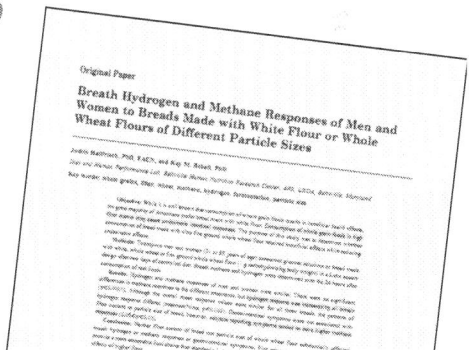

Nutrition & FxMed for chronic immune-inflammatory disorders

Food, Diet

1. Food-induced inflammation

2. Oxidative stress

3. Immune suppression

4. Phytonutrient deficiency

5. Sugar/insulin excess

6. GI dysbiosis & the need for probiotics

7. Deficiencies of vitamins, minerals, ALA, GLA, EPA, DHA

Healthy diets alleviate inflammation by improving quality & reducing quantity of intestinal bacteria

▸ "43 RA patients were randomized into two groups: the test group to receive living food, a form of uncooked vegan diet rich in lactobacilli, and the control group to continue their ordinary omnivorous diets."

▸ "We conclude that a vegan diet changes the fecal microbial flora in RA patients, and **changes in the fecal flora are associated with improvement in RA activity.**"

Peltonen, *Br J Rheumatol*, 1997 Jan

Food, Diet

1. Food-induced inflammation

2. Oxidative stress

3. Immune suppression

4. Phytonutrient deficiency

5. Sugar/insulin excess

6. GI dysbiosis & the need for probiotics

7. Deficiencies of vitamins, minerals, ALA, GLA, EPA, DHA

Healthy diets alleviate inflammation by improving quality & reducing quantity of intestinal bacteria

▶ "Significant alteration in the intestinal flora was observed when the patients changed from omnivorous to vegan diet.

▶ This finding of an association between intestinal flora and disease activity may have implications for our understanding of how diet can affect RA."

Toivanen. *Rheumatology.* 2002 Aug

Nutrition & FxMed for chronic immune-inflammatory disorders

Food, Diet

1. Food-induced inflammation

2. Oxidative stress

3. Immune suppression

4. Phytonutrient deficiency

5. Sugar/insulin excess

6. **GI dysbiosis & the need for probiotics**

7. Deficiencies of vitamins, minerals, ALA, GLA, EPA, DHA

8. Allergens

Excess exposure to (SIBO) and/or absorption (leaky gut) of bacterial debris promotes diabetes:

▸ **"bacterial components in blood predicts the onset of diabetes mellitus in a large general population."** Koch *Nature Reviews Endocrinology* 2012 Jan

▸ **Blood levels of the bacterial marker (16S rDNA) predict the onset of diabetes and abdominal adiposity in a large general population (n= 3,280) followed for 9 years.** The adjusted OR (95% CIs) for incident diabetes and for abdominal adiposity were 1.35 and 1.18, respectively. **16S rDNA was shown to be an independent marker of the risk of diabetes. These findings are evidence for the concept that tissue** <u>**bacteria are involved in the onset of diabetes in humans**</u>. Amar. *Diabetologia.* 2011 Dec

Nutrition & FxMed for chronic immune-inflammatory disorders

Food, Diet

1. Food-induced inflammation

2. Oxidative stress

3. Immune suppression

4. Phytonutrient deficiency

5. Sugar/insulin excess

6. GI dysbiosis & the need for probiotics

7. Deficiencies of vitamins, minerals, ALA, GLA, EPA, DHA

8. Allergens

Nutritional deficiencies = inflammation, oxidative stress, low-grade immune activation

▸ Vitamin and mineral deficiencies are epidemic in the general population and are pandemic among patients with chronic diseases due to disease effects, malabsorption-maldigestion-hyperexcretion (due to disease or drugs), hypermetabolism and oxidative stress due to inflammation.

   ▸ My research: Vitamin D deficiency was found in 156/157 rheumatology patients in Texas in the southern USA, a region with abundant sunshine,

   ▸ Magnesium deficiency has been noted in ~40% of general and patient populations internationally, with some studies as large as 16,000 subjects.

▸ Fatty acid deficiencies of ALA, GLA, EPA, and DHA are commonplace: the average intake of n3 fatty acids has historically been 7 grams per day and in industrialized nations is currently 1 gram per day; thus patients should be assumed to be deficient in n3 fatty acids.

Nutritional supplementation should be routine

▶ **Most people do not consume an optimal amount of all vitamins by diet alone.**

▶ ...it appears prudent for all adults to take vitamin supplements.

▶ **Physicians should make specific efforts to...ensure that patients are taking the vitamins they should..."**

Fletcher, Fairfield. *JAMA*. 2002 Jun

Nutritional supplementation alleviates inflammation

▸ "RESULTS: At 6 months, C-reactive protein levels were significantly lower in the multivitamin group than in the placebo group (between-group difference = -0.91 mg/L).

▸ CONCLUSION: In a post hoc analysis of a randomized, double-blind, placebo-controlled study, **multivitamin use was associated with lower C-reactive protein levels**."

Church. *Am J Med.* 2003 Dec

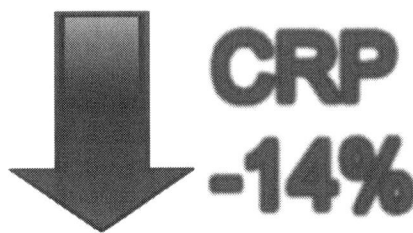

CRP -14%

Nutrition & FxMed for chronic immune-inflammatory disorders

Food, Diet

1. Food-induced inflammation

2. Oxidative stress

3. Immune suppression

4. Phytonutrient deficiency

5. Sugar/insulin excess

6. GI dysbiosis & the need for probiotics

7. Deficiencies of vitamins, minerals, ALA, GLA, EPA, DHA

8. Allergens

Vitamin D is an anti-autoimmune agent and antiinflammatory treatment

▸ "Several observations have shown that **vitamin D inhibits proinflammatory processes** by **suppressing the enhanced activity of immune cells that take part in the autoimmune reaction.**"

▸ "…vitamin D…has become a significant factor in a number of physiological functions, specifically as **a biological inhibitor of inflammatory hyperactivity.**"

Ann Rheum Dis. 2007 Sep

Nutrition & FxMed for chronic immune-inflammatory disorders

Food, Diet

1. Food-induced inflammation

2. Oxidative stress

3. Immune suppression

4. Phytonutrient deficiency

5. Sugar/insulin excess

6. GI dysbiosis & the need for probiotics

7. Deficiencies of vitamins, minerals, ALA, GLA, EPA, DHA

8. Allergens

Vitamin D3 supplementation— correction of vitamin D deficiency— causes clinically important reductions in systemic inflammatory activity:

- MMP9 (-68%),
- TIMP-1 (-38%)
- CRP (-23%)

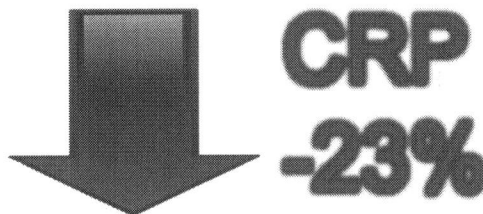

CRP -23%

Timms, *QJM*. 2002 Dec

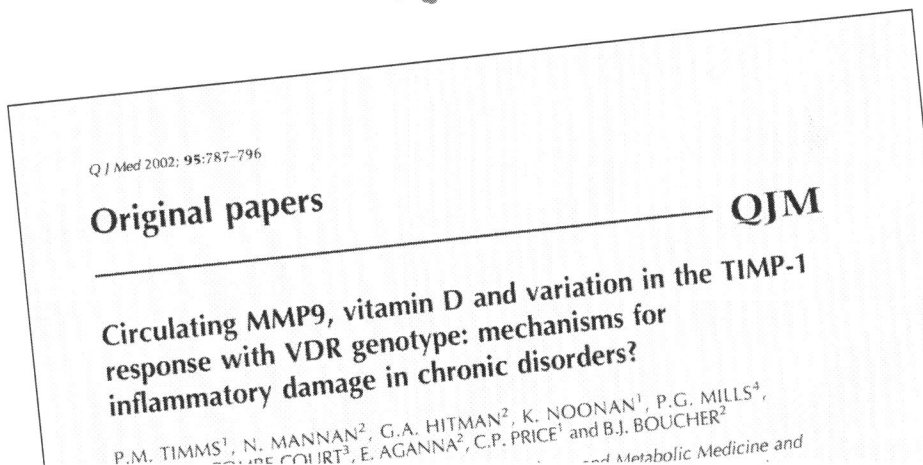

Q J Med 2002; **95**:787–796

Original papers ———— QJM

Circulating MMP9, vitamin D and variation in the TIMP-1 response with VDR genotype: mechanisms for inflammatory damage in chronic disorders?

P.M. TIMMS[1], N. MANNAN[2], G.A. HITMAN[2], K. NOONAN[1], P.G. MILLS[4], ...RE COURT[3], E. AGANNA[2], C.P. PRICE[1] and B.J. BOUCHER[2] ...nd Metabolic Medicine and

Mechanisms of vitamin D immunomodulation:

1. VDR is a member of the steroid/thyroid/retinoid receptor gene superfamily of transcription factors and regulates the expression of many genes.

2. **VDR have been detected in over 30 different tissues including circulating monocytes, dendritic cells and activated T cells—"...the highest concentration is in immature immune cells within the thymus and in mature CD8 T lymphocytes..."**

3. Vitamin D "has direct effects on T and B cells and shapes their responses to activation"

4. **Vitamin D inhibits T lymphocyte proliferation, particularly inhibits Th1 cell proliferation and cytokine production.**

5. Vitamin D "decreased secretion of interleukin (IL)-2 and IFNγ by CD4 T cells and promotes IL-5 & IL-10 production.

Mechanisms of vitamin D immunomodulation:

6. 1,25(OH)2D3 downregulates IL-6, an important stimulator of Th17 cells, which are a critical component of autoimmunity.

7. "In B cells, **vitamin D has been shown to inhibit antibody secretion and autoantibody production**.

8. "1,25(OH)2D3 is one of the most powerful blockers of dendritic cell differentiation and of IL-12 secretion.

9. "interferes with the NFκB-induced transcription of IL-12.

10. "decrease in IL-12 and IFNγ **while IL-10 and transforming growth factor β production is enhanced**, resulting in inhibition of T cell activation.

11. 1,25(OH)2D3 increased the macrophage-specific surface antigens and the lysosomal enzyme acid phosphatase while stimulating the "oxidative burst" function.

Nutrition & FxMed for chronic immune-inflammatory disorders

Food, Diet

Deficiencies of vitamins, minerals, fatty acids: Most vitamins and minerals and "healthy" fatty acids have an anti-inflammatory effect.

Vitamin D has important anti-autoimmune effects:

Novel role of the vitamin D receptor in maintaining the integrity of the intestinal mucosal barrier.

Kong J. *Am J Physiol Gastrointest Liver Physiol.* 2008 Jan

In summary, in this report we presented evidence suggesting that the VDR plays a critical role in preserving the integrity of the intestinal mucosal barrier. VDR is able to enhance the intercellular junctions; it is also required for mucosal wound healing. Mice lacking VDR are much more susceptible to DSS-induced mucosal injury, leading to extensive ulceration and early death. In vitro experiments demonstrate that VDR mediates the activity of $1{,}25(OH)_2D_3$ that induces junction protein expression and strengthens the tight junction complex. These data are consistent with, and explain at least in part, the observation reported in the literature that vitamin D deficiency is linked to increased incidence of IBD in human population.

Vitamin D deficiency probably → leaky gut → microbe/food antigen absorption → immune stimulation → immune activation → inflammation/allergy/autoimmunity

Deficiencies of vitamins, minerals, fatty acids: Vitamin C has anti-allergy and enjoyment-enhancing benefits ☺

▸ Antihistamine effect of supplemental ascorbic acid: "...[blood] histamine levels were depressed 38% following VC supplementation. ...These data indicate that VC may indirectly enhance chemotaxis by detoxifying histamine in vivo." *J Am Coll Nutr.* 1992 Apr

▸ High-dose ascorbic acid increases intercourse frequency and improves mood. *Biol Psychiatry.* 2002 Aug

BRIEF REPORT

High-Dose Ascorbic Acid Increases Intercourse Frequency and Improves Mood: A Randomized Controlled Clinical Trial

Stuart Brody

Background: *Ascorbic acid (AA) modulates catecholaminergic activity, decreases stress reactivity, approaches anxiety and prolactin release, improves vascular*... *These processes*... *anxiety and*... *oxytocin*... *mood.*

al 1994, Gulley and Rebec 1999; Nurse et al 1985, Pierce et al 1995, Seitz et al 1998; Sershen et al 1987) and noradrenergic (Kimelberg and Goderie 1993; Paterson and Hertz 1989) activity, potentiate dopamine's inhibitory effect on prolactin release (Shin et al 1990), and increase oxytocin secretion (Luck and Jungclas 1987). All of these ... enhance frequency of penile-vaginal ... the effect of high-dose double-

These fatty acids are anti-inflammatory

▸ These fatty acids are notably missing from many modern "convenience" diets, and each of these has antiinflammatory effects; thus, "combination fatty acid deficiency" contributes to a pro-inflammatory condition, and supplementation has a clinically proven antiinflammatory effect.:

1. <u>ALA</u>—n3 alpha linolenic acid from flax oil,

2. <u>GLA</u>—n6 gamma linolenic acid, borage oil,

3. <u>EPA</u>—n3 eicosapentaenoic acid from cold water fatty fish,

4. <u>DHA</u>—n3 docosahexaenoic acid from cold water fatty fish, also algae,

5. <u>Oleic acid</u>: n9 mostly in olive oil.

Historical Paleolithic intake of n3 fatty acids was **seven** grams per day; Western/American intake of n3 fatty acids is **one** gram per day. Thus, by definition, nearly everyone is deficient in n3 anti-inflammatory fatty acids.

Health-promoting fatty acids (ALA, GLA, EPA, DHA, oleic acid) provide clinically meaningful antiinflammatory benefits:

▸ GLA—dose 500-**1,000**-4,000 mg/d for proven clinical benefits in RA via activation of PPAR-g and reductions in NFkB and leukotrienes,

▸ EPA and DHA—therapeutic benefits start at 1,000 mg/d but are more significant at **3,000 mg/d** via activation of PPAR-a and reductions in NFkB and prostaglandins, increases in docosatrienes and resolvins.

http://OptimalHealthResearch.com/reprints/series/

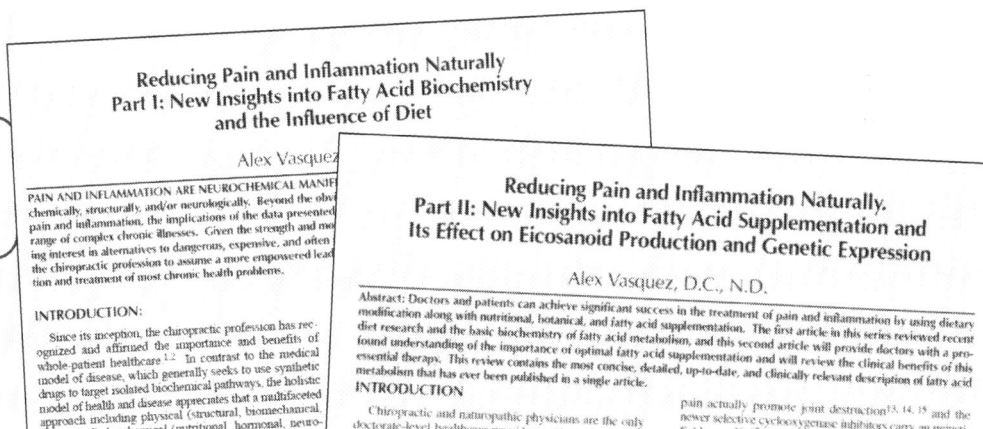

Reducing Pain and Inflammation Naturally
Part I: New Insights into Fatty Acid Biochemistry and the Influence of Diet

Alex Vasquez

PAIN AND INFLAMMATION ARE NEUROCHEMICAL MANIFE chemically, structurally, and/or neurologically. Beyond the obvi pain and inflammation, the implications of the data presented range of complex chronic illnesses. Given the strength and mo ing interest in alternatives to dangerous, expensive, and often the chiropractic profession to assume a more empowered lead tion and treatment of most chronic health problems.

INTRODUCTION:

Since its inception, the chiropractic profession has rec ognized and affirmed the importance and benefits of whole-patient healthcare [1,2] In contrast to the medical model of disease, which generally seeks to use synthetic drugs to target isolated biochemical pathways, the holistic model of health and disease appreciates that a multifaceted approach including physical (structural, biomechanical,

Reducing Pain and Inflammation Naturally.
Part II: New Insights into Fatty Acid Supplementation and Its Effect on Eicosanoid Production and Genetic Expression

Alex Vasquez, D.C., N.D.

Abstract: Doctors and patients can achieve significant success in the treatment of pain and inflammation by using dietary modification along with nutritional, botanical, and fatty acid supplementation. The first article in this series reviewed recent diet research and the basic biochemistry of fatty acid metabolism, and this second article will provide doctors with a pro- found understanding of the importance of optimal fatty acid supplementation and will review the clinical benefits of this essential therapy. This review contains the most concise, detailed, up-to-date, and clinically relevant description of fatty acid metabolism that has ever been published in a single article.

INTRODUCTION

Chiropractic and naturopathic physicians are the only doctorate-level healthcare

pain actually promote joint destruction [13, 14, 15] and the newer selective cyclooxygenase inhibitors carry an

Fish oil [EPA & DHA] supplementation allows patients with inflammatory diseases such as **rheumatoid arthritis** to reduce their need for anti-inflammatory drugs.

Br J Rheumatol. 1993 Nov

"CONCLUSION: A diet low in arachidonic acid ameliorates clinical signs of inflammation in patients with RA and augments the **beneficial effect of fish oil supplementation**."

Rheumatol Int. 2003 Jan

"The children (**mean age, 11.4 months**) with atopic dermatitis (mean duration, 8.56 months) were openly treated with **3 g/day gamma-linolenic acid**, for 28 days... A gradual improvement in erythema, excoriations and lichenification was seen; significant differences were shown for itching, and the use of antihistamines."

J Int Med Res. 1994 Jan-Feb

Food, Diet

1. Food-induced inflammation

2. Oxidative stress

3. Immune suppression

4. Phytonutrient deficiency

5. Sugar/insulin excess

6. GI dysbiosis & the need for probiotics

7. Deficiencies of vitamins, minerals, ALA, GLA, EPA, DHA

8. Allergens

Allergenic foods (foods to which the patient is immunologically sensitized) can contribute to systemic inflammation and musculoskeletal pain by many mechanisms:

1. Formation of immune complexes (chains of antigens and antibodies) that can deposit in the joints/vessels/kidneys to cause a localized inflammatory response.

2. Triggering migraine headaches: (neurogenic switching?)

3. Increasing intestinal permeability, which then increases antigen load and systemic inflammation.

4. Adversely altering gastrointestinal flora, which can then promote systemic inflammation, particularly if the intestinal mucosa is compromised by the allergic inflammation.

Inman, *Rheum Dis Clin North Am.* 1991

Allergens: Many patients unknowingly consume foods that promote their allergic reactions—wheat is the best example.

- "60 migraine patients, elimination diets after a 5-day period of withdrawal from their normal diet.

- **The commonest foods causing reactions were:**
  - wheat (78%)—look out for celiac disease,
  - orange (65%),
  - eggs (45%),
  - tea and coffee (40% each),
  - chocolate and milk (37%) each),
  - beef (35%),
  - corn, cane sugar, and yeast (33% each).

- When **an average of ten common foods were avoided** there was a dramatic fall in the number of headaches per month, 85% of patients becoming headache-free.

  Grant. *Lancet.* 1979 May

Nutrition & FxMed for chronic immune-inflammatory disorders

Food, Diet

1. Food-induced inflammation

2. Oxidative stress

3. Immune suppression

4. Phytonutrient deficiency

5. Sugar/insulin excess

6. GI dysbiosis & the need for probiotics

7. Deficiencies of vitamins, minerals, ALA, GLA, EPA, DHA

8. Allergens

Allergens: Many patients unknowingly consume foods that promote their allergic reactions—wheat is the best example. Mechanisms include increased intestinal permeability (progressive panallergy), exacerbation of dysbiosis-mediated disorders) formation of immune complexes. Inman, *Rheum Dis Clin North Am.* 1991

Scandinavian Journal of Gastroenterology, 2009; 44: 168–171

informa
healthcare

ORIGINAL ARTICLE

Gliadin IgG antibodies and circulating immune complexes

ALEXANDER EISENMANN[1], CHRISTIAN MURR[2], DIETMAR FUCHS[2] & MAXIMILIAN LEDOCHOWSKI[1]

[1]*Department of Clinical Nutrition, Medical University of Innsbruck, Austria, and* [2]*Division of Biological Chemistry, Biocentre, Medical University of Innsbruck, Austria*

Abstract
Objective. Circulating immune complexes (CICs) in blood are associated with autoimmune-diseases such as systemic lupus erythematosus, immune complex glomerulonephritis, rheumatoid arthritis and vasculitis. However, slightly increased serum concentrations of such CICs are sometimes also found in healthy individuals. The objective of the current study was to assess whether food antigens could play a role in the formation of CICs. *Material and methods.* A total of 352 (265 F, 87 M), so far, healthy individuals were tested for CICs containing C1q and immunoglobulin G (IgG) as well as for gliadin IgG antibodies using the ELISA technique. Additionally, fructose and lactose malabsorption was assessed using hydrogen

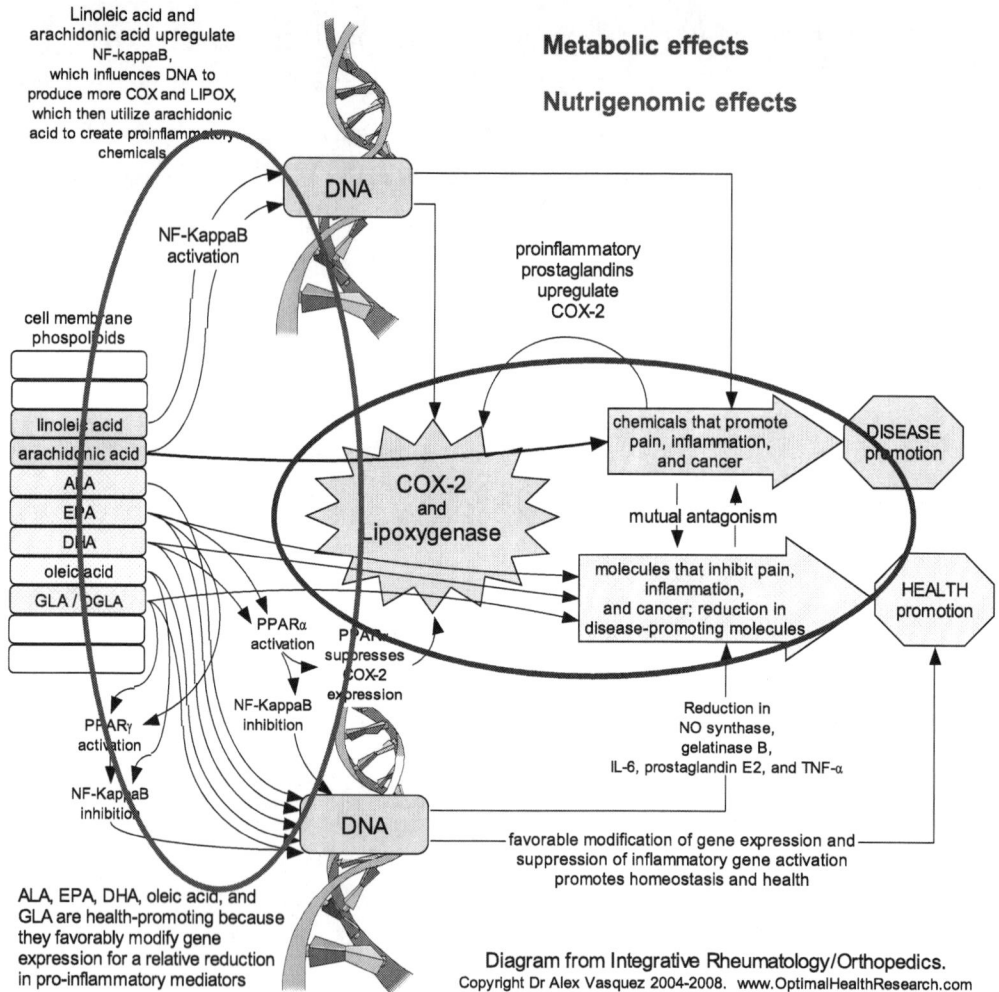

Nutrigenomics

Diet and nutrition affect gene expression and thus directly impact on health/disease phenotype

Vasquez A. *Nutritional Perspectives* 2005; Jan: 5-16

Physiol Genomics. 2004;16(2):166-7

Linoleic acid and arachidonic acid upregulate NF-kappaB, which influences DNA to produce more COX and LIPOX, which then utilize arachidonic acid to create proinflammatory chemicals.

Metabolic effects

Nutrigenomic effects

NF-KappaB activation

DNA

proinflammatory prostaglandins upregulate COX-2

cell membrane phospolipids

linoleic acid

arachidonic acid

ALA

EPA

DHA

oleic acid

GLA / DGLA

chemicals that promote pain, inflammation, and cancer

DISEASE promotion

COX-2 and Lipoxygenase

mutual antagonism

molecules that inhibit pain, inflammation, and cancer; reduction in disease-promoting molecules

HEALTH promotion

PPARα activation

PPARγ suppresses COX-2 expression

NF-KappaB inhibition

PPARγ activation

NF-KappaB inhibition

Reduction in NO synthase, gelatinase B, IL-6, prostaglandin E2, and TNF-α

DNA

favorable modification of gene expression and suppression of inflammatory gene activation promotes homeostasis and health

ALA, EPA, DHA, oleic acid, and GLA are health-promoting because they favorably modify gene expression for a relative reduction in pro-inflammatory mediators

Diagram from Integrative Rheumatology/Orthopedics.
Copyright Dr Alex Vasquez 2004-2008. www.OptimalHealthResearch.com

Nutrition & FxMed for chronic immune-inflammatory disorders

Causes of Inflammation-Immune-Metabolic Imbalance:

1. Food, Diet

2. Infection, Dysbiosis

3. Nutritional Immunomodulation

4. Dysfunctional mitochondria

5. Stress, Emotions, Psychology, Sociology

6. Endocrine, Hormones

7. Xenobiotics, Toxins

Infections & Dysbiosis = inflammation

Important concepts:

 ▹ Subclinical infections are common in patients with chronic inflammatory diseases, especially autoimmunity.

 ▹ Remember, the microbe(s) alone are not the problem; the patient's total inflammatory load (TIL) must also be addressed, as well as immunorestoration to prevent recurrence of the colonization.

Clinical assessments:

 ▹ Culture/sensitivity are helpful; DNA-based assessments are also used,

 ▹ **Response to treatment is most compelling and meaningful.**

Therapeutic implementation:

 ▹ Antimicrobials,

 ▹ Immunorestoration,

 ▹ Enhance inflammatory tolerance.

Often what we find when working with autoimmune/inflammatory patients is that they are having a *pathogenic inflammatory response* to a *nonpathogenic* microbe:

▶ Wegener's granulomatosis
▶ Rheumatoid arthritis
▶ Ankylosing spondylitis
▶ Dermatomyositis/PM
▶ Sjogren's syndrome
▶ Psoriasis
▶ SLE

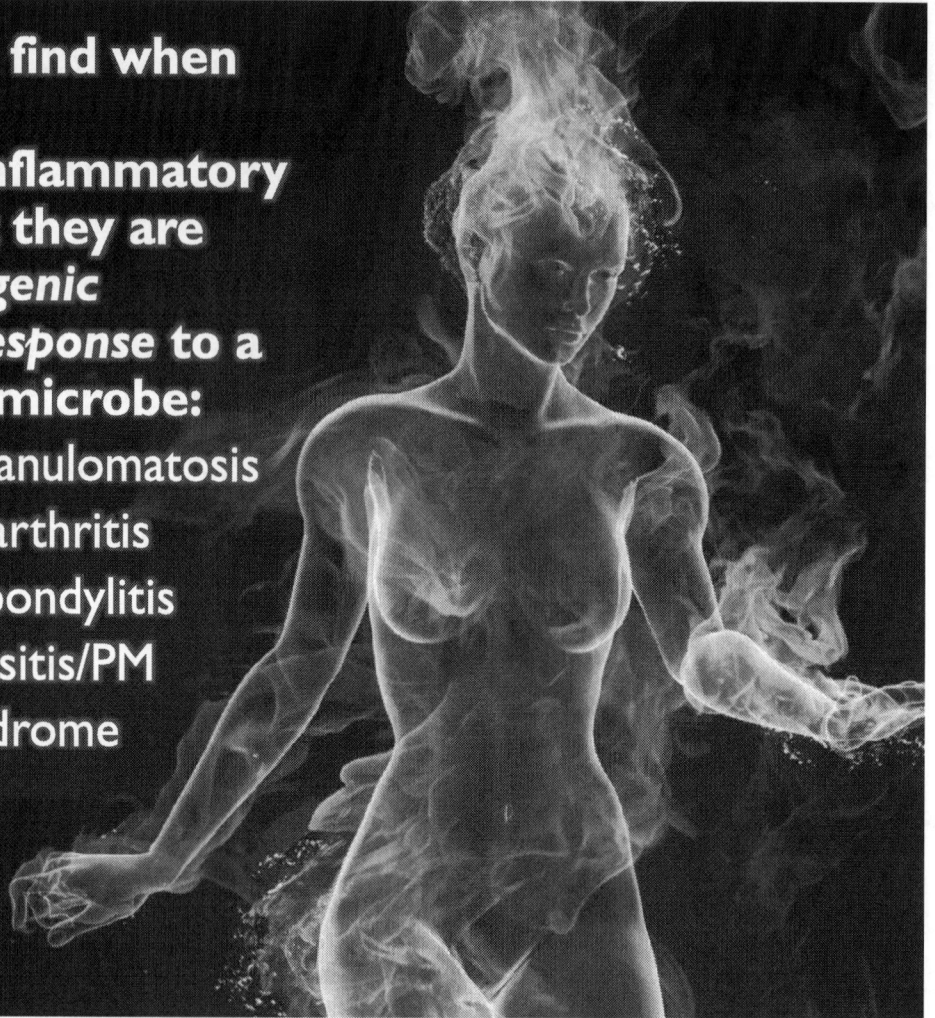

Causes of Inflammation-Immune-Metabolic Imbalance:

1. Food, Diet

2. Infection, Dysbiosis

3. Nutritional Immunomodulation

4. Dysfunctional mitochondria

5. Stress, Emotions, Psychology, Sociology

6. Endocrine, Hormones

7. Xenobiotics, Toxins

Often what we find when working with autoimmune/inflammatory patients is that they are having a *pathogenic inflammatory response* to a *nonpathogenic* microbe.

▸ **Remember, we are not looking for classic "infection" here; we are looking to determine which <u>underlying disruptions</u> may be exacerbating inflammation and the patient's symptomatology.**

▸ We have to look beyond the *disease-associated characteristics of the microbe* to see *the <u>patient's individualized response</u>* to the microbe.

  ▸ Dysbiosis in one patient may present with dermatitis, while [what appears to be] the same microbial imbalance in another patient can present as peripheral neuropathy or inflammatory arthritis.

Dysbiosis → "*multi*focal *poly*dysbiosis"

Location Subtypes:

1. **Gastrointestinal**
2. **Orodental**
3. **Sinorespiratory**
4. **Parenchymal**
5. **Genitourinary**
6. **Cutaneous**
7. **Environmental**

Problematic GI Microbes Include:

Aeromonas hydrophila, Blastocystis hominis, Candida albicans and other yeasts, *Citrobacter rodentium, Citrobacter freundii, Dientamoeba fragilis, Endolimax nana, Entamoeba histolytica,* Gamma strep, *Enterococcus, Giardia lamblia, Hafnia alvei, Helicobacter pylori, Klebsiella pneumoniae, Proteus mirabilis, Pseudomonas aeruginosa, Staphylococcus aureus, Staphylococcus epidermidis, Streptococcus pyogenes,* Group A streptococci

Molecular Mechanisms

1. **Molecular mimicry**
2. Superantigens
3. Enhanced processing of autoantigens
4. **Bystander activation**
5. Peptidoglycans and exotoxins
6. Endotoxins (LPS)
7. Immunostimulation by bacterial DNA
8. Activation of Toll-like receptors and NF-kappaB
9. **Immune complex formation and deposition**
10. Haptenization and Neoantigen formation
11. Damage to the intestinal mucosa
12. Inhibition/alteration of detoxification
13. Antimetabolites
14. Autointoxication, hepatic encephalopathy, intestinal arthritis-dermatitis syndrome
15. Impairment of mucosal and systemic defenses
16. Impairment of mucosal digestion by microbial proteases and inflammation
17. Inflammation-induced endocrine dysfunction

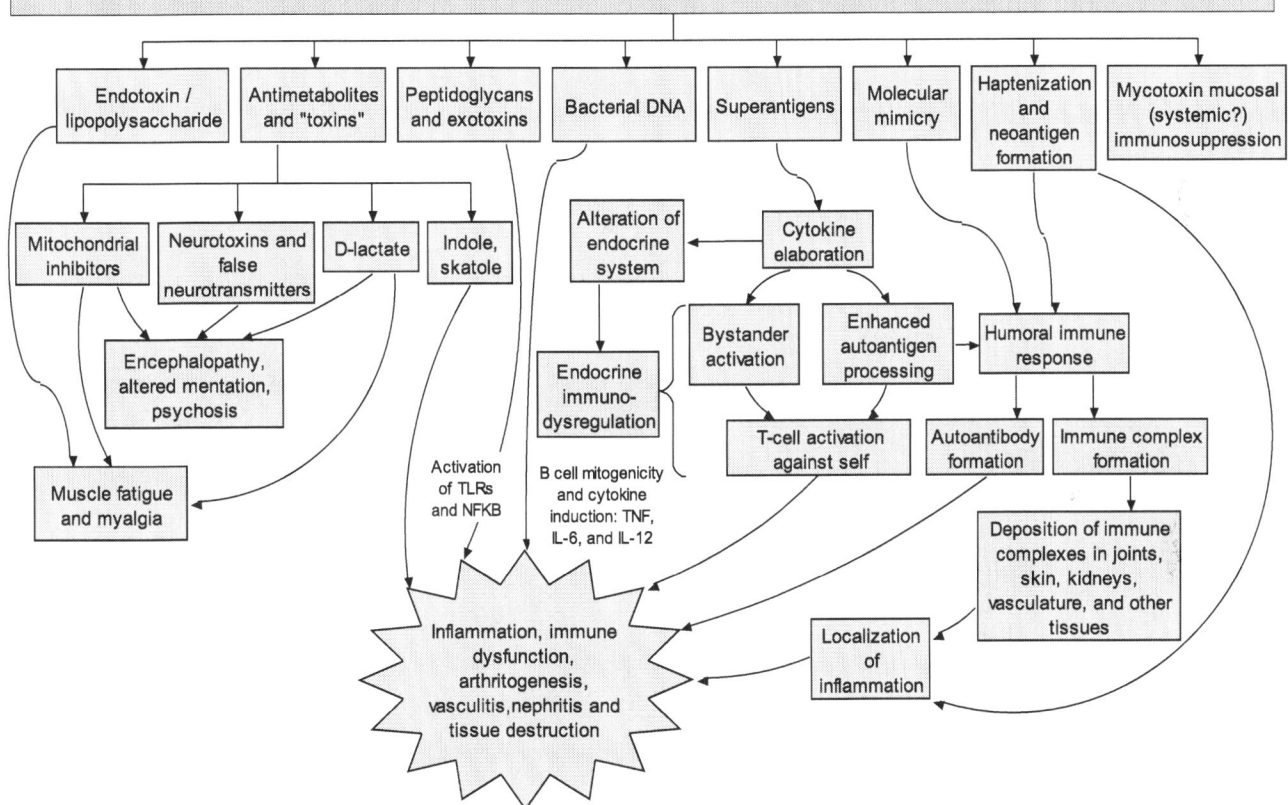

Pro-inflammatory [additive/synergistic] Consequences of Exposure to Microbial Antigens, Superantigens, and Antimetabolites

Endotoxin / lipopolysaccharide

Antimetabolites and "toxins"

Peptidoglycans and exotoxins

Bacterial DNA

Superantigens

Molecular mimicry

Haptenization and neoantigen formation

Mycotoxin mucosal (systemic?) immunosuppression

Mitochondrial inhibitors

Neurotoxins and false neurotransmitters

D-lactate

Indole, skatole

Alteration of endocrine system

Cytokine elaboration

Bystander activation

Enhanced autoantigen processing

Humoral immune response

Encephalopathy, altered mentation, psychosis

Endocrine immuno-dysregulation

T-cell activation against self

Autoantibody formation

Immune complex formation

Muscle fatigue and myalgia

Activation of TLRs and NFKB

B cell mitogenicity and cytokine induction: TNF, IL-6, and IL-12

Deposition of immune complexes in joints, skin, kidneys, vasculature, and other tissues

Localization of inflammation

Inflammation, immune dysfunction, arthritogenesis, vasculitis, nephritis and tissue destruction

Copyright © by Vasquez A. *Integrative Rheumatology*. www.OptimalHealthResearch.com

Causes of Inflammation-Immune-Metabolic Imbalance:

1. Food, Diet

2. Infection, Dysbiosis

3. Nutritional Immunomodulation

4. Dysfunctional mitochondria

5. Stress, Emotions, Psychology, Sociology

6. Endocrine, Hormones

7. Xenobiotics, Toxins

Dysbiosis subtypes by location:

1. **Gastrointestinal**: at least 7 different subtypes of gastrointestinal dysbiosis.

2. **Orodental**: Noted in rheumatoid arthritis.

3. **Sinorespiratory**: Noted in Wegener's vasculitis.

4. **Parenchymal**: Occult infections in liver, joints.

5. **Genitourinary**: Classic in reactive arthritis.

6. **Cutaneous**: Eczema and more.

7. **Environmental**: Exposure to microbial debris/toxins and bioaerosols can induce a pro-inflammatory state that triggers autoimmunity and systemic inflammation.

8. **Microbial**: Yes, es posible que a vezes [it is possible that at times] microbes such as amoeba may be infected with smaller microbes and that one can have environmental dysbiosis induced by a microbe-within-a-microbe. *Eur J Clin Microbiol Infect Dis.* 2005 Mar

Dysbiosis Location Subtypes: Gastrointestinal, Orodental, Sinorespiratory, ***Parenchymal***, Genitourinary, Cutaneous, Environmental, Microbial

Date and Time Collected	Date Entered	Date and Time Reported	Physician Name	NPI	Physician ID
08/29/11 09:41	08/29/11	09/03/11 01:35ET	VASQUEZ , A		

Tests Ordered
FSH+TestT+LH+DHEA S+Prog+E2...; CBC With Differential/Platelet; Comp. Metabolic Panel (14); Chlamydia pneumoniae(IgG/M); Thyroxine (T4) Free, Direct, S; TSH; Prolactin; IGF-1; C-Reactive Protein, Cardiac; Homocyst(e)ine, Plasma; Triiodothyronine (T3); Reverse T3; Magnesium, RBC; Cortisol - AM; Venipuncture

```
Chlamydia pneumoniae(IgG/M)
  Chlamydia pneumoniae IgG      >1:256    High          Neg:<1:16
  Chlamydia pneumoniae IgM       <1:10                   Neg:<1:10
  Test Information:
```

▸ "*Chlamydia trachomatis* and *Chlamydophila (Chlamydia) pneumoniae* are known triggers of reactive arthritis (ReA) and exist in a persistent metabolically active infection state in the synovium..." *Arthritis Rheum* 2010 May

▸ "These studies confirm our previous reports concerning the high prevalence of C. pneumoniae in the CSF of MS patients." *Clin Diagn Lab Immunol.* 2002 Nov

▸ "Because there is as yet no standardisation of serological criteria for persistent infection, we considered antibody titers of > 1/20 in the IgA fraction, together with **IgG titers of 1/64 to 1/256, to be indicative of persistent infection**." *J Clin Pathol.* 2002 May

▸ Thank you, Bill Beakey DOM, from www.professionalco-op.com for provision of these lab tests.

Causes of Inflammation-Immune-Metabolic Imbalance:

1. Food, Diet

2. Infection, Dysbiosis

3. Nutritional Immunomodulation

4. Dysfunctional mitochondria

5. Stress, Emotions, Psychology, Sociology

6. Endocrine, Hormones

7. Xenobiotics, Toxins

Case report: 40yo white male with a 5-y history of "idiopathic" peripheral neuropathy (numbness, weakness, tingling)…exacerbated by consumption of shellfish, associated with fever.

1. Some evidence of autoimmunity (slightly elevated ANA) and a family history of autoimmunity.

2. Has already spent $10,000 on neurological consultations, MRIs, CT scans, lab tests, CSF analysis.

3. Desires cure and preventive healthcare.

4. Refuses parasitology pending LM test for "leaky gut."

Patient:

Age: 40
Sex: M
MRN: 0000345768

Order Number: 40220637
Completed: April 24, 2003
Received: April 22, 2003
Collected: April 21, 2003

ALEX VASQUEZ DC ND
2217 ____th Street
Houston, TX 77098

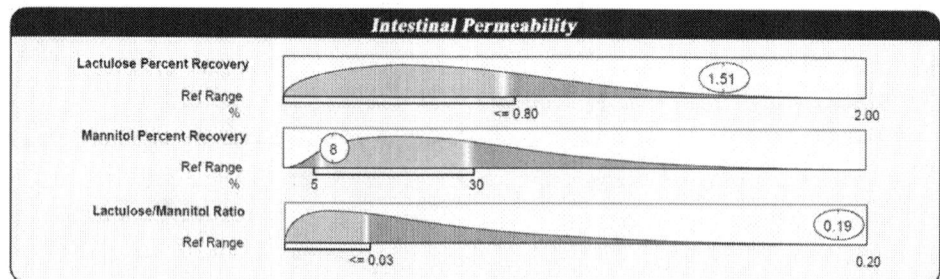

Intestinal Permeability

Lactulose Percent Recovery	Ref Range %	1.51
		<= 0.80 · 2.00
Mannitol Percent Recovery	Ref Range %	8
		5 · 30
Lactulose/Mannitol Ratio	Ref Range	0.19
		<= 0.03 · 0.20

Causes of Inflammation-Immune-Metabolic Imbalance:

1. Food, Diet

2. Infection, Dysbiosis

3. Nutritional Immunomodulation

4. Dysfunctional mitochondria

5. Stress, Emotions, Psychology, Sociology

6. Endocrine, Hormones

7. Xenobiotics, Toxins

Case report: 40yo white male with a 5-y history of peripheral neuropathy (numbness, weakness, tingling)

Comprehensive Stool Analysis / Parasitology x3

MICROBIOLOGY

Bacteriology Culture

Beneficial flora		Imbalances		Dysbiotic flora	
Bifidobacter	4+	Haemolytic E. coli	4+	Pseudomonas sp.	4+
E. coli	4+	Gamma strep	2+		
Lactobacillus	2+				

Mycology (Yeast) Culture

Normal flora		Dysbiotic flora
Candida glabrata	1+	
Rhodotorula sp.	1+	

ELSEVIER

Journal of Neuroimmunology 144 (2003) 105 - 115

Journal of
Neuroimmunology

www.elsevier.com/locate/jneuroim

Cross-reactivity between related sequences found in *Acinetobacter* sp., *Pseudomonas aeruginosa*, myelin basic protein and myelin oligodendrocyte glycoprotein in multiple sclerosis

L.E. Hughes[a], P.A. Smith[b], S. Bonell[a], R.S. Natt[a], C. Wilson[a], T. Rashid[a], S. Amor[b,c], E.J. Thompson[d], J. Croker[e], A. Ebringer[a,*]

Causes of Inflammation-Immune-Metabolic Imbalance:

1. Food, Diet

2. Infection, Dysbiosis

3. Nutritional Immunomodulation

4. Dysfunctional mitochondria

5. Stress, Emotions, Psychology, Sociology

6. Endocrine, Hormones

7. Xenobiotics, Toxins

Consumption of food allergens + GI dysbiosis = 2 causes of "leaky gut" and (progressive) systemic inflammation

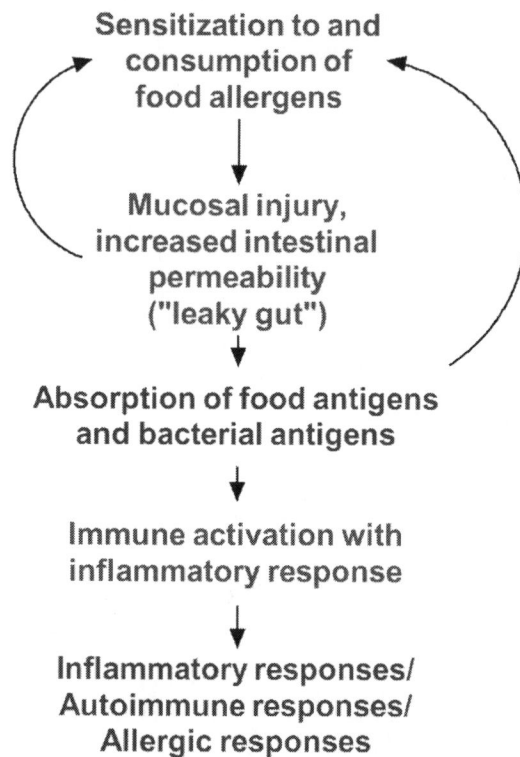

Sensitization to and consumption of food allergens

↓

Mucosal injury, increased intestinal permeability ("leaky gut")

↓

Absorption of food antigens and bacterial antigens

↓

Immune activation with inflammatory response

↓

Inflammatory responses/ Autoimmune responses/ Allergic responses

Dysbiosis → "*multi*focal *poly*dysbiosis"

Location Subtypes:

1. **Gastrointestinal**

2. **Orodental**

3. **Sinorespiratory**

4. **Parenchymal**

5. **Genitourinary**

6. **Cutaneous**

7. **Environmental**

Problematic GI Microbes Include:

Aeromonas hydrophila, Blastocystis hominis, Candida albicans and other yeasts, *Citrobacter rodentium, Citrobacter freundii, Dientamoeba fragilis, Endolimax nana, Entamoeba histolytica,* Gamma strep, *Enterococcus, Giardia lamblia, Hafnia alvei, Helicobacter pylori, Klebsiella pneumoniae, Proteus mirabilis, Pseudomonas aeruginosa, Staphylococcus aureus, Staphylococcus epidermidis, Streptococcus pyogenes,* Group A streptococci

Molecular Mechanisms

1. **Molecular mimicry**
2. Superantigens
3. Enhanced processing of autoantigens
4. **Bystander activation**
5. Peptidoglycans and exotoxins
6. Endotoxins (LPS)
7. Immunostimulation by bacterial DNA
8. Activation of Toll-like receptors and NF-kappaB
9. **Immune complex formation and deposition**
10. Haptenization and Neoantigen formation
11. Damage to the intestinal mucosa
12. Inhibition/alteration of detoxification
13. Antimetabolites
14. Autointoxication, hepatic encephalopathy, intestinal arthritis-dermatitis syndrome
15. Impairment of mucosal and systemic defenses
16. Impairment of mucosal digestion by microbial proteases and inflammation
17. Inflammation-induced endocrine dysfunction

Causes of Inflammation-Immune-Metabolic Imbalance:

1. Food, Diet

2. Infection, Dysbiosis

3. Nutritional Immunomodulation

4. Dysfunctional mitochondria

5. Stress, Emotions, Psychology, Sociology

6. Endocrine, Hormones

7. Xenobiotics, Toxins

Often what we find when working with autoimmune/inflammatory patients is that they are having a _pathogenic inflammatory response_ to a _nonpathogenic_ microbe.

▶ **Remember, we are not looking for classic "infection" here; we are looking to determine which <u>underlying disruptions</u> may be exacerbating inflammation and the patient's symptomatology.**

▶ We have to look beyond the _disease-associated characteristics of the microbe_ to see _the <u>patient's individualized response</u>_ to the microbe. **Dysbiosis = relationship**

▶ Dysbiosis in one patient may present with dermatitis, while [what appears to be] the same microbial imbalance in another patient can present as peripheral neuropathy or inflammatory arthritis.

Nutrition & FxMed for chronic immune-inflammatory disorders

Causes of Inflammation-Immune-Metabolic Imbalance:

1. Food, Diet

2. Infection, Dysbiosis

3. Nutritional Immunomodulation

4. Dysfunctional mitochondria

5. Stress, Emotions, Psychology, Sociology

6. Endocrine, Hormones

7. Xenobiotics, Toxins

Nutritional Immunomodulation

Important concept: We can favorably influence the number and function of immune cell populations by using nutrients.

▶ Our clinical goal: to reduce inflammation, allergy, autoimmunity.

▶ Our mechanistic goal: to increase number-activity of T-regulatory (Treg) cells and to decrease number-activity of Th1 (cell-mediated inflammation), Th2 (humoral inflammation, autoimmunity), and Th-17 (autoimmunity) cells.

Causes of Inflammation-Immune-Metabolic Imbalance:

1. Food, Diet

2. Infection, Dysbiosis

3. Nutritional Immunomodulation

4. Dysfunctional mitochondria

5. Stress, Emotions, Psychology, Sociology

6. Endocrine, Hormones

7. Xenobiotics, Toxins

Nutritional Immunomodulation

How does this work?

▸ Naïve/undifferentiated T-cells (Th0) born in the bone marrow, move to the thymus (and tonsils[?]) and then to the gut-associated lymphoid tissue (GALT).

▸ In the GALT, Th0 cells are programmed to become "effector cells" capable of action:

  ▸ Th0 = undifferentiated,

  ▸ Th1 = cell-mediated inflammation,

  ▸ Th2 = antibodies (allergy, autoimmunity)

  ▸ Th17 = autoimmune inflammation

  ▸ T-regulatory, Treg = promote tolerance, suppress inflammation, allergy, and autoimmunity.

▸ Epigenetic: Changes in gene expression, phenotype, and cell activity

97

Nutritional induction of regulatory T-cells

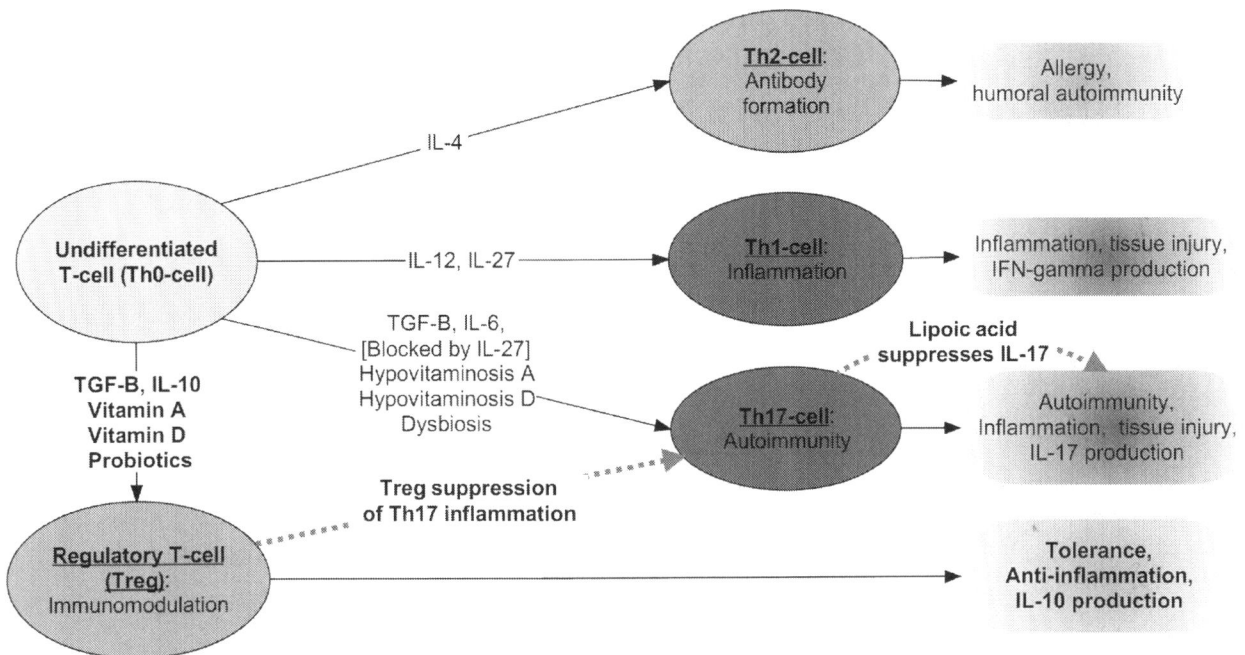

Th2-cell: Antibody formation → Allergy, humoral autoimmunity

Th1-cell: Inflammation → Inflammation, tissue injury, IFN-gamma production

Th17-cell: Autoimmunity → Autoimmunity, Inflammation, tissue injury, IL-17 production

Regulatory T-cell (Treg): Immunomodulation → Tolerance, Anti-inflammation, IL-10 production

Undifferentiated T-cell (Th0-cell)

IL-4

IL-12, IL-27

TGF-B, IL-6, [Blocked by IL-27] Hypovitaminosis A Hypovitaminosis D Dysbiosis

Lipoic acid suppresses IL-17

TGF-B, IL-10 Vitamin A Vitamin D Probiotics

Treg suppression of Th17 inflammation

Excerpted from Copyright 2011-2012 Vasquez A. *Nutritional and Functional Immunology: An Introduction to the Modifiable Factors in Chronic Inflammation, Allergy, and Autoimmunity*. 2012

Causes of Inflammation-Immune-Metabolic Imbalance:

1. Food, Diet

2. Infection, Dysbiosis

3. Nutritional Immunomodulation

4. Dysfunctional mitochondria

5. Stress, Emotions, Psychology, Sociology

6. Endocrine, Hormones

7. Xenobiotics, Toxins

Therapeutic implementation, mechanisms, dose

1. **Vitamin A**: epigenetic, more Treg, enhanced gut health and immunity. *Dose*: at least 10,000 IU/d of "preformed" vitamin A, not beta-carotene. 27-47% of patients cannot effectively convert beta-carotene to vitamin A; they must have pre-formed vitamin A.

2. **Vitamin D**: epigenetic, more Treg, enhanced gut health and immunity. *Dose*: average 4,000 IU/d for adults.

3. **Probiotics, elimination of GI dysbiosis**: create a non-inflammatory climate in the gastrointestinal tract. *Method*: use probiotics; also use plant-based diet, herbal and drug antimicrobials to promote eubiosis.

4. **Green tea**: epigenetic, more Treg. *Dose*: tea & capsules.

5. **Lipoic acid**: suppresses IL-17 by 35-50%. *Dose*: average 200-400 mg 3 times per day.

6. **N3 fatty acids**: activation of PPAR-g = Treg

Nutrition & FxMed for chronic immune-inflammatory disorders

Causes of Inflammation-Immune-Metabolic Imbalance:

1. Food, Diet

2. Infection, Dysbiosis

3. Nutritional Immunomodulation

4. Dysfunctional mitochondria

5. Stress, Emotions, Psychology, Sociology

6. Endocrine, Hormones

7. Xenobiotics, Toxins

<u>Vitamin A</u>: necessary for Treg induction

PLoS one

Characterization of Protective Human CD4⁺CD25⁺ FOXP3⁺ Regulatory T Cells Generated with IL-2, TGF-β and Retinoic Acid

Ling Lu[1,2], Xiaohui Zhou[1,3], Julie Wang[1], Song Guo Zheng[1*], David A. Horwitz[1*]

1 Division of Rheumatology, Department of Medicine, Keck School of Medicine at University of Southern California, Los Angeles, California, United States of America. 2 Department of Liver Transplantation, First Affiliated Hospital of Nanjing Medical University, Nanjing, China, 3 Immune Tolerance Center Shanghai East Hospital, Tonji University of Medicine, Shanghai, China

Abstract

Background: Protective CD4+CD25+ regulatory T cells bearing the Forkhead Foxp3 transcription factor can now be divided into three subsets: Endogenous thymus-derived cells, those induced in the periphery, and another subset induced ex-vivo with pharmacological amounts of IL-2 and TGF-β. Unfortunately, endogenous CD4+CD25+ regulatory T cells are unstable and can be converted to effector cells by pro-inflammatory cytokines. Although protective Foxp3+CD4+CD25+ cells resistant to proinflammatory cytokines have been generated in mice, in humans this result has been elusive. Our objective, therefore, was to induce human naïve CD4+ cells to become stable, functional CD25+ Foxp3+ regulatory cells that were also resistant to the inhibitory effects of proinflammatory cytokines.

Methodology/Principal Findings: The addition of the vitamin A metabolite, all-trans retinoic acid (atRA) to human naïve CD4+ cells suboptimally activated with IL-2 and TGF-β enhanced and stabilized FOXP3 expression, and accelerated their maturation to protective regulatory T cells. AtRA, by itself, accelerated conversion of naïve to mature cells but did not induce FOXP3 or suppressive activity. The combination of atRA and TGF-β enabled CD4+CD45RA+ cells to express a phenotype and trafficking receptors similar to natural Tregs. AtRA/TGF-β-induced CD4+ regs were anergic and low producers of IL-2. They had potent *in vitro* suppressive activity and protected immunodeficient mice from a human-anti-mouse GVHD as well as expanded endogenous Tregs. However, treatment of endogenous Tregs with IL-1β and IL-6 decreased FOXP3 expression and diminished their protective effects *in vivo* while atRA-induced iTregs were resistant to these inhibitory effects.

Conclusions/Significance: We have developed a methodology that induces human CD4⁺ cells to rapidly become stable, fully functional suppressor cells that are also resistant to proinflammatory cytokines. This methodology offers a practical novel strategy to treat human autoimmune diseases and prevent allograft rejection without the use of agents that kill cells or interfere with signaling pathways.

Vitamin A: NIH Guidelines

Office of
Dietary Supplements
National Institutes of Health

Table 3: Recommended Dietary Allowances (RDAs) for vitamin A

Age (years)	Children (mcg RAE)	Males (mcg RAE)	Females (mcg RAE)	Pregnancy (mcg RAE)	Lactation (mcg RAE)
1-3	300 (1,000 IU)				
4-8	400 (1,320 IU)				
9-13	600 (2,000 IU)				
14-18		900 (3,000 IU)	700 (2,310 IU)	750 (2,500 IU)	1,200 (4,000 IU)
19+		900 (3,000 IU)	700 (2,310 IU)	770 (2,565 IU)	1,300 (4,300 IU)

In Table 3, RDAs for vitamin A are listed as micrograms (mcg) of Retinol Activity Equivalents (RAE) to account for the different biological activities of retinol and provitamin A carotenoids. Table 3 also lists RDAs for vitamin A in International Units (IU), which are used on food and supplement labels (1 RAE = 3.3 IU).

http://ods.od.nih.gov/factsheets/vitamina/ Accessed August 2011

Causes of Inflammation-Immune-Metabolic Imbalance:

1. Food, Diet

2. Infection, Dysbiosis

3. Nutritional Immunomodulation

4. Dysfunctional mitochondria

5. Stress, Emotions, Psychology, Sociology

6. Endocrine, Hormones

7. Xenobiotics, Toxins

Vitamin D induces regulatory T-cells

Vitamin D is epigenetically active. Burrell. *Discov Med.* 2011

▸ Most "healthy" subjects were vitamin D deficient at the start of this study.

▸ Participants received one dose of vitamin D 140,000 IU (nonphysiologic dosing)

▸ Most patients were not corrected to optimal vitamin D status.

▸ **Benefit: Significant increase in Treg cells.**

Prietl, *Isr Med Assoc J.* 2010 Mar

ORIGINAL ARTICLES   IMAJ • VOL 12 • MARCH 2010

Vitamin D Supplementation and Regulatory T Cells in Apparently Healthy Subjects: Vitamin D Treatment for Autoimmune Diseases?

Barbara Prietl Msc[1]*, Stefan Pilz MD[1]*, Michael Wolf[1], Andreas Tomaschitz MD[1], Barbara Obermayer-Pietsch MD[1], Winfried Graninger MD[2] and Thomas R. Pieber MD[1,3]

[1]Division of Endocrinology and Nuclear Medicine, and [2]Division of Rheumatology and Immunology, Department of Internal Medicine, Medical University of Graz, and [3]Institute of Medical Technologies and Health Management, Joanneum Research, Graz, Austria

Causes of Inflammation-Immune-Metabolic Imbalance:

1. Food, Diet

2. Infection, Dysbiosis

3. Nutritional Immunomodulation

4. Dysfunctional mitochondria

5. Stress, Emotions, Psychology, Sociology

6. Endocrine, Hormones

7. Xenobiotics, Toxins

Vitamin D induces regulatory T-cells

- 15 patients with MS given Vitamin D3 20,000 IU per day for 3 months: Reasonable dose, short duration

- **Treg suppressive function improved** in several subjects, this effect was not significant in the total cohort (P = 0.143).

- **Increased suppressor T-cells**: an increased proportion of IL-10+CD4+T cells was found after supplementation (P = 0.021) =

- Note the lack of vitamin A, which must be administered with vitamin D to achieve benefit.

Safety and T Cell Modulating Effects of High Dose Vitamin D$_3$ Supplementation in Multiple Sclerosis

Joost Smolders[1,2,3], Evelyn Peelen[1,2,3], Mariëlle Thewissen[2], Jan Willem Cohen Tervaert[1,2,5], Paul Menheere[4], Raymond Hupperts[1,3], Jan Damoiseaux[2,5]

1 School for Mental Health and Neuroscience, Maastricht University Medical Center, Maastricht, The Netherlands. 2 Division of Clinical and Experimental Immunology, Department of Internal Medicine, Maastricht University Medical Center, Maastricht, The Netherlands. 3 Academic MS Center Limburg, Orbis Medical Center, Sittard, The Netherlands, 4 Department of Clinical Chemistry, Maastricht University Medical Center, Maastricht, The Netherlands, 5 Laboratory for Clinical Immunology, Maastricht University Medical Center, Maastricht, The Netherlands

Abstract

Background: A poor vitamin D status has been associated with a high disease activity of multiple sclerosis (MS). Recently, we described associations between vitamin D status and peripheral T cell characteristics in relapsing remitting MS (RRMS) patients. In the present study, we studied the effects of high dose vitamin D$_3$ supplementation on safety and T cell related outcome measures.

Methodology/Principal Findings: Fifteen RRMS patients were supplemented with 20 000 IU/d vitamin D$_3$ for 12 weeks. Vitamin D and calcium metabolism were carefully monitored, and T cell characteristics were studied by flowcytometry. All patients finished the protocol without side-effects, hypercalcaemia, or hypercalciuria. The median vitamin D status increased from 50 nmol/L (31–175) at week 0 to 380 nmol/L (151–535) at week 12 (P<0.001). During the study, 1 patient experienced a relapse of MS and was censored from the T cell analysis. The proportions of (naïve and memory) CD4+ Tregs improved in several subjects, this effect was not significant in the total supplementation. (P = 0.021)

Vitamin D3: optimize serum levels

Overview of Clinical Approach, Assessments, and Therapeutics

Proof of the cause-and-effect relationship between vitamin D deficiency and chronic musculoskeletal pain comes from clinical trials among deficient patients showing that vitamin D monotherapy alleviates pain. The exemplary study by Al Faraj and Al Mutairi[55] showed that among patients with "idiopathic chronic low back pain," 83% (n = 299) were vitamin D deficient, and supplementation with 5000 to 10 000 IU/d of cholecalciferol for 3 months alleviated or cured the low back pain in more than 95% of patients. The authors concluded that, in the evaluation of chronic musculoskeletal pain among populations with a sufficiently high prevalence of vitamin D deficiency, "screening for vitamin D deficiency and treatment with supplements should be mandatory in this setting."

Vitamin D has a wide range of safety according to an extensive review of the literature performed by Vieth.[225] Doses of 2000 IU/d of vitamin D3 have been given to children starting at 1 year of age and were not associated with toxicity but led to a reduction in the incidence of type 1 diabetes by 80%, consistent with the vitamin's anti-infective and immunomodulatory roles.[226] A 2004 review[56] on the clinical importance of vitamin D proposed that optimal vitamin D status is defined as 40 ng/mL to 65 ng/mL (100-160 nmol/L) and that "until proven otherwise, the balance of the research indicates that oral supplementation in the range of 1600 IU per day for infants, 2000 IU per day for children and 4000 IU per day for adults is safe and reasonable to meet physiological requirements, to promote optimal health, and to reduce the risk of several serious diseases. Safety and effectiveness of supplementation are assured by periodic monitoring of serum 25(OH)D and serum calcium." Current data and laboratory reference ranges support a higher top limit for serum 25(OH)D of approximately 100 ng/mL (250 nmol/L). Vitamin D hypersensitivity is seen with primary hyperparathyroidism, granulomatous diseases (such as sarcoidosis, Crohn's disease, and tuberculosis), adrenal insufficiency, hyperthyroidism, hypothyroidism, and various forms of cancer, as well as adverse drug effects, particularly with thiazide diuretics. Thiazide diuretics are known to potentiate hypercalcemia.

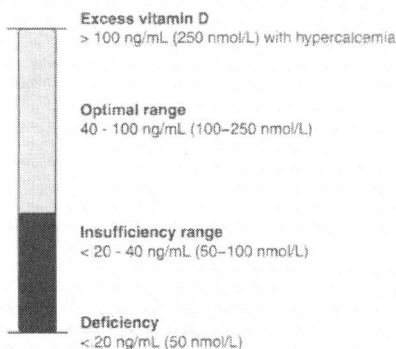

Excess vitamin D
> 100 ng/mL (250 nmol/L) with hypercalcemia

Optimal range
40 - 100 ng/mL (100–250 nmol/L)

Insufficiency range
< 20 - 40 ng/mL (50–100 nmol/L)

Deficiency
< 20 ng/mL (50 nmol/L)

Figure 2.1—Interpretation of Serum 25(OH)D Levels
Adapted from Vasquez A, Manso G, Cannell J. Altern Ther Health Med. 2004;10:28-37;36

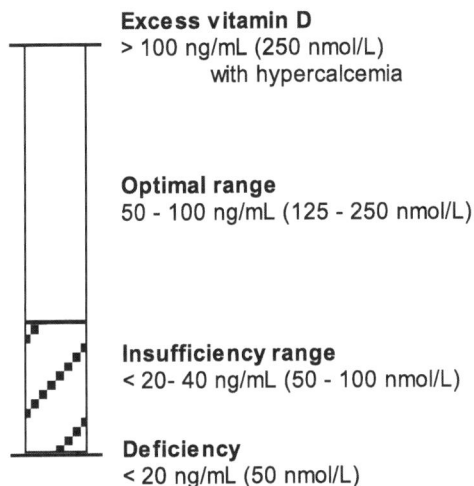

Excess vitamin D
> 100 ng/mL (250 nmol/L)
  with hypercalcemia

Optimal range
50 - 100 ng/mL (125 - 250 nmol/L)

Insufficiency range
< 20- 40 ng/mL (50 - 100 nmol/L)

Deficiency
< 20 ng/mL (50 nmol/L)

Interpretation of serum 25(OH) vitamin D levels.
Modified from Vasquez et al, *Alternative Therapies in Health and Medicine* 2004 and Vasquez A. *Musculoskeletal Pain: Expanded Clinical Strategies* (Institute for Functional Medicine) 2008.

http://optimalhealthresearch.com/cholecalciferol.html

Vitamin D3: clinical implementation protocol

BIOTICS RESEARCH CORPORATION

6801 Biotics Research Drive
Rosenberg, TX 77471
Toll Free: 1-800-231-5777
www.bioticsresearch.com

CME
CONTINUING MEDICAL EDUCATION

THE CLINICAL IMPORTANCE OF VITAMIN D (CHOLECALCIFEROL): A PARADIGM SHIFT WITH IMPLICATIONS FOR ALL HEALTHCARE PROVIDERS

Alex Vasquez, DC, ND, Gilbert Manso, MD, John Cannell, MD

Alex Vasquez, DC, ND, is a licensed naturopathic physician in Washington and Oregon, and licensed chiropractic doctor in Texas, where he maintains a private practice and is a member of the Research Team at Biotics Research Corporation. He is a former Adjunct Professor of Orthopedics and Rheumatology for the Naturopathic Medicine Program at Bastyr University. Gilbert Manso, MD, is a medical doctor practicing integrative medicine in Houston, Texas. In practice for more than 35 years, he is Board Certified in Family Practice and is Associate Professor of Family Medicine at University of Texas Medical School in Houston. John Cannell, MD, is a medical physician practicing in Atascadero, California, and is president of the Vitamin D Council (Cholecalciferol-Council.com), a non-profit, tax-exempt organization working to promote awareness of the manifold adverse effects of vitamin D deficiency.

THE LANCET.com   May 6, 2005

Subphysiologic Doses of Vitamin D are Subtherapeutic: Comment on the Study by The Record Trial Group

bmj.com

Calcium and vitamin D in preventing fractures

Data are not sufficient to show inefficacy

We provided six guidelines for interventional studies with vitamin D.[5] Dosages of vitamin D must reflect physiological requirements and natural endogenous production and should therefore be in the range of 3000-10 000 IU daily. Vitamin D supplementation must be continued for at least five to nine months. The form of vitamin D should be D_3 rather than D_2. Supplements should be assayed for potency. Effectiveness of supplementation must include measurement of serum 25-hydroxyvitamin D. Serum 25(OH)D concentrations must enter the optimal range, which is 40-65 ng/ml (100-160 nmol/l).

1. Appreciate and identify the manifold clinical presentations and consequences of vitamin D deficiency
2. Identify patient groups that are predisposed to vitamin D hypersensitivity
3. Know how to implement vitamin D supplementation in proper doses and with appropriate laboratory monitoring

the 5 10,000 IU that can be produced endogenously with full-body sun exposure.[2] With the discovery of vitamin D receptors in tissues other than the gut and bone—especially the brain, breast, prostate, and lymphocytes— and the recent research suggesting that higher vitamin D levels provide protection from diabetes mellitus, osteoporosis, osteoarthritis, hypertension, cardiovascular disease, metabolic syndrome, depression, several autoimmune diseases, and cancers of the breast, prostate, and colon, we can now utilize vitamin D for a wider range of preventive and therapeutic applications to maintain and improve our patients' health.[1] Based on the research reviewed in this article, the current authors believe that assessment of vitamin D status and treatment of vita-

http://optimalhealthresearch.com/cholecalciferol.html

Vitamin D3: clinical implementation

▸ <u>Rationale</u>: Benefits heart, glucose/insulin/diabetes, anti-inflammatory, immunomodulatory, anti-cancer, mood enhancement.

▸ <u>Dosing</u>: Infants and children 2,000 IU/d, Adults 4,000-10,000 IU/d to optimize serum 25-OH-vitamin D.

▸ <u>Safety margin</u>: Very wide.

▸ <u>Toxicity</u>: Mediated exclusively via hypercalcemia. Periodically monitor serum calcium.

▸ <u>Cautions/contraindications/considerations</u>: Use lower dose and frequent monitoring in patients with hypercalcemic states, sarcoidosis, and granulomatous diseases (lymphoma).

   ▹ <u>Hepatic/renal insufficiency</u>: Renal insufficiency reduces conversion to 1,25-di-OH-vitamin D; severe ESRD promotes hypercalcemia due to reduced renal excretion.

   ▹ <u>Drugs</u>: HCTZ (hydrochlorothiazide, used for HTN) reduces renal excretion of calcium and promotes hypercalcemia.

   http://optimalhealthresearch.com/cholecalciferol.html

Nutrition & FxMed for chronic immune-inflammatory disorders

Causes of Inflammation-Immune-Metabolic Imbalance:

1. Food, Diet

2. Infection, Dysbiosis

3. Nutritional Immunomodulation

4. Dysfunctional mitochondria

5. Stress, Emotions, Psychology, Sociology

6. Endocrine, Hormones

7. Xenobiotics, Toxins

Probiotics

▸ Rationale: "Probiotics" in general have been shown/suggested/correlated to have anti-inflammatory and anti-allergy anti-autoimmune activities, and recently two mechanistic explanations have been provided 1) direct via microbe-specific effects, and 2) indirect via the probiotic metabolite butyric acid.

▸ Dosing: Per product, per diet, billions/trillions organisms.

▸ Safety/Risks: Very safe; however, legitimate concern exists for exacerbation of SIBO, which can cause D-lactic acidosis and other inflammatory complications; probiotic-induced abscess/sepsis is rare but has been reported.

▸ Cautions/contraindications/considerations:

  ▸ Pregnancy/lactation: No special precautions.

  ▸ Hepatic/renal insufficiency: No special precautions; benefit shown in these groups.

  ▸ Drugs: Probiotic supplementation should be used nearly anytime antibiotics/antibacterials are administered.

Generation of regulatory dendritic cells and CD4+Foxp3+ T cells by probiotics administration suppresses immune disorders

PNAS 2010, J Nutr 2007

Ho-Keun Kwon[a], Choong-Gu Lee[a], Jae-Seon So[a], Chang-Suk Chae[a], Ji-Sun Hwang[a], Anupama Sahoo[a], Jong Hee Nam[b], Joon Haeng Rhee[b], Ki-Chul Hwang[c], and Sin-Hyeog Im[a,d,1]

[a]Department of Life Sciences, Gwangju Institute of Science and Technology, Gwangju 500-712, Korea; [b]Chonnam National University Medical School, Gwangju 501-749, Korea; [c]Cardiovascular Research Institute, Yonsei University College of Medicine, Seoul 120-752, Korea; and [d]Center for Distributed Sensor Network, Gwangju Institute of Science and Technology, Gwangju 500-712, Korea

Edited by Anjana Rao, Harvard Medical School, Boston, MA, and approved December 8, 2009 (received for review April 15, 2009)

The beneficial effects of probiotics have been described in many diseases, but the mechanism by which they modulate the immune system is poorly understood. In this study, we identified a m of probiotics that up-regulates CD4+Foxp3+ regulatory (Tregs). Administration of the probiotics mixture induced b cell and B-cell hyporesponsiveness and down-regulated T (Th) 1, Th2, and Th17 cytokines without apoptosis induction. induced generation of CD4+Foxp3+ Tregs from the CD4+CD25 ulation and increased the suppressor activity of naturally occ CD4+CD25+ Tregs. Conversion of T cells into Foxp3+ Tregs is d mediated by regulatory dendritic cells (rDCs) that express hi els of IL-10, TGF-β, COX-2, and indoleamine 2,3-dioxygenas ministration of probiotics had therapeutical effects in experi inflammatory bowel disease, atopic dermatitis, and rheum arthritis. The therapeutical effect of the probiotics is asso with enrichment of CD4+Foxp3+ Tregs in the inflamed regior lectively, the administration of probiotics that enhance the ation of rDCs and Tregs represents an applicable treatm inflammatory immune disorders.

regulatory T cell | inflammation | atopic dermatitis | inflammatory b disease | rheumatoid arthritis

dritic cells (rDCs) that express increased levels of IL-10, TGF-β, COX-2, and indoleamine 2,3-dioxygenase (iDO). Administration

Gastrointestinal microorganisms affect host phys through diverse mechanisms, including modulation host immune system. Probiotics are nonpathogenic

Antiallergic Effects of Probiotics[1,2]

Arthur C. Ouwehand*

Department of Biochemistry and Food Chemistry and Functional Foods Forum, University of Turku, 20014 Turku, Finland and Danisco Innovation, 02460 Kantvik, Finland

Abstract

A considerable part of the Western population suffers from some form of allergy, and the incidence is still rising with no sign of an end to this trend. Reduced exposure to microbial allergens as a result of our hygienic lifestyle has been suggested as one of the possible causes. It has also been suggested that probiotics may provide safe alternative microbial stimulation needed for the developing immune system in infants. This idea is supported by the fact that allergic infants have been observed to have an aberrant intestinal microbiota. They were shown to have more clostridia and fewer bifidobacteria and, in addition, to have an adult-like *Bifidobacterium* microbiota. Clinical trials have shown that the standard treatment of infants with atopic eczema, extensively hydrolyzed infant formula, can be significantly improved through the addition of *Lactobacillus rhamnosus* GG or *Bifidobacterium lactis* Bb-12. It has also been shown possible to halve the incidence of allergy in at-risk infants through administration of *L. rhamnosus* GG to expecting mothers and subsequently to their infants during the first half-year of life. Many mechanisms have been proposed for these beneficial effects, ranging from improved mucosal barrier function to direct influences on the immune system. However, the exact model(s) of action are not yet known. For the future, elucidation of these mechanisms will be an important target. Another important area will be the investigation of interactions between probiotics and other food components that influence allergies. This will enable optimization of probiotic use for the allergic subject. J Nutr. 137: 794S–797S, 2007.

Nutrition & FxMed for chronic immune-inflammatory disorders

Causes of Inflammation-Immune-Metabolic Imbalance:

1. Food, Diet

2. Infection, Dysbiosis

3. Nutritional Immunomodulation

4. Dysfunctional mitochondria

5. Stress, Emotions, Psychology, Sociology

6. Endocrine, Hormones

7. Xenobiotics, Toxins

Lipoic acid reduces IL-17 by 35-50% in vitro in patients with multiple sclerosis.

Salinthone, *PLoS One*. 2010 Sep

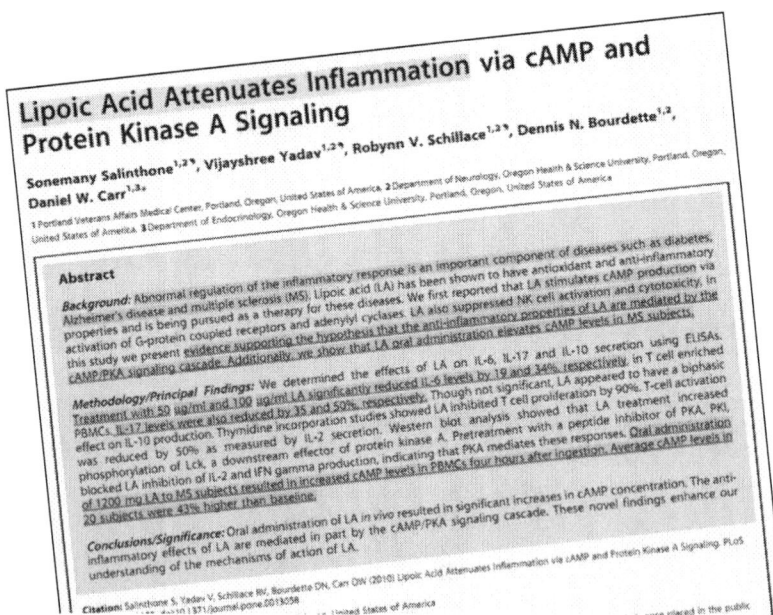

Lipoic Acid Attenuates Inflammation via cAMP and Protein Kinase A Signaling

Sonemany Salinthone[1,2*], Vijayshree Yadav[1,2*], Robynn V. Schillace[1,2*], Dennis N. Bourdette[1,2], Daniel W. Carr[1,3*]

1 Portland Veterans Affairs Medical Center, Portland, Oregon, United States of America. 2 Department of Neurology, Oregon Health & Science University, Portland, Oregon, United States of America. 3 Department of Endocrinology, Oregon Health & Science University, Portland, Oregon, United States of America.

Abstract

Background: Abnormal regulation of the inflammatory response is an important component of diseases such as diabetes, Alzheimer's disease and multiple sclerosis (MS). Lipoic acid (LA) has been shown to have antioxidant and anti-inflammatory properties and is being pursued as a therapy for these diseases. We first reported that LA stimulates cAMP production via activation of G-protein coupled receptors and adenylyl cyclases. LA also suppressed NK cell activation and cytotoxicity. In this study we present evidence supporting the hypothesis that the anti-inflammatory properties of LA are mediated by the cAMP/PKA signaling cascade. Additionally, we show that LA oral administration elevates cAMP levels in MS subjects.

Methodology/Principal Findings: We determined the effects of LA on IL-6, IL-17 and IL-10 secretion using ELISAs. Treatment with 50 µg/ml and 100 µg/ml LA significantly reduced IL-6 levels by 19 and 34%, respectively, in T cell enriched PBMCs. IL-17 levels were also reduced by 35 and 50%, respectively. Though not significant, LA appeared to have a biphasic effect on IL-10 production. Thymidine incorporation studies showed LA inhibited T cell proliferation by 90%. T-cell activation was reduced by 50% as measured by IL-2 secretion. Western blot analysis showed that LA treatment increased phosphorylation of Lck, a downstream effector of protein kinase A. Pretreatment with a peptide inhibitor of PKA, PKI, blocked LA inhibition of IL-2 and IFN gamma production, indicating that PKA mediates these responses. Oral administration of 1200 mg LA to MS subjects resulted in increased cAMP levels in PBMCs four hours after ingestion. Average cAMP levels in 20 subjects were 43% higher than baseline.

Conclusions/Significance: Oral administration of LA in vivo resulted in significant increases in cAMP concentration. The anti-inflammatory effects of LA are mediated in part by the cAMP/PKA signaling cascade. These novel findings enhance our understanding of the mechanisms of action of LA.

Citation: Salinthone S, Yadav V, Schillace RV, Bourdette DN, Carr DW (2010) Lipoic Acid Attenuates Inflammation via cAMP and Protein Kinase A Signaling. PLoS

Causes of Inflammation-Immune-Metabolic Imbalance:

1. Food, Diet

2. Infection, Dysbiosis

3. Nutritional Immunomodulation

4. Dysfunctional mitochondria

5. Stress, Emotions, Psychology, Sociology

6. Endocrine, Hormones

7. Xenobiotics, Toxins

N3 fatty acids have an anti-inflammatory (metabolic, nutrigenomic) and anti-autoimmune (epigenetic) effect that is mediated in part via induction of Treg cells.

▹ ## N3 fatty acids protect against autoimmune diabetes

▹ Subjects: 1770 children at increased risk for type 1 diabetes. Results: 1) omega-3 fatty acid intake was inversely associated with risk of IA (hazard ratio [HR], 0.45), 2) omega-3 fatty acid content of erythrocyte membranewas also inversely associated with IA risk (HR, 0.63

▹ **Conclusion: Dietary intake of omega-3 fatty acids is associated with reduced risk of [islet autoimmunity] in children at increased genetic risk for type 1 diabetes.**

Norris. *JAMA*. 2007 Sep

Nutri-immuno-epigenomics: GLA activates PPAR-gamma

DCs from other sites. In the present studies, using in vitro and in vivo approaches, we now demonstrate that PPARγ activation enhances iTreg generation through increased RA synthesis from murine splenic DCs and that endogenous PPARγ ligands may play a critical role in regulating iTreg generation.

Es probable que, some of the anti-inflammatory benefit of GLA is derived from GLA's activation of PPAR-gamma with works with/via retinol (vitamin A) for the induction of immunomodulating anti-allergy and anti-inflammatory Treg cells.

Housley. PPARgamma regulates retinoic acid-mediated DC induction of Tregs. *J Leukoc Biol.* 2009 Aug
Vasquez A. New Insights into Fatty Acid Supplementation and Its Effect on Eicosanoid Production and Genetic Expression. *Nutr Perspect* 2005; Jan

G Model
IMLET 5103 1–7

ARTICLE IN PRESS

Immunology Letters xxx (2011) xxx–xxx

Contents lists available at ScienceDirect

Immunology Letters

ELSEVIER

journal homepage: www.elsevier.com/locate/immlet

Induction of regulatory T cells by green tea polyphenol EGCG

Carmen P. Wong[a], Linda P. Nguyen[a], Sang K. Noh[b,c], Tammy M. Bray[a,b],
Richard S. Bruno[b], Emily Ho[a,d,*]

[a] Department of Nutrition and Exercise Sciences, Oregon State University, Corvallis, OR, USA
[b] Department of Nutritional Sciences, University of Connecticut, Storrs, CT, USA
[c] Department of Food and Nutrition, Changwon National University, Changwon, South Korea
[d] Linus Pauling Institute, Oregon State University, Corvallis, OR, USA

ARTICLE INFO

Article history:
Received 29 December 2010
Received in revised form 7 April 2011
Accepted 21 April 2011
Available online xxx

Keywords:
Regulatory T cells
Foxp3
DNA methylation
Green tea polyphenols

ABSTRACT

Regulatory T cells (Treg) are critical in maintaining immune tolerance and suppressing autoimmunity. The transcription factor Foxp3 serves as a master switch that controls the development and function of Treg. Foxp3 expression is epigenetically regulated by DNA methylation, and DNA methyltransferase

"Our data suggested that EGCG can induce Foxp3 expression and increase Treg frequency via a novel epigenetic mechanism."
Wong, *Immunol Lett.* 2011 Sep

1. Introduction

Regulatory T cells (Treg) play a pivotal role in the maintenance of immune tolerance and the suppression of autoimmunity [1,2]. Disruption of Treg development and function results in immune

CD4+ T cells using DNA methyltransferase (DNMT) inhibitors such as 5-aza-2′-deoxycytidine (Aza) results in de-repressed and stable expression of Foxp3, and the subsequent differentiation of naïve CD4+ T cells into Treg [4]. The epigenetic regulation of Foxp3 can be potentially exploited in generating suppressive Treg for ther-

Nutritional induction of regulatory T-cells

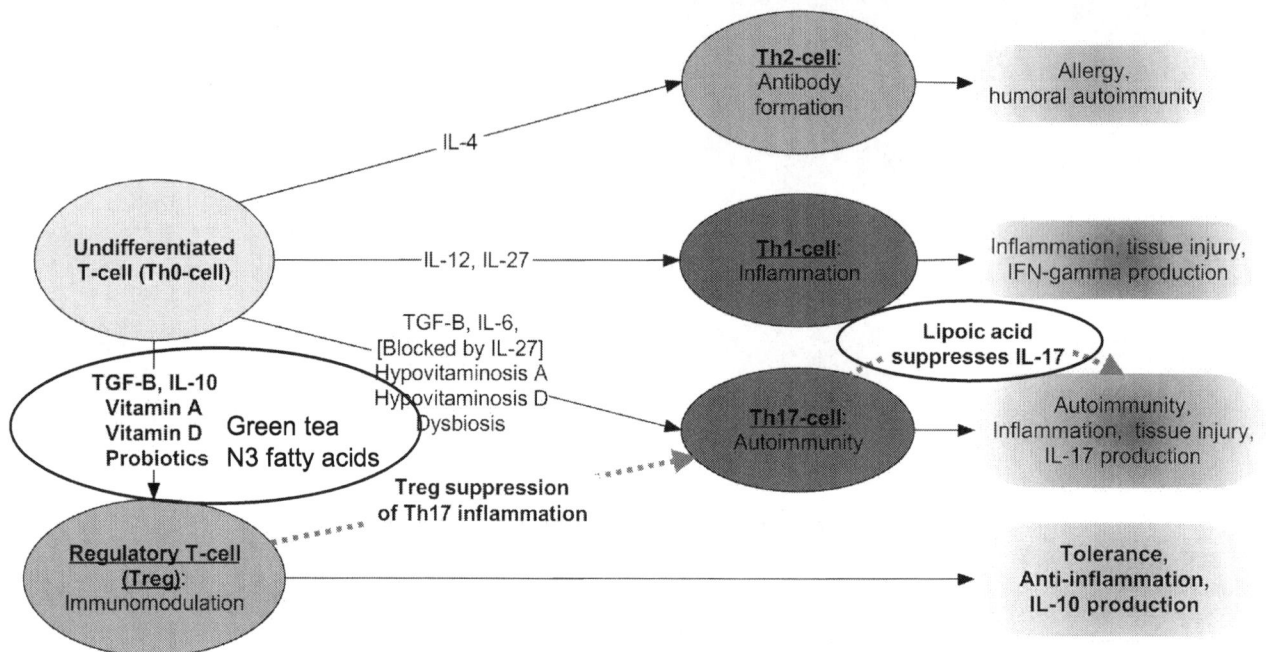

Excerpted Copyright 2012 Vasquez A. *Textbook of Nutritional and Functional Immunology: An Introduction to the Modifiable Factors in Chronic Inflammation, Allergy, and Autoimmunity.* http://**OptimalHealthResearch.com**/

Nutrition & FxMed for chronic immune-inflammatory disorders

Causes of Inflammation-Immune-Metabolic Imbalance:

1. Food, Diet

2. Infection, Dysbiosis

3. Nutritional Immunomodulation

4. Dysfunctional mitochondria

5. Stress, Emotions, Psychology, Sociology

6. Endocrine, Hormones

7. Xenobiotics, Toxins

Nutritional Immunomodulation: the nutrients

1. **Vitamin A**: *Dose*: at least 10,000 IU/d of "preformed" vitamin A, not beta-carotene.

2. **Vitamin D**: *Dose*: average 4,000 IU/d for adults.

3. **Probiotics, elimination of GI dysbiosis**: *Method*: use probiotics, plant-based diet, herbal and drug antimicrobials.

4. **Green tea**: *Dose*: tea & capsules.

5. **Lipoic acid**: *Dose*: 200-400 mg 3 times per day.

6. **N3 fatty acids**: activation of PPAR-g = Treg

Causes of Inflammation-Immune-Metabolic Imbalance:

1. Food, Diet

2. Infection, Dysbiosis

3. Nutritional Immunomodulation

4. Dysfunctional mitochondria

5. Stress, Emotions, Psychology, Sociology

6. Endocrine, Hormones

7. Xenobiotics, Toxins

Mitochondrial Dysfunction = Inflammation: Vasquez, *Mitochondrial Nutrition* 2012

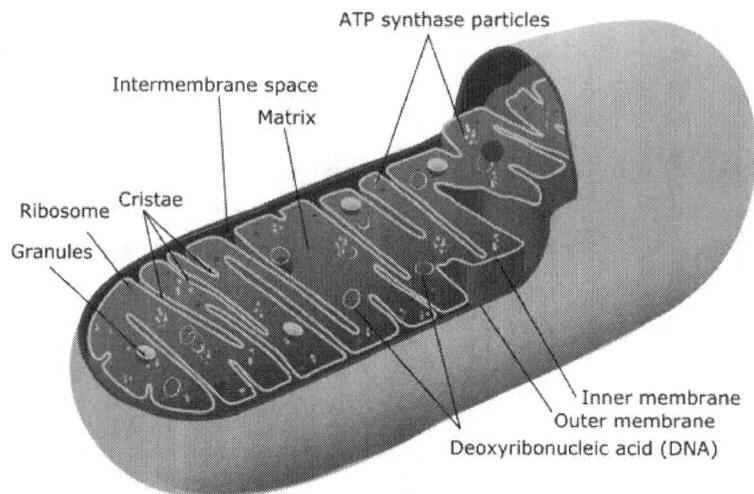

ATP synthase particles

Intermembrane space

Matrix

Ribosome   Cristae

Granules

Inner membrane
Outer membrane
Deoxyribonucleic acid (DNA)

Image from Wikimedia Commons: http://en.wikipedia.org/wiki/Mitochondrion

Causes of Inflammation-Immune-Metabolic Imbalance:

1. Food, Diet

2. Infection, Dysbiosis

3. Nutritional Immunomodulation

4. Dysfunctional mitochondria

5. Stress, Emotions, Psychology, Sociology

6. Endocrine, Hormones

7. Xenobiotics, Toxins

Mitochondrial dysfunction = disease

1. Inflammation: mitochondrial dysfunction contributes to cell senescence, chronic inflammation, and "inflammaging"

2. Allergy: especially asthma,

3. Autoimmunity: especially SLE and RA,

4. Metabolic Syndrome, Diabetes Type-2, Hypertension: mitochondria are required for insulin secretion and reception,

5. Heart failure: failure of energy production,

6. Fibromyalgia: histologic and biochemical evidence of mitochondrial failure, mitophagy,

7. Migraine: biochemical evidence of mitochondrial impairment,

8. Neurodegeneration—Parkinson's and Alzheimer's, et al: I think pretty much everyone should know this by now, especially regarding Parkinson's disease.

Mitochondrial dysfunction = disease (new)

1. Mitochondrial dysfunction increases allergic airway inflammation. *J Immunol* 2009 Oct

2. Mitochondrial dysfunction increases the inflammatory responsiveness to cytokines in normal human chondrocytes. *Arthritis Rheum* 2012 May

3. Mitochondrial dysfunction activates cyclooxygenase 2 expression in cultured normal human chondrocytes. *Arthritis Rheum* 2008 Aug

4. Age-Related Mitochondrial Dysfunction Sensitizes Human Synoviocytes to Inflammatory Response [abstract]: "The present study identifies for the first time mitochondria as organelles implicated in the proinflammatory response in human synoviocytes, since **mitochondrial dysfunction sensitizes these cells amplifying the inflammatory response induced by cytokines.**" *Arthritis Rheum* 2011

5. Mitochondrial dysfunction and biogenesis: do ICU patients die from mitochondrial failure? "Collectively the data discussed in this review suggest that appropriate diagnosis and **specific treatment of mitochondrial dysfunction in ICU patients may significantly improve the clinical outcome.**" *Ann Intensive Care* 2011 Sept

6. Effects of mitochondrial dysfunction on the immunological properties of microglia. *Journal of Neuroinflammation* 2010

Mitochondrial Dysfunction = Inflammation:

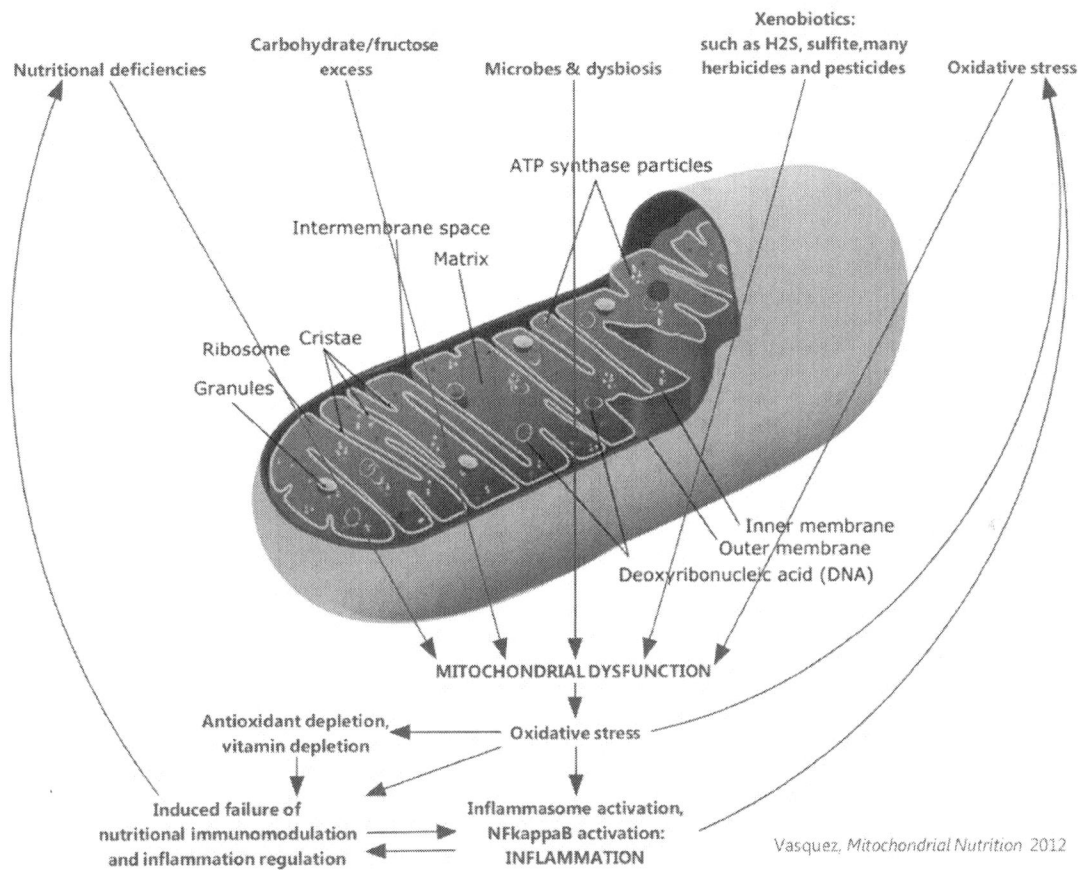

Nutritional deficiencies

Carbohydrate/fructose excess

Microbes & dysbiosis

Xenobiotics:
such as H2S, sulfite, many
herbicides and pesticides

Oxidative stress

ATP synthase particles

Intermembrane space

Matrix

Ribosome

Cristae

Granules

Inner membrane

Outer membrane

Deoxyribonucleic acid (DNA)

MITOCHONDRIAL DYSFUNCTION

Antioxidant depletion,
vitamin depletion

Oxidative stress

Induced failure of
nutritional immunomodulation
and inflammation regulation

Inflammasome activation,
NFkappaB activation:
INFLAMMATION

Vasquez, *Mitochondrial Nutrition* 2012

Nutrition & FxMed for chronic immune-inflammatory disorders

Causes of Inflammation-Immune-Metabolic Imbalance:

1. Food, Diet

2. Infection, Dysbiosis

3. Nutritional Immunomodulation

4. Dysfunctional mitochondria

5. Stress, Emotions, Psychology, Sociology

6. Endocrine, Hormones

7. Xenobiotics, Toxins

Mitochondria cause Inflammation: important concepts:

▸ "Mitochondria participate in the detection of infectious microorganisms and cellular damage to activate innate immune responses."

▸ "...likely that accumulation of damaged mitochondria is an important cause of inflammation."

▸ "...the removal of mitochondria that have a rather low threshold for permeabilization (mitochondrial "purging")."

▸ **"Exercise and caloric restriction stimulate autophagy** in most tissues..."

Green, *Science*. 2011 Aug

Causes of Inflammation-Immune-Metabolic Imbalance:

1. Food, Diet

2. Infection, Dysbiosis

3. Nutritional Immunomodulation

4. Dysfunctional mitochondria

5. Stress, Emotions, Psychology, Sociology

6. Endocrine, Hormones

7. Xenobiotics, Toxins

Mitochondrial Dysfunction: a self-perpetuating vicious cycle

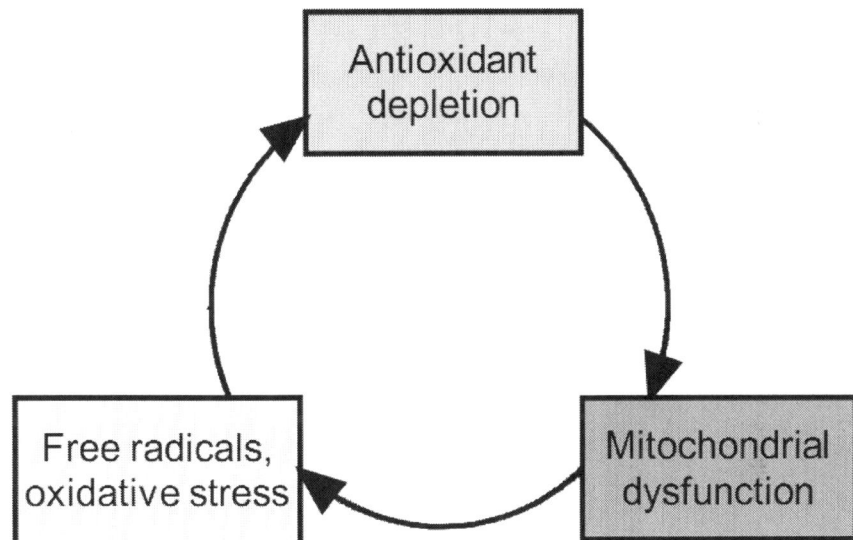

Causes of Inflammation-Immune-Metabolic Imbalance:

1. Food, Diet

2. Infection, Dysbiosis

3. Nutritional Immunomodulation

4. <u>Dysfunctional mitochondria</u>

5. Stress, Emotions, Psychology, Sociology

6. Endocrine, Hormones

7. Xenobiotics, Toxins

<u>Mitochondria cause Inflammation: important concepts:</u>

▸ Mitochondria have the ability to sense microbial (especially viral) infections and also to contribute to chronic inflammation.

▸ Dysfunctional mitochondria can be "purged" with **exercise** and **fasting**, and/or their function can be improved with nutritional supplementation, especially **CoQ-10, actyl-carnitine, lipoic acid**.

<u>Therapeutic implementation:</u>

> ▸ **Exercise:**

> ▸ **Therapeutic fasting and caloric restriction:**

> ▸ **Mitochondrial nutritional support: CoQ-10, acetyl-carnitine, resveratrol, and other nutrients**

Causes of Inflammation-Immune-Metabolic Imbalance:

1. Food, Diet

2. Infection, Dysbiosis

3. Nutritional Immunomodulation

4. Dysfunctional mitochondria

5. Stress, Emotions, Psychology, Sociology

6. Endocrine, Hormones

7. Xenobiotics, Toxins

Mitochondrial myopathy = ragged red fibers (seen in fibromyalgia):

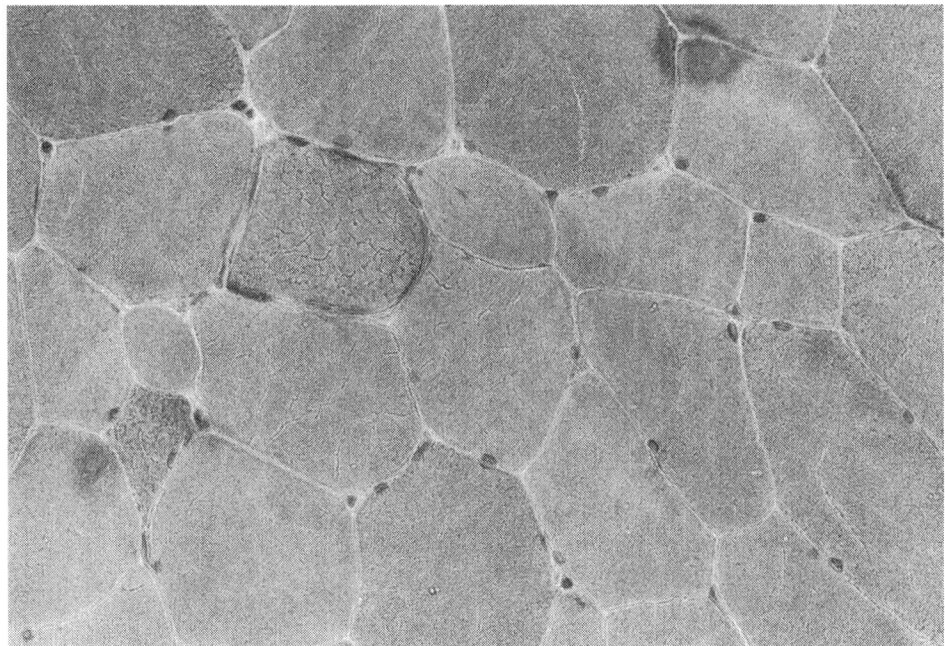

Muscle biopsy micrograph showing ragged red fibers, a finding seen in mitochondrial diseases. en.wikipedia.org/wiki/Ragged_red_fibres
Pongratz in *Z Rheumatol*. 1998;57 Suppl 2
Pongratz *Scand J Rheumatol* Suppl. 2000;113:3-7

Causes of Inflammation-Immune-Metabolic Imbalance:

1. Food, Diet

2. Infection, Dysbiosis

3. Nutritional Immunomodulation

4. Dysfunctional mitochondria

5. Stress, Emotions

6.

7.

Mitochondrial dysfunction: details and clinical applications:

▸ Mitochondrial dysfunction contributes to chronic inflammation, diabetes, hypertension, asthma, Parkinson's/Alzheimer's diseases, and fibromyalgia. *Exp Mol Pathol.* 2007 Aug

▸ We have at least 26 interventions to improve mitochondrial function, summarized in *Mitochondrial Nutrition* (July 2012).

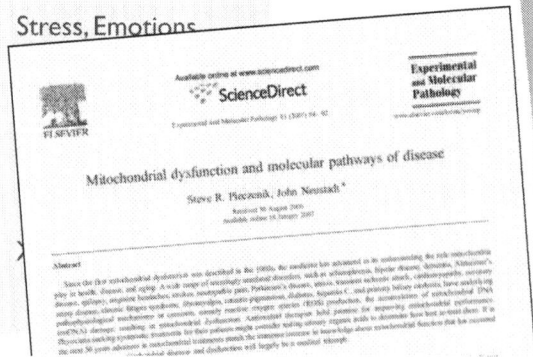

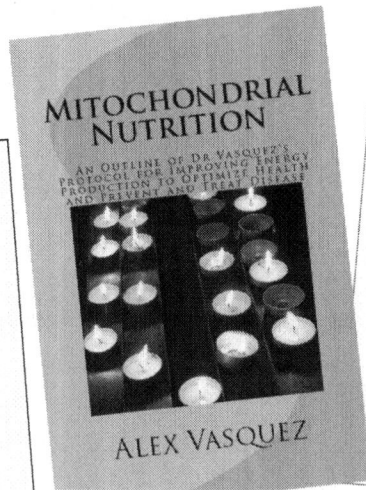

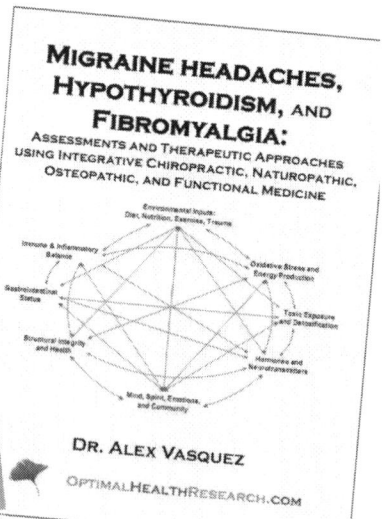

Causes of Inflammation-Immune-Metabolic Imbalance:

1. Food, Diet

2. Infection, Dysbiosis

3. Nutritional Immunomodulation

4. Mitochondrial dysfunctional

5. Stress, E

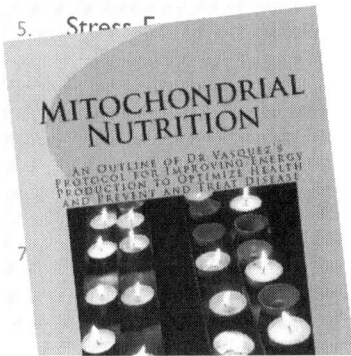

7

MitoDys treatments: We have at least 26 interventions to improve mitochondrial function, summarized in _Mitochondrial Nutrition_ (July 2012).

1. Fasting
2. Exercise
3. _____
4. _____
5. Lipoic acid
6. CoQ10
7. Acetyl-carnitine
8. _____
9. _____
10. _____
11. _____
12. _____
13. _____

14. _____
15. _____
16. _____
17. _____
18. _____
19. Herpes viruses kill mitochondrial DNA
20. _____
21. _____
22. _____
23. _____
24. _____
25. _____
26. _____

Stress, Emotions, Psychology, Sociology:

▸ We live in a fast-paced stressful world where we paradoxically have more "networks" and activities, yet less meaningful connection with people. "Problems of existence" are generally ignored in preference for entertainment/distraction, shopping, alcohol, drugs. I think many of these issues were best addressed by Fredrich Nietzsche PhD (*Twilight of the Idols*, and *Human, All to Human**) and Nathaniel Branden PhD (*Six Pillars of Self-Esteem*)

* http://video.google.com/videoplay?docid=-1842405914611103528

Mechanisms:

1. Mucosal immune suppression: reductions in sIgA
2. "Stress eating": people eat more wheat, sugar, alcohol when stressed; these promote inflammation, immune suppression, nutrient loss, oxidative stress, and increased gut permeability.
3. Microbial endocrinology: norepinephrine promotes microbial pathogenicity.
4. Sleep deprivation: promotes inflammation.

Nutrition & FxMed for chronic immune-inflammatory disorders

Causes of Inflammation-Immune-Metabolic Imbalance:

1. Food, Diet
2. Infection, Dysbiosis
3. Nutritional Immunomodulation
4. Dysfunctional mitochondria
5. Stress, Psychology, Sociology, Lifestyle
6. Endocrine, Hormones
7. Xenobiotics, Toxins

Causes of Inflammation-Immune-Metabolic Imbalance:

1. Food, Diet

2. Infection, Dysbiosis

3. Nutritional Immunomodulation

4. Dysfunctional mitochondria

5. Stress, Psychology, Sociology, Lifestyle

6. Endocrine, Hormones

7. Xenobiotics, Toxins

Stress, Sociology, Psychology, Lifestyle:

▶ RESULTS: **Participants categorized as poor sleepers on the basis of Pittsburgh Sleep Quality Index scores had significantly larger IL-6 responses to the cognitive stressors** than good sleepers. The association between poor sleep and **heightened IL-6 response** to acute stress was not explained by other psychosocial factors previously linked to immune Dysregulation, including depressive symptoms, perceived stress, and loneliness.

▶ CONCLUSIONS: Findings add to the growing evidence for poor sleep as an independent risk factor for poor mental and physical health. Older adults may be particularly vulnerable to effects of sleep disturbance due to significant age-related changes in sleep and inflammatory regulation."

Heffner. *Am J Geriatr Psychiatry.* 2012 Feb

Causes of Inflammation-Immune-Metabolic Imbalance:

1. Food, Diet

2. Infection, Dysbiosis

3. Nutritional Immunomodulation

4. Dysfunctional mitochondria

5. Stress, Emotions, Psychology, Sociology

6. Endocrine, Hormones

7. Xenobiotics, Toxins

Patients with inflammatory and autoimmune disorders have hormonal imbalances:

▸ Hormones modulate immune and inflammation balance; thus, **hormone imbalances cause immune imbalances**. Anti-inflammatory eumetabolic benefits are derived from optimization of hormone levels and correction of the underlying imbalances:

1. **Prolactin—high**: promotes inflammation, lymphocyte proliferation,

2. **Estradiol—high, imbalanced**: drives inflammation, lymphocyte proliferation, autoantibodies, DNA mutation.

3. **Fasting glucose <85 mg/dL, HgbA1c 4-5%, Insulin <5 microIU/mL,**: Hyperinsulinemia is a marker for chronic hyperglycemia and insulin resistance, which correlate directly with inflammation, oxidative stress, atherosclerosis, visceral adiposity, hypertension, hypercoagulability. Lindeberg *Metabolism* 1999 Oct, Brewer *Diabetes Care* 2008 Jun and discussion with Bill Beakey, Todd LePine, Umahro Cadogan, Maelan Fontes, Kara Fitzgerald, Pedro Bastos.

1. **Low DHEA**: immunomodulatory,

2. **Low cortisol**: immunomodulatory,

3. **Low testosterone**: immunomodulatory.

Vasquez A. *Integrative Rheumatology, Second Edition*, chapter 4

34yoM presented for consultation on "possible psoriatic arthritis"

▶ <u>Presentation</u>: several years of debilitating joint pain; additional complaints.

▶ <u>US Dermatologist</u>: "classic psoriatic flare" following use of penicillin for dental procedure,

▶ <u>Two US rheumatologists</u>: "uncertain of exact diagnosis", positive response to prednisone, recommended to start so-called "biologic" drug infliximab/Remicade,

▶ <u>Physicians in Mexico</u>: prescribed the usual gamut of anti-inflammatory drugs; to their credit they found that the patient is CCP+ and RF+ and that the patient shows exposure to *Proteus*.

▶ <u>Physical examination</u>:

  ▷ One psoriatic patch measuring 2x2 inches, no pitting of nails,

  ▷ Obesity at BMI 42 = Obese Class III (very severely obese, morbid obesity),

  ▷ Hypertension 145/95

Patients with inflammatory and autoimmune disorders often have multiple hormonal imbalances, metabolic disturbances, and autoimmune disorders:

▸ This 34yoM presented for consultation on "possible psoriatic arthritis" and was also found to have conjugate seropositivity for RA, as well as thyroiditis.

Date and Time Collected	Date Entered	Date and Time Reported	Physician Name	NPI	Physician ID
05/24/12 14:42	05/24/12	05/30/12 15:39ET	VASQUEZ , A		

TESTS	RESULT	FLAG	UNITS	REFERENCE INTERVAL	LAB
Testosterone, F Eqlib+T LC/MS					
Testosterone, Total, LC/MS	**334.1**	Low	ng/dL	348.0 - 1197.0	Low
Testosterone, Free	7.85		ng/dL	5.00 - 21.00	testosterone
% Free Testosterone	2.35		%	1.50 - 4.20	
Thyroid Antibodies					
Thyroid Peroxidase (TPO) Ab	**235**	High	IU/mL	0 - 34	Thyroid
		Please note reference interval change			autoimmunity
Antithyroglobulin Ab	<20		IU/mL	0 - 40	
Siemens (DPC) ICMA Methodology					
Hemoglobin A1c	5.4		%	4.8 - 5.6	Glucose acceptable but slight insulin resistance
Increased risk for diabetes: 5.7 - 6.4					
Diabetes: >6.4					
Glycemic control for adults with diabetes: <7.0					
Thyroxine (T4) Free, Direct, S					
T4,Free(Direct)	1.12		ng/dL	0.82 - 1.77	
DHEA-Sulfate	267.7		ug/dL	160.0 - 449.0	
TSH	3.510		uIU/mL	0.450 - 4.500	Slight high TSH
Prolactin	5.6		ng/mL	4.0 - 15.2	
Estradiol	28.4		pg/mL	7.6 - 42.6	Test./Est. imbalance
Roche ECLIA methodology					
Reverse T3, Serum	25.5		ng/dL	13.5 - 34.2	Vitamin D deficiency
Vitamin D, 25-Hydroxy	**19.4**	Low	ng/mL	30.0 - 100.0	

Patients with inflammatory and autoimmune disorders often have multiple hormonal imbalances, metabolic disturbances, and autoimmune disorders:

▸ This 34yoM presented for consultation on "possible psoriatic arthritis" and was also found to have conjugate seropositivity for RA, as well as thyroiditis.

Date and Time Collected	Date Entered	Date and Time Reported	Physician Name	NPI	Physician ID
05/24/12 14:42	05/24/12	05/30/12 15:39ET	VASQUEZ , A		

Account Number	Patient ID	Control Number	Date and Time Collected	Date Reported	Sex	Age(Y/M/D)	Date of Birth
			05/24/12 14:42	05/30/12	M	34/05/02	

TESTS	RESULT	FLAG	UNITS	REFERENCE INTER

1. IOM (Institute of Medicine). 2010. Dietary reference intakes for calcium and D. Washington DC: The National Academies Press.
2. Holick MF, Binkley NC, Bischoff-Ferrari HA, et al. Evaluation, treatment, and prevention of vitamin D deficiency: an Endocrine Society clinical practice guideline. JCEM. 2011 Jul; 96(7):1911-30.

```
t-Transglutaminase (tTG) IgA        <2              U/mL            0 - 3
                                                    Negative        0 - 3
                                                    Weak Positive   4 - 10
                                                    Positive        >10
```

> Probably no celiac disease unless pt has selective sIgA deficiency. Regardless, this pt must avoid wheat and other grains (rice acceptable).

Tissue Transglutaminase (tTG) has been identified as the endomysial antigen. Studies have demonstrated that endomysial IgA antibodies have over 99% specificity for gluten sensitive enteropathy.

```
Triiodothyronine (T3)               128             ng/dL           71 - 180
Ferritin, Serum                     234             ng/mL           30 - 400
```

> Ferritin slightly elevated but probably secondary to inflammation along with quite probable hemochromatosis heterozysity. Vasquez. *Arthritis Rheum.* 1996 Oct

> Thyroid hormone prescribed per autoimmunity, fatigue, et al.

Patients with inflammatory and autoimmune disorders often have multiple hormonal imbalances, metabolic disturbances, and autoimmune disorders:

▸ This 34yoM presented for consultation on "possible psoriatic arthritis" and was also found to have conjugate seropositivity for RA, as well as thyroiditis.

EXAMEN GENERAL DE ORINA

EDAD   33 AÑOS   Sexo M

PRUEBA	RESULTADO		REFERENCIA	
Densidad	+1.030		1.01 - 1.03	
pH	5.5		5.00 8.00	
Proteinas	0	mg/dl	0	mg/dl
Glucosa	0	mg/dl	0	mg/dl
Cetonas	0	mg/dl	0	mg/dl
Bilirrubinas	0		0	
Urobilinogeno	NORMAL		0.2	E.U./dl.
Hemoglobina	0		0	
Nitritos	NEGATIVO		Negativo	

> **Chronic mild metabolic acidosis promotes hypertension, insulin resistance, chronic inflammation.** *Clin Nutr 2011 Aug*

Examen Microscopico 40x

Leucocitos:	0 A 1 POR 3 CAMPOS	Piocitos:	0
Eritrocitos:	0	Cilindros:	0
Cristales:	0	Bacterias:	MODERADAS
Filamento Moco:	MODERADO	Levaduras:	0
Cels. Epiteliales:	ESCASAS		

> **Probable genitourinary dysbiosis.** *Br J Rheumatol 1995 Sep*

Patients with inflammatory and autoimmune disorders often have multiple hormonal imbalances, metabolic disturbances, and autoimmune disorders:

▸ This 34yoM presented for consultation on "possible psoriatic arthritis" and was also found to have conjugate seropositivity for RA, as well as thyroiditis.

QUIMICA CLINICA

Equipo: ARCHITECT CI8200

ESTUDIO	RESULTADO	UNIDAD	REFERENCIA
QUIMICA SANGUINEA			
GLUCOSA	91	mg/dL	70.00-105.00
NITROGENO UREICO	17	mg/dL	9.00-21.00
UREA	36	mg/dL	19.00-45.00
CREATININA	1.07	mg/dL	0.70-1.30
COLESTEROL TOTAL	190	mg/dL	50.00-200.00
TRIGLICERIDOS	126	mg/dL	45.00-150.00
ACIDO URICO	4.7	mg/dL	3.50-7.20
FACTOR REUMATOIDE	*98.7	IU/ml	0.00-30.00

** RESULTADO VERIFICADO

Mild metabolic syndrome: pt is also obese and hypertensive

Rheumatoid factor is positive

Patients with inflammatory and autoimmune disorders often have multiple hormonal imbalances, metabolic disturbances, and autoimmune disorders:

▸ This 34yoM presented for consultation on "possible psoriatic arthritis" and was also found to have conjugate seropositivity for RA, as well as thyroiditis.

FECHA 24/08/2011 **#** 200037

EDAD 33 AÑOS **Sexo** M

REFERENCIAS

ESTUDIO	RESULTADO	UNIDAD	REFERENCIA
Acs. ANTI PEPTIDO CICLICO CITRULINADO (Ac. CCP) IgG	*200.0	U/mL	0.00-5.00
Ac. ANTI-NUCLEARES	NEGATIVOS		NEGATIVOS

Anti-CCP antibodies are highly positive, correlating with aggressive rheumatoid arthritis.

Note that rheumatoid factor is also positive; thus, this patient has "conjugate seropositivity" for rheumatoid arthritis which correlates with aggressive disease.

Patients with inflammatory and autoimmune disorders often have multiple hormonal imbalances, metabolic disturbances, and autoimmune disorders:

▸ This 34yoM presented for consultation on "possible psoriatic arthritis" and was also found to have conjugate seropositivity for RA, as well as thyroiditis.

FECHA   20/08/2011   # 200037

EDAD   33 AÑOS   **Sexo** M

INMUNOLOGIA

ESTUDIO   RESULTADO

REACCIONES FEBRILES

ESTUDIO	RESULTADO
PARATIFICO A	**NEGATIVO**
PARATIFICO B	**NEGATIVO**
TIFICO O	**NEGATIVO**
TIFICO H	**NEGATIVO**
PROTEUS OX - 19	**POSITIVO 1:80**
BRUCELLA HUDDLESON	**NEGATIVO**

Método: Aglutinación en placa.

> *Proteus mirabilis* and *Proteus vulgaris* are both strongly correlated with both rheumatoid arthritis and psoriasis.
>
> Vasquez, *Integrative Rheumatology, Second Edition*.

Causes of Inflammation-Immune-Metabolic Imbalance:

1. Food, Diet

2. Infection, Dysbiosis

3. Nutritional Immunomodulation

4. Dysfunctional mitochondria

5. Stress, Emotions, Psychology, Sociology

6. Endocrine, Hormones

7. Xenobiotics, Toxins

Xenobiotic/toxin (mercury, lead, chemical persistent organic pollutants [POPs]) cause inflammation:

▸ <u>Toxins impair metabolic function</u>: mercury and lead promote hypertension; mercury promotes drug-resistance by bacteria.

▸ <u>Toxins promote insulin resistance</u>: well-established in diabetes: "…any effort to reduce the external and internal exposure to POPs would be necessary to decrease the social burden of type 2 diabetes. Lee, *Epidemiol Health.* 2012

▸ <u>Toxins lower immunity</u>: Lower IgG

▸ <u>Toxins promote autoimmunity</u>: Higher levels of ANA—antinuclear antibodies. Cooper, *Environ Health Perspect.* 2004 Jul

Toxin awareness / detoxification support are necessary!

Causes of Inflammation-Immune-Metabolic Imbalance:

1. Food, Diet

2. Infection, Dysbiosis

3. Nutritional Immunomodulation

4. Dysfunctional mitochondria

5. Stress, Emotions, Psychology, Sociology

6. Endocrine, Hormones

7. Xenobiotics, Toxins

13 pesticides in body of average American:

▸ "A comprehensive survey of more than 1,300 Americans has found traces of **weed- and bug-killers [herbicides and pesticides] in the bodies of everyone tested**, leading environmentalists in both Canada and the United States to call for far tighter controls on pesticides."

▸ "The survey, conducted by the U.S. Centers for Disease Control and Prevention, found that **the body of the average American contained 13 of these chemicals**.

The Globe and Mail, Friday May 21, 2004, Page A17
http://www.theglobeandmail.com/life/article927534.ece

Toxin awareness / detoxification support are necessary!

Nutrition & FxMed for chronic immune-inflammatory disorders

Causes of Inflammation-Immune-Metabolic Imbalance:

1. Food, Diet

2. Infection, Dysbiosis

3. Nutritional Immunomodulation

4. Dysfunctional mitochondria

5. Stress, Emotions, Psychology, Sociology

6. Endocrine, Hormones

7. Xenobiotics, Toxins

Everyone in the world has hexachlorobenzene/ perchlorobenzene:
fungicide (banned?), industrial pollution continues at 4,000 tons/y in USA.

▶ **This probably includes *you*.**

▶ **"world-wide detectable levels are approaching 100% and average residue levels tend to increase with age.** World-wide HCB levels are higher in females...."

An evaluation of hexachlorobenzene body-burden levels in the general population of the USA. *IARC Sci Publ.* 1986

Toxin awareness / detoxification support are necessary!

Causes of Inflammation-Immune-Metabolic Imbalance:

1. Food, Diet

2. Infection, Dysbiosis

3. Nutritional Immunomodulation

4. Dysfunctional mitochondria

5. Stress, Emotions, Psychology, Sociology

6. Endocrine, Hormones

7. Xenobiotics, Toxins

Everyone in the world has hexachlorobenzene/perchlorobenzene:

▸ "Persistent environmental pollutant,

▸ "HCB has **immunotoxic properties** in laboratory animals and probably also in man,

▸ "**Stimulatory effects** on spleen and lymph node weights and histology,

▸ "increased serum IgM levels, and an enhancement of several parameters of immune function.

▸ "Moreover, more recent studies indicate that HCB-induced effects in the rat may be related to **autoimmunity**.

▸ "In Wistar rats exposed to HCB, IgM **antibodies against several autoantigens were elevated**; in the Lewis rat, HCB differently modulated two experimental models of autoimmune disease.

▸ "Such a thymus-independent immunopathology is remarkable, as HCB strongly modulates T-cell-mediated immune parameters. This points at a very complex mechanism and possible involvement of multiple factors in the immunopathology of HCB.

Environ Health Perspect. 1999 Oct

Toxin awareness / detoxification support are necessary!

Causes of Inflammation-Immune-Metabolic Imbalance:

1. Food, Diet

2. Infection, Dysbiosis

3. Nutritional Immunomodulation

4. Dysfunctional mitochondria

5. Stress, Emotions, Psychology, Sociology

6. Endocrine, Hormones

7. Xenobiotics, Toxins

Diabetes mellitus type-2 is linked to accumulation of dioxins/toxins—epidemiology and biologic plausibility:

▸ "Specifically, we suggest that **aryl hydrocarbon (Ah) receptor functions may antagonize peroxisome proliferator-activated receptor (PPAR) functions**, and hence that the Ah receptor may promote diabetogenesis through a mechanism of PPAR antagonism."

Environ Health Perspect. 2002 Sep;110(9):853-8

http://www.ncbi.nlm.nih.gov/pmc/articles/PMC1240982

Toxin awareness / detoxification support are necessary!

Causes of Inflammation-Immune-Metabolic Imbalance:

1. Food, Diet

2. Infection, Dysbiosis

3. Nutritional Immunomodulation

4. Dysfunctional mitochondria

5. Stress, Emotions, Psychology, Sociology

6. Endocrine, Hormones

7. Xenobiotics, Toxins

Parkinson's disease strongly linked to persistent organic pollutants (POPs):

▸ "These findings are not inconsistent [ie, they *are consistent*] with the hypothesis derived from epidemiological work and animal studies that **organochlorine insecticides produce a direct toxic action on the dopaminergic tracts of the substantia nigra** and may contribute to the **development of PD in those rendered susceptible by virtue of cytochrome P-450 polymorphism, excessive exposure,** or other factors."

J Toxicol Environ Health. 2000 Feb 25

Toxin awareness / detoxification support are necessary!

Causes of Inflammation-Immune-Metabolic Imbalance:

1. Food, Diet

2. Infection, Dysbiosis

3. Nutritional Immunomodulation

4. Dysfunctional mitochondria

5. Stress, Emotions, Psychology, Sociology

6. Endocrine, Hormones

7. Xenobiotics. Toxins

Xenobiotics & toxic metals:

▸ Toxins lower immunity (lower IgG) and promote autoimmunity via higher levels of ANA—antinuclear antibodies. Cooper, *Environ Health Perspect.* 2004 Jul

▸ **Mercury**: known to increase ANA production, promote colonization by drug-resistant bacteria, and to increase IgE-mediated allergies.

  ▸ Mercury and acute eczema: "The results of this population-based case-control study in children with **acute eczema** show a strong association between the body burden of mercury and disease state, indicating a possible role for mercury as triggering factor."

  ▸ clear-cut relation between body burdens of mercury and acute but not chronic AE.

  ▸ Children with amalgam fillings = higher urinary mercury,

  ▸ Significantly higher risk for acute eczematous lesions with higher urinary mercury concentrations,

  ▸ **positive and linear association between mercury and serum levels of total IgE.**

  ▸ Perhaps mercury exacerbates allergic disorders by promoting a TH2-cytokine profile and facilitating production of IgE against yet unknown antigens, such as autoantigens.

Weidinger, *J Allergy Clin Immunol,* 2004 Oct

Toxin awareness / detoxification support

are necessary!

Nutrition & FxMed for chronic immune-inflammatory disorders

Causes of Inflammation-Immune-Metabolic Imbalance:

1. Food, Diet

2. Infection, Dysbiosis

3. Nutritional Immunomodulation

4. Dysfunctional mitochondria

5. Stress, Emotions, Psychology, Sociology

6. Endocrine, Hormones

7. Xenobiotics, Toxins

Accumulation of "persistent organic pollutants" (POPs) = insulin resistance = MetSyn

▸ <u>Mechanism</u>: Exposure to and accumulation of toxic chemicals leads to activation of the Aryl hydrocarbon receptor, which causes downregulation (suppressed expression) of GLUT-4 insulin receptors, thus leading to insulin resistance. (*J Med Toxicol* 2010; 6:275. *Lancet* 2008 Jan)

▸ <u>Solution</u>: Detoxification programs, or—better yet—*detoxification as a lifestyle.*

Toxicant Exposures and the Obesity Epidemic

William J. Meggs · Kori L. Brewer

Published online: 13 April 2010
© American College of Medical Toxicology 201

Environmental pollution and diabetes: a neglected association

Using cross-sectional data from the 1999-2002 US National Health and Examination Survey, Duk-Hee Lee and colleagues[1,2] reported a strong correlation between insulin resistance and serum concentrations of persistent organic pollutants, especially for organochlorine compounds. This result was a surprise for many people and fatty liver.[5] The versatility of high-throughput screening in metabolomics and metabonomics is an especially useful way of monitoring metabolic changes caused by disease or exposure to toxicants (eg, heavy metals) in animal models.[10] Although most studies have tested acute exposure (ie, less than 2 weeks) in the few

The Art of Therapeutic Detoxification

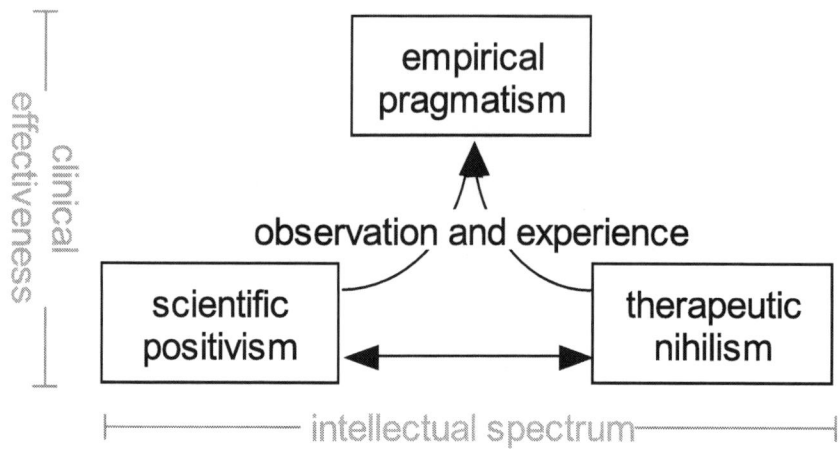

Nutrition & FxMed for chronic immune-inflammatory disorders

Causes of Inflammation-Immune-Metabolic Imbalance:

1. Food, Diet

2. Infection, Dysbiosis

3. Nutritional Immunomodulation

4. Dysfunctional mitochondria

5. Stress, Emotions, Psychology, Sociology

6. Endocrine, Hormones

7. Xenobiotics, Toxins

Vasquez A. *Integrative Rheumatology*, chap 4

Causes of Inflammation-Immune-Metabolic Imbalance:

1. Food, Diet

2. Infection, Dysbiosis

3. Nutritional Immunomodulation

4. Dysfunctional mitochondria

5. Stress, Emotions, Psychology, Sociology

6. Endocrine, Hormones

7. Xenobiotics, Toxins

Common problems in "detoxification"

1. Oxidation: Phase 1
   - Inhibition: too slow
   - Imbalanced: too fast relative to phase 2
2. Conjugation
   - Too slow
   - Unsupported
3. Urinary excretion
   - Hydration
   - Urinary pH
4. Biliary-colonic excretion
   - Insufficient bile flow
   - Enterohepatic recirculation
   - Deconjugation by microflora
   - Constipation
5. Failure to limit/reduce exposure

Vasquez A. *Integrative Rheumatology*, chap 4

Causes of Inflammation-Immune-Metabolic Imbalance:

1. Food, Diet

2. Infection, Dysbiosis

3. Nutritional Immunomodulation

4. Dysfunctional mitochondria

5. Stress, Emotions, Psychology, Sociology

6. Endocrine, Hormones

7. Xenobiotics, Toxins

Detoxification: from exposure to excretion

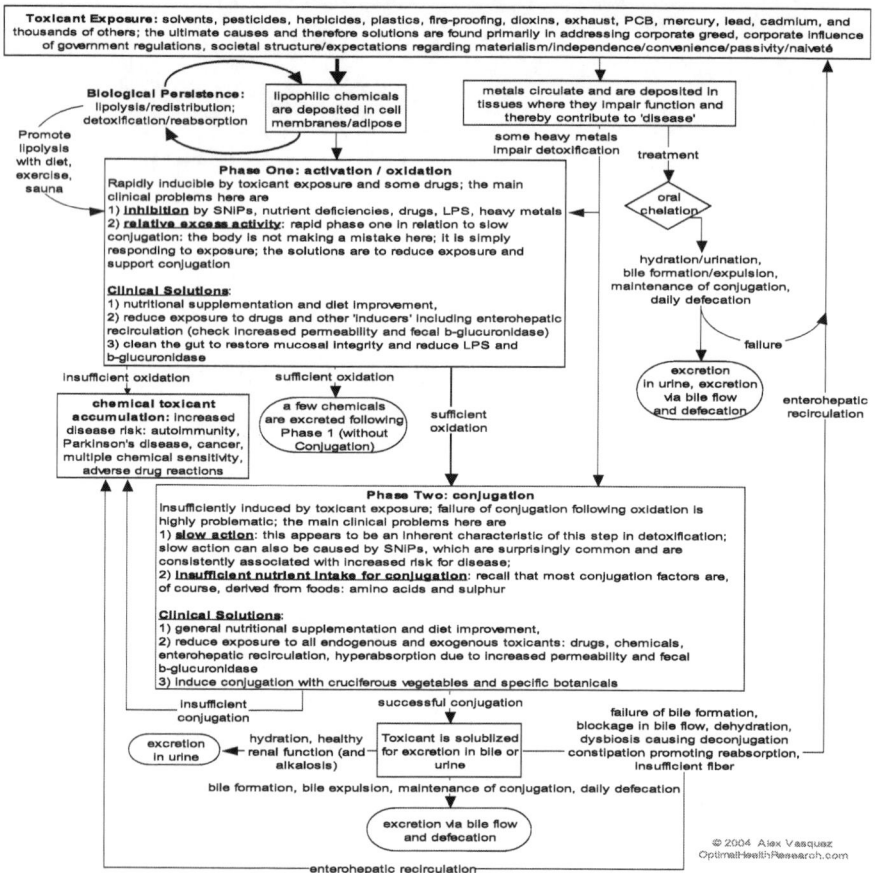

Toxicant Exposure: solvents, pesticides, herbicides, plastics, fire-proofing, dioxins, exhaust, PCB, mercury, lead, cadmium, and thousands of others; the ultimate causes and therefore solutions are found primarily in addressing corporate greed, corporate influence of government regulations, societal structure/expectations regarding materialism/independence/convenience/passivity/naiveté

Biological Persistence: lipolysis/redistribution; detoxification/reabsorption

lipophilic chemicals are deposited in cell membranes/adipose

metals circulate and are deposited in tissues where they impair function and thereby contribute to 'disease'

some heavy metals impair detoxification

treatment

Promote lipolysis with diet, exercise, sauna

oral chelation

Phase One: activation / oxidation
Rapidly inducible by toxicant exposure and some drugs; the main clinical problems here are
1) **inhibition** by SNIPs, nutrient deficiencies, drugs, LPS, heavy metals
2) **relative excess activity**: rapid phase one in relation to slow conjugation: the body is not making a mistake here; it is simply responding to exposure; the solutions are to reduce exposure and support conjugation

Clinical Solutions:
1) nutritional supplementation and diet improvement,
2) reduce exposure to drugs and other 'inducers' including enterohepatic recirculation (check increased permeability and fecal b-glucuronidase)
3) clean the gut to restore mucosal integrity and reduce LPS and b-glucuronidase

hydration/urination, bile formation/expulsion, maintenance of conjugation, daily defecation

failure

excretion in urine, excretion via bile flow and defecation

enterohepatic recirculation

insufficient oxidation

sufficient oxidation

chemical toxicant accumulation: increased disease risk: autoimmunity, Parkinson's disease, cancer, multiple chemical sensitivity, adverse drug reactions

a few chemicals are excreted following Phase 1 (without Conjugation)

sufficient oxidation

Phase Two: conjugation
Insufficiently induced by toxicant exposure; failure of conjugation following oxidation is highly problematic; the main clinical problems here are
1) **slow action**: this appears to be an inherent characteristic of this step in detoxification; slow action can also be caused by SNIPs, which are surprisingly common and are consistently associated with increased risk for disease;
2) **insufficient nutrient intake for conjugation**: recall that most conjugation factors are, of course, derived from foods: amino acids and sulphur

Clinical Solutions:
1) general nutritional supplementation and diet improvement,
2) reduce exposure to all endogenous and exogenous toxicants: drugs, chemicals, enterohepatic recirculation, hyperabsorption due to increased permeability and fecal b-glucuronidase
3) induce conjugation with cruciferous vegetables and specific botanicals

insufficient conjugation

successful conjugation

failure of bile formation, blockage in bile flow, dehydration, dysbiosis causing deconjugation constipation promoting reabsorption, insufficient fiber

excretion in urine

hydration, healthy renal function (and alkalosis)

Toxicant is solubilized for excretion in bile or urine

bile formation, bile expulsion, maintenance of conjugation, daily defecation

excretion via bile flow and defecation

enterohepatic recirculation

© 2004 Alex Vasquez
OptimalHealthResearch.com

Vasquez A. *Integrative Rheumatology*, chap 4

The new approach to disease treatment

Treat the Causes of Inflammation-Immune-Metabolic Imbalance:

1. Food, Diet
2. Infection, Dysbiosis
3. Nutritional Immunomodulation
4. Dysfunctional mitochondria
5. Stress, Emotions, Psychology, Sociology
6. Endocrine, Hormones
7. Xenobiotics, Toxins

Today, we have a massive task in front of us.

▸ Learn a new approach to clinical diseases.

▸ **Much new information to be integrated into a model that we can use clinically with patients.**

▸ In order to present this large amount of information in a short amount of time, I have had to be very efficient with references and words; please review this information after the seminar in order to learn it at a deeper level.

Clinical protocol

▸ **Subjective**—patient's concerns and complaints

▸ **Objective**—clinical findings

▸ **Assessment**—diagnoses

▸ **Plan**—treatments, tests, referral, follow-up

1. Food and lifestyle
2. Infection and dysbiosis
3. Nutritional immunomodulation
4. Dysfunctional mitochondria
5. Stress, Sociology-psychology, Lifestyle
6. Endocrine/hormones
7. Toxins/Xenobiotics

Clinical protocol—chart note

S.
O.
A.
P.
F.
I.
N.
D.
S.
E.
T.

Clinical protocol: recitation and implementation

▸ **Plan**—treatments, tests, referral, follow-up

1. **Food and lifestyle**: 5-part supplemented Paleo diet with allergy avoidance,

2. **Infection/dysbiosis**: eliminate problematic microbes (antimicrobials, immunonutrition) and promote inflammatory tolerance (anti-inflammatory nutrients, hormones, immunomodulation for Treg, not Th17)

3. **Nutritional immunomodulation**: more Treg, less Th17.

4. **Dysfunctional mitochondria**: carbohydrate restriction, exercise, nutritional supplementation.

5. **Stress, Sociology-psychology, Lifestyle**: confront and accept problems of human existence; avoid toxic relationships, jobs, and lifestyles; live strong.

6. **Endocrine/hormones**: create hormonal balance.

7. **Toxins/Xenobiotics**: promote detoxification daily.

Clinical protocol

▸ **S**ubjective—patient's concerns and complaints

▸ **O**bjective—clinical findings

▸ **A**ssessment—diagnoses

▸ **Pl**an—treatments, tests, referral, follow-up

1. **F**ood and lifestyle
2. **I**nfection and dysbiosis
3. **N**utritional immunomodulation
4. **D**ysfunctional mitochondria
5. **S**tress, Sociology-psychology, Lifestyle
6. **E**ndocrine/hormones
7. **T**oxins/**X**enobiotics

THANK YOU!

<u>Published books</u>

1. Integrative Orthopedics
2. Integrative Rheumatology
3. Musculoskeletal Pain
4. Chiropractic and Naturopathic Mastery of Common Clinical Disorders
5. Integrative Medicine and Functional Medicine for Chronic Hypertension
6. Integrative Chiropractic Management of High Blood Pressure & Chronic Hypertension
7. Migraine Headaches, Hypothyroidism, and Fibromyalgia

<u>Upcoming books</u>

▶ Fibromyalgia in a Nutshell

▶ Mitochondrial Nutrition—26 interventions and counting!

▶ Textbook of Functional Immunology and Nutritional Immunomodulation

▶ Psoriasis and Psoriatic Arthritis

<u>Audio files, Mp3 downloads, Podcasts:</u>

▶ **OptimalHealthResearch.com/action**

▶ InternationalCMEonline.com: USA, Spain, Colombia, France, Holland, Canada, UK,…

Revisiting the Five-Part Nutritional Wellness Protocol: The Supplemented Paleo-Mediterranean Diet

Alex Vasquez, DC, ND, DO

ABSTRACT: This article reviews the five-part nutritional protocol that incorporates a health-promoting nutrient-dense diet and essential supplementation with vitamins/minerals, specific fatty acids, probiotics, and physiologic doses of vitamin D3. This foundational nutritional protocol has proven benefits for disease treatment, disease prevention, and health maintenance and restoration. Additional treatments such as botanical medicines, additional nutritional supplements, and pharmaceutical drugs can be used atop this foundational protocol to further optimize clinical effectiveness. The rationale for this five-part protocol is presented, and consideration is given to adding iodine-iodide as the sixth component of the protocol.

INTRODUCTION:

In 2004 and 2005 I first published a "five-part nutrition protocol"[1, 2] that provides the foundational treatment plan for a wide range of health disorders. This protocol served and continues to serve as the foundation upon which other treatments are commonly added, and without which those other treatments are likely to fail, or attain suboptimal results at best.[3] Now as then, I will share with you what I consider a basic foundational protocol for wellness promotion and disease treatment. I have used this protocol in my own self-care for many years and have used it in the treatment of a wide range of health-disease conditions in clinical practice.

REVIEW:

This nutritional protocol is validated by biochemistry, physiology, experimental research, peer-reviewed human trials, and the clinical application of common sense. It is the most nutrient-dense diet available, satisfying nutritional needs and thereby optimizing metabolic processes while promoting satiety and weight loss/optimization. Nutrients are required in the proper amounts, forms, and approximate ratios for critical and innumerable physiologic functions; if nutrients are lacking, the body cannot function *normally,* let alone *optimally.* Impaired function results in subjective and objective manifestations of what is eventually labeled as "disease." Thus, a powerful and effective alternative to treating diseases with drugs is to re-establish normal/optimal physiologic function by replenishing the body with essential nutrients, reestablishing hormonal balance ("orthoendocrinology"), promoting detoxification of environmental toxins, and by reestablishing the optimal microbial milieu, especially the eradication of (multifocal) dysbiosis; this multifaceted approach can be applied to several diseases, especially those of the inflammatory and autoimmune varieties.[4]

Of course, most diseases are multifactorial and therefore require multicomponent treatment plans, and some diseases actually require the use of drugs in conjunction with assertive interventional nutrition. However, while only a smaller portion of patients actually need drugs for the long-term management their problems, all clinicians should agree that everyone needs a foundational nutrition plan because nutrients—not drugs—are universally required for life and health. This five-part nutrition protocol is briefly outlined below; a much more detailed substantiation of the underlying science and clinical application of this protocol was recently published in a review of more than 650 pages and approximately 3,500 citations.[5]

1. Health-promoting Paleo-Mediterranean diet: Following an extensive review of the research literature, I developed what I call the "supplemented Paleo-Mediterranean diet." In essence, this diet plan combines the best of the Mediterranean diet with the best of the Paleolithic diet, the latter of which has been best distilled by Dr. Loren Cordain in his book "The Paleo Diet"[6] and his numerous scientific articles.[7, 8, 9] The Paleolithic diet is superior to the Mediterranean diet in nutrient density for promoting satiety, weight loss, and improvements/normalization in overall metabolic function.[10, 11] This diet places emphasis on fruits, vegetables, nuts, seeds, and berries that meet the body's needs for fiber, carbohydrates, and most importantly, the 8,000+ phytonutrients that have additive and synergistic health effects[12]—including immunomodulating, antioxidant, anti-inflammatory, and anti-cancer benefits. High-quality protein sources such as fish, poultry, eggs, and grass-fed meats are emphasized. Slightly modifying Cordain's paleo diet, I also advocate soy and whey protein isolates for their high-quality protein and their anticancer, cardioprotective, and mood-enhancing (due to the high tryptophan content) benefits. Potatoes and other starchy vegetables, wheat and other grains including rice are discouraged due to their high glycemic indexes and high glycemic loads, and their relative insufficiency of fiber and phytonutrients compared to fruits and vegetables. Grains such as wheat, barley, and rye are discouraged due to the high glycemic loads/indexes of most breads, pastries, and other grain-derived products, as well as due to the

immunogenicity of constituents such as gluten, a protein composite (consisting of a prolamin and a glutelin) that can contribute to disorders such as migraine, epilepsy, eczema, arthritis, celiac disease, psoriasis and other types of autoimmunity. Sources of simple sugars and foreign chemicals such as colas/sodas (which contain artificial colors, flavors, and high-fructose corn syrup, which contains mercury[13] and which can cause the hypertensive-diabetic metabolic syndrome[14]) and processed foods (e.g., "TV dinners" and other manufactured snacks and convenience foods) are strictly forbidden. Chemical preservatives, colorants, sweeteners, flavor-enhancers such as monosodium glutamate and carrageenan are likewise avoided. In summary, this diet plan provides plenty of variety, as most dishes comprised of poultry, fish, lean meats, soy, eggs, fruits, vegetables, nuts, berries, and seeds are allowed. The diet provides an abundance of fiber, phytonutrients, carbohydrates, potassium, and protein, while simultaneously being low in fat, sodium, arachidonic acid, and "simple sugars." The diet must be customized with regard to total protein and calorie intake, as determined by the size, status, and activity level of the patient; individual per-patient food allergens should be avoided. Regular consumption of this diet has shown the ability to reduce hypertension, alleviate diabetes, ameliorate migraine headaches, and result in improvement of overall health and a lessening of the severity of many common "diseases", particularly those with an autoimmune or inflammatory component. This Paleo-Mediterranean diet is supplemented with vitamins, minerals, fatty acids, and probiotics—making it the "supplemented Paleo-Mediterranean diet" as described below.

2. Multivitamin and multimineral supplementation: Vitamin and mineral supplementation has been advocated for decades by the chiropractic/naturopathic professions while being scorned by so-called "mainstream medicine." Vitamin and mineral supplementation finally received bipartisan endorsement when researchers from Harvard Medical School published a review article in *Journal of the American Medical Association* that concluded, "Most people do not consume an optimal amount of all vitamins by diet alone. ...it appears prudent for all adults to take vitamin supplements."[15] Long-term nutritional insufficiencies experienced by "most people" promote the development of "long-latency deficiency diseases"[16] such as cancer, neuroemotional deterioration, and cardiovascular disease. Impressively, the benefits of multivita-

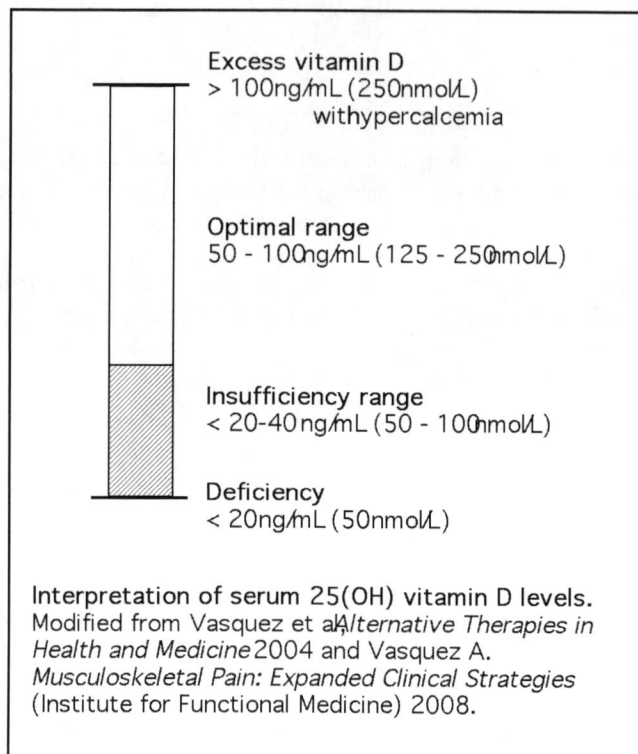

Excess vitamin D
> 100ng/mL (250nmol/L)
with hypercalcemia

Optimal range
50 - 100ng/mL (125 - 250nmol/L)

Insufficiency range
< 20-40ng/mL (50 - 100nmol/L)

Deficiency
< 20ng/mL (50nmol/L)

Interpretation of serum 25(OH) vitamin D levels. Modified from Vasquez et al *Alternative Therapies in Health and Medicine* 2004 and Vasquez A. *Musculoskeletal Pain: Expanded Clinical Strategies* (Institute for Functional Medicine) 2008.

min/multimineral supplementation have been demonstrated in numerous clinical trials. Multivitamin/multimineral supplementation has been shown to improve nutritional status and reduce the risk for chronic diseases[17], improve mood[18], potentiate antidepressant drug treatment[19], alleviate migraine headaches (when used with diet improvement and fatty acids[20]), improve immune function and infectious disease outcomes in the elderly[21] (especially diabetics[22]), reduce morbidity and mortality in patients with HIV infection[23, 24], alleviate premenstrual syndrome[25, 26] and bipolar disorder[27], reduce violence and antisocial behavior in children[28] and incarcerated young adults (when used with essential fatty acids[29]), and improve scores of intelligence in children.[30] Multivitamin and multimineral supplementation provides anti-inflammatory benefits, as evidenced by significant reduction in C-reactive protein (CRP) in a double-blind, placebo-controlled trial.[31] The ability to safely and affordably deliver these benefits makes multimineral-multivitamin supplementation an essential component of any and all health-promoting and disease-prevention strategies. A few cautions need to be observed; for example, vitamin A can (rarely) result in liver damage with chronic consumption of 25,000 IU or more, and intake should generally not exceed 10,000 IU per day in women of childbearing age. Also, iron should not be supplemented except in patients diagnosed with iron deficiency by a blood test (serum ferritin).

3. Physiologic doses of vitamin D3: The prevalence of vitamin D deficiency varies from 40-80 percent (general population) to almost 100 percent (patients with musculoskeletal pain) among Americans and Europeans. Vasquez, Manso, and Cannell described the many benefits of vitamin D3 supplementation in an assertive review published in 2004.[32] Our publication showed that vitamin D deficiency causes or contributes to depression, hypertension, seizures, migraine, polycystic ovary syndrome, inflammation, autoimmunity, and musculoskeletal pain, particularly low-back pain. Clinical trials using vitamin D supplementation have proven the cause-and-effect relationship between vitamin D deficiency and most of these conditions by showing that each could be cured or alleviated with vitamin D supplementation. In our review of the literature, we concluded that daily vitamin D doses should be 1,000 IU for infants, 2,000 IU for children, and 4,000 IU for adults, although some adults respond better to higher doses of 10,000 IU per day. Cautions and contraindications include the use of thiazide diuretics (e.g., hydrochlorothiazide) or any other medications that promote hypercalcemia, as well as granulomatous diseases such as sarcoidosis, tuberculosis, and certain types of cancer, especially lymphoma. Effectiveness is monitored by measuring serum 25-OH-vitamin D, and safety is monitored by measuring serum calcium. Dosing should be tailored for the attainment of optimal serum levels of 25-hydroxy-vitamin D3, generally 50-100 ng/ml (125-250 nmol/l) as illustrated.

4. Balanced and complete fatty acid supplementation: A detailed survey of the literature shows that five fatty acids have major health-promoting disease-preventing benefits and should therefore be incorporated into the daily diet and/or regularly consumed as dietary supplements.[33] These are alpha-linolenic acid (ALA; omega-3, from flaxseed oil), eicosapentaenoic acid (EPA; omega-3, from fish oil), docosahexaenoic acid (DHA; omega-3, from fish oil and algae), gamma-linolenic acid (GLA; omega-6, most concentrated in borage oil but also present in evening primrose oil, hemp seed oil, black currant seed oil), and oleic acid (omega-9, most concentrated in olive oil, which contains in addition to oleic acid many anti-inflammatory, antioxidant, and anticancer phytonutrients). Supplementing with one fatty acid can exacerbate an insufficiency of other fatty acids; hence the impor-

tance of balanced combination supplementation. Each of these fatty acids has health benefits that cannot be fully attained from supplementing a different fatty acid; hence, again, the importance of balanced combination supplementation. The benefits of GLA are not attained by consumption of EPA and DHA; in fact, consumption of fish oil can actually promote a deficiency of GLA.[34] Likewise, consumption of GLA alone can reduce EPA levels while increasing levels of proinflammatory arachidonic acid; both of these problems are avoided with co-administration of EPA any time GLA is used because EPA inhibits delta-5-desaturase, which converts dihomo-GLA into arachidonic acid. Using ALA alone only slightly increases EPA but generally leads to no improvement in DHA status and can lead to a reduction of oleic acid; thus, DHA and oleic acid should be supplemented when flaxseed oil is used.[35] Obviously, the goal here is physiologically-optimal (i.e., "balanced") intake of all of the health-promoting fatty acids; using only one or two sources of fatty acids is not balanced and results in suboptimal improvement. In clinical practice, I routinely use combination fatty acid therapy comprised of ALA, EPA, DHA, and GLA for essentially all patients; when one appreciates that the average daily Paleolithic intake of n-3 fatty acids was 7 grams per day contrasted to the average daily American intake of 1 gram per day, we can see that—by using combination fatty acid therapy emphasizing n-3 fatty acids—we are simply meeting physiologic expectations via supplementation, rather than performing an act of recklessness or heroism. The product I use also contains a modest amount of oleic acid that occurs naturally in flax and borage seed oils, and I encourage use of olive oil for salads and cooking. This approach results in complete and balanced fatty acid intake, and the clinical benefits are impressive. Benefits are to be expected in the treatment of premenstrual syndrome, diabetic neuropathy, respiratory distress syndrome, Crohn's disease, lupus, rheumatoid arthritis, cardiovascular disease, hypertension, psoriasis, eczema, migraine headaches, bipolar disorder, borderline personality disorder, mental depression, schizophrenia, osteoporosis, polycystic ovary syndrome, multiple sclerosis, and musculoskeletal pain. The discovery in September 2010 that the G protein-coupled receptor 120 (GPR120) functions as an n-3 fatty acid receptor that, when stimulated with EPA or DHA, exerts broad anti-inflammatory effects (in cell experiments) and enhances systemic insulin sensitivity (in animal study) confirms a new mechanism of action of fatty acid supplementation and shows that we as clinician-researchers are still learning the details of the beneficial effects of commonly used treatments.[36]

5. Probiotics /gut flora modification: Proper levels of good bacteria promote intestinal health, support proper immune function, and encourage overall health. Excess bacteria or yeast, or the presence of harmful bacteria, yeast, or "parasites" such as amoebas and protozoas, can cause "leaky gut," systemic inflammation, and a wide range of clinical problems, especially autoimmunity. Intestinal flora can become imbalanced by poor diets, excess stress, immunosuppressive drugs, and antibiotics, and all of these factors are common among American patients. Thus, as a rule, I reinstate the good bacteria by the use of probiotics (good bacteria and yeast), prebiotics (fiber, arabinogalactan, and inulin), and the use of fermented foods such as kefir and yogurt for patients not allergic to milk. Harmful yeast, bacteria, and other "parasites" can be eradicated with the combination of dietary change, antimicrobial drugs, and/or herbal extracts. For example, oregano oil in an emulsified, time-released form has proven safe and effective for the elimination of various parasites encountered in clinical practice.[37] Likewise, the herb Artemisia annua (sweet wormwood) commonly is used to eradicate specific bacteria and has been used for thousands of years in Asia for the treatment and prevention of infectious diseases, including drug-resistant malaria.[38] Restoring microbial balance by providing probiotics, restoring immune function (immunorestoration) and eliminating sources of dysbiosis, especially in the gastrointestinal tract, genitourinary tract, and oropharynx, is a very important component in the treatment plan of autoimmunity and systemic inflammation.[39]

Should combinations of iodine and iodide be the Sixth Component of the Protocol?: Both iodine and iodide have biological activity in humans. An increasing number of clinicians are using combination iodine-iodide products to provide approximately 12 mg/d; this is consistent with the average daily intake of iodine-iodide in countries such as Japan with a high intake of seafood, including fish, shellfish, and seaweed. Collectively, iodine and iodide provide antioxidant, antimicrobial, mucolytic, immunosupportive, antiestrogen, and anticancer benefits that extend far beyond the mere incorporation of iodine into thyroid hormones.[5] Benefits of iodine/iodide in the treatment of asthma[40,41] and systemic fungal infections[42,43] have been documented, and many clinicians use combination iodine/iodide supplementation for the treatment of estrogen-driven conditions such as fibrocystic breast disease.[44] While additional research is needed and already underway to further establish the role of iodine-iodide as a routine component of clinical care, clinicians should begin incorporating this nutrient into their protocols based on the above-mentioned physiologic roles and clinical benefits.

SUMMARY AND CONCLUSIONS:

In this brief review, I have described and substantiated a fundamental protocol that can serve as effective therapy for patients with a wide range of diseases and health disorders. Customizing the Paleo-Mediterranean diet to avoid patient-specific food allergens, using vitamin-mineral supplements along with physiologic doses of vitamin D and broad-spectrum balanced fatty acid supplementation, and ensuring "immunomicrobial" health with the skillful use of probiotics, prebiotics, immunorestoration, and antimicrobial treatments provides an excellent health-promoting and disease-eliminating foundation and lifestyle for many patients. Often, this simple protocol is all that is needed for the effective treatment of a wide range of clinical problems, even those that have been "medical failures" for many years. For other patients with more complex illnesses, of course, additional interventions and laboratory assessments can be used to optimize and further customize the treatment plan. Clinicians should avoid seeking "silver bullet" treatments that ignore overall metabolism, immune function, and inflammatory balance, and we must always remember that the attainment and preservation of health requires that we first meet the body's basic nutritional and physiologic needs. This five-step protocol begins the process of meeting those needs. With it, health can be restored and the need for disease-specific treatment is obviated or reduced; without it, fundamental physiologic needs are not met, and health cannot be obtained and maintained. Addressing core physiologic needs empowers doctors to deliver the most effective healthcare possible, and it allows patients to benefit from such treatment.

Dr Alex Vasquez is a Director of the Medical Board of Advisors for Biotics Research Corporation and is the author of many articles and books for doctors. His professional degrees include Doctor of Chiropractic, (University of Western States, March 1996), Doctor of Naturopathic Medicine (Bastyr University, September 1999), and Doctor of Osteopathic Medicine (University of North Texas Health Science Center, May 2010).

REFERENCES

1. Vasquez A. Integrative Orthopedics: The Art of Creating Wellness While Managing Acute and Chronic Musculoskeletal Disorders. 2004, 2007
2. Vasquez A. A Five-Part Nutritional Protocol that Produces Consistently Positive Results. Nutritional Wellness 2005 September Available in the printed version and on-line at http://www.nutritionalwellness.com/archives/2005/sep/09_vasquez.php
3. Vasquez A. Common Oversights and Shortcomings in the Study and Imple-

mentation of Nutritional Supplementation. Naturopathy Digest 2007 June. http://www.naturopathydigest.com/archives/2007/jun/vasquez.php

4. Vasquez A. Integrative Rheumatology. IBMRC: 2006, 2009. http://optimal-healthresearch.com/rheumatology.html

5. Vasquez A. Chiropractic and Naturopathic Mastery of Common Clinical Disorders. IBMRC: 2009. http://optimalhealthresearch.com/clinical_mastery.html

6. Cordain L. The Paleo Diet. John Wiley and Sons, 2002

7. O'Keefe JH Jr, Cordain L. Cardiovascular disease resulting from a diet and lifestyle at odds with our Paleolithic genome: how to become a 21st-century hunter-gatherer. Mayo Clin Proc. 2004 Jan;79(1):101-8

8. Cordain L. Cereal grains: humanity's double edged sword. World Rev Nutr Diet 1999;84:19-73

9. Cordain L, Eaton SB, Sebastian A, Mann N, Lindeberg S, Watkins BA, O'Keefe JH, Brand-Miller J. Origins and evolution of the Western diet: health implications for the 21st century. Am J Clin Nutr. 2005 Feb;81(2):341-54

10. "A high micronutrient density diet mitigates the unpleasant aspects of the experience of hunger even though it is lower in calories. Hunger is one of the major impediments to successful weight loss. Our findings suggest that it is not simply the caloric content, but more importantly, the micronutrient density of a diet that influences the experience of hunger. It appears that a high nutrient density diet, after an initial phase of adjustment during which a person experiences "toxic hunger" due to withdrawal from pro-inflammatory foods, can result in a sustainable eating pattern that leads to weight loss and improved health." Fuhrman J, Sarter B, Glaser D, Acocella S. Changing perceptions of hunger on a high nutrient density diet. Nutr J. 2010 Nov 7;9:51 http://www.nutritionj.com/content/9/1/51

11. "The Paleolithic group were as satiated as the Mediterranean group but consumed less energy per day (5.8 MJ/day vs. 7.6 MJ/day, Paleolithic vs. Mediterranean, p=0.04). Consequently, the quotients of mean change in satiety during meal and mean consumed energy from food and drink were higher in the Paleolithic group (p=0.03). Also, there was a strong trend for greater Satiety Quotient for energy in the Paleolithic group (p=0.057). Leptin decreased by 31% in the Paleolithic group and by 18% in the Mediterranean group with a trend for greater relative decrease of leptin in the Paleolithic group." Jonsson T, Granfeldt Y, Erlanson-Albertsson C, Ahren B, Lindeberg S. A Paleolithic diet is more satiating per calorie than a Mediterranean-like diet in individuals with ischemic heart disease. Nutr Metab (Lond). 2010 Nov 30;7(1):85.

12. Liu RH. Health benefits of fruit and vegetables are from additive and synergistic combinations of phytochemicals. Am J Clin Nutr 2003;78(3 Suppl):517S-520S

13. "With daily per capita consumption of HFCS in the US averaging about 50 grams and daily mercury intakes from HFCS ranging up to 28 µg, this potential source of mercury may exceed other major sources of mercury especially in high-end consumers of beverages sweetened with HFCS." Dufault R, LeBlanc B, Schnoll R, Cornett C, Schweitzer L, Wallinga D, Hightower J, Patrick L, Lukiw WJ. Mercury from chlor-alkali plants: measured concentrations in food product sugar. Environ Health. 2009 Jan 26;8:2 http://www.ehjournal.net/content/8/1/2

14. Vasquez A. Integrative Medicine and Functional Medicine for Chronic Hypertension: An Evidence-based Patient-Centered Monograph for Advanced Clinicians. IBMRC; 2011. http://optimalhealthresearch.com/hypertension_functional_integrative_medicine.html See also: Reungjui S, Roncal CA, Mu W, Srinivas TR, Sirivongs D, Johnson RJ, Nakagawa T. Thiazide diuretics exacerbate fructose-induced metabolic syndrome. J Am Soc Nephrol. 2007 Oct;18(10):2724-31 http://jasn.asnjournals.org/content/18/10/2724.full.pdf

15. Fletcher RH, Fairfield KM. Vitamins for chronic disease prevention in adults: clinical applications. JAMA 2002;287:3127-9

16. Heaney RP. Long-latency deficiency disease: insights from calcium and vitamin D. Am J Clin Nutr 2003;78:912-9

17. McKay DL, Perrone G, Rasmussen H, Dallal G, Hartman W, Cao G, Prior RL, Roubenoff R, Blumberg JB. The effects of a multivitamin/mineral supplement on micronutrient status, antioxidant capacity and cytokine production in healthy older adults consuming a fortified diet. J Am Coll Nutr 2000;19(5):613-21

18. Benton D, Haller J, Fordy J. Vitamin supplementation for 1 year improves mood. Neuropsychobiology 1995;32(2):98-105

19. Coppen A, Bailey J. Enhancement of the antidepressant action of fluoxetine by folic acid: a randomised, placebo controlled trial. J Affect Disord 2000;60:121-30

20. Wagner W, Nootbaar-Wagner U. Prophylactic treatment of migraine with gamma-linolenic and alpha-linolenic acids. Cephalalgia 1997;17:127-30

21. Langkamp-Henken B, Bender BS, Gardner EM, Herrlinger-Garcia KA, Kelley MJ, Murasko DM, Schaller JP, Stechmiller JK, Thomas DJ, Wood SM. Nutritional formula enhanced immune function and reduced days of symptoms of upper respiratory tract infection in seniors. J Am Geriatr Soc 2004;52:3-12

22. Barringer TA, Kirk JK, Santaniello AC, Foley KL, Michielutte R. Effect of a multivitamin and mineral supplement on infection and quality of life. A randomized, double-blind, placebo-controlled trial. Ann Intern Med 2003;138:365-71

23. Fawzi WW, Msamanga GI, Spiegelman D, et al. A randomized trial of multivitamin supplements and HIV disease progression and mortality. N Engl J Med 2004;351:23-32

24. Burbano X, Miguez-Burbano MJ, McCollister K, Zhang G, Rodriguez A, Ruiz P, Lecusay R, Shor-Posner G. Impact of a selenium chemoprevention clinical trial on hospital admissions of HIV-infected participants. HIV Clin Trials 2002;3:483-91

25. Abraham GE. Nutritional factors in the etiology of the premenstrual tension syndromes. J Reprod Med 1983;28(7):446-64

26. Stewart A. Clinical and biochemical effects of nutritional supplementation on the premenstrual syndrome. J Reprod Med 1987;32:435-41

27. Kaplan BJ, Simpson JS, Ferre RC, Gorman CP, McMullen DM, Crawford SG. Effective mood stabilization with a chelated mineral supplement: an open-label trial in bipolar disorder. J Clin Psychiatry 2001;62:936-44

28. Kaplan BJ, Crawford SG, Gardner B, Farrelly G. Treatment of mood lability and explosive rage with minerals and vitamins: two case studies in children. J Child Adolesc Psychopharmacol 2002;12(3):205-19

29. Gesch CB, Hammond SM, Hampson SE, Eves A, Crowder MJ. Influence of supplementary vitamins, minerals and essential fatty acids on the antisocial behaviour of young adult prisoners. Randomised, placebo-controlled trial. Br J Psychiatry 2002;181:22-8

30. Benton D. Micro-nutrient supplementation and the intelligence of children. Neurosci Biobehav Rev 2001;25:297-309

31. Church TS, Earnest CP, Wood KA, Kampert JB. Reduction of C-reactive protein levels through use of a multivitamin. Am J Med 2003;115:702-7

32. Vasquez A, Manso G, Cannell J. The clinical importance of vitamin D (cholecalciferol): a paradigm shift with implications for all healthcare providers. Alternative Therapies in Health and Medicine 2004;10:28-37 http://optimal-healthresearch.com/cholecalciferol.html

33. Vasquez A. Reducing Pain and Inflammation Naturally - Part 1: New Insights into Fatty Acid Biochemistry and the Influence of Diet. Nutritional Perspectives 2004; October: 5, 7-10, 12, 14 http://optimalhealthresearch.com/reprints/series/

34. Cleland LG, Gibson RA, Neumann M, French JK. The effect of dietary fish oil supplement upon the content of dihomo-gammalinolenic acid in human plasma phospholipids. Prostaglandins Leukot Essent Fatty Acids 1990 May;40(1):9-12

35. Jantti J, Nikkari T, Solakivi T, Vapaatalo H, Isomaki H. Evening primrose oil in rheumatoid arthritis: changes in serum lipids and fatty acids. Ann Rheum Dis 1989;48(2):124-7

36. Oh da Y, Talukdar S, Bae EJ, Imamura T, Morinaga H, Fan W, Li P, Lu WJ, Watkins SM, Olefsky JM. GPR120 is an omega-3 fatty acid receptor mediating potent anti-inflammatory and insulin-sensitizing effects. Cell. 2010 Sep 3;142(5):687-98 http://www.cell.com/abstract/S0092-8674%2810%2900888-3?switch=standard

37. Force M, Sparks WS, Ronzio RA. Inhibition of enteric parasites by emulsified oil of oregano in vivo. Phytother Res 2000;14:213-4

38. Schuster BG. Demonstrating the validity of natural products as anti-infective drugs. J Altern Complement Med 2001;7 Suppl 1:S73-82

39. Vasquez A. Integrative Rheumatology. IBMRC: 2006, 2009. http://optimal-healthresearch.com/rheumatology.html

40. Tuft L. Iodides in bronchial asthma. J Allergy Clin Immunol. 1981 Jun;67(6):497

41. Falliers CJ, McCann WP, Chai H, Ellis EF, Yazdi N. Controlled study of iodotherapy for childhood asthma. J Allergy. 1966 Sep;38(3):183-92

42. Tripathy S, Vijayashree J, Mishra M, Jena DK, Behera B, Mohapatra A. Rhinofacial zygomycosis successfully treated with oral saturated solution of potassium iodide: a case report. J Eur Acad Dermatol Venereol. 2007 Jan;21(1):117-9

43. Bonifaz A, Saúl A, Paredes-Solis V, Fierro L, Rosales A, Palacios C, Araiza J. Sporotrichosis in childhood: clinical and therapeutic experience in 25 patients. Pediatr Dermatol. 2007 Jul-Aug;24(4):369-72

44. Ghent WR, Eskin BA, Low DA, Hill LP. Iodine replacement in fibrocystic disease of the breast. Can J Surg. 1993 Oct;36(5):453-60

Made in the USA
Charleston, SC
27 June 2012